JOURNEYS IN NARRATIVE INQUIRY

Organized around a metaphor of an academic journey, D. Jean Clandinin offers published tracings of an unfolding journey over 40 years that, at its outset, appeared to focus only on questions of epistemology. However, the book illuminates how that apparent beginning focus shape-shifted to questions of methodology, ethics, ontology, and subsequently, political concerns.

Clandinin shows that, even at the outset, her research wonders were grounded in relational understandings of experience, understandings that were simultaneously ontological, methodological, epistemological, and ethical. Jean's work is collaborative, an engagement alongside others and within the contexts in which they and she lived and worked, including those who were participants in the research. She continues to acknowledge that narrative inquiry changes people's ways of being in the world, and those changes have ethical significance. While what she and her colleagues now call relational ethics has always been central, recently her sense of ethics has become more explicitly political. She shows the development of ideas over time, beginning as she entered doctoral work and continuing through 2019 and onward.

Jean's work, centered on relational understandings of experience, highlights ethical dimensions and has come to define narrative understandings for generations of researchers. This book will be an invaluable resource for researchers and graduate students and professional researchers in both educational and healthcare settings.

D. Jean Clandinin is Professor Emeritus and Founding Director of the Centre for Research for Teacher Education and Development at the University of Alberta. A former teacher, counsellor, and psychologist, she is author or co-author of 17 books and many articles and book chapters. She is affiliated with Griffith University and Royal Roads University, and has worked at the Universities of Alberta, Calgary, and Toronto.

World Library of Educationalists series

The *World Library of Educationalists* celebrates the important contributions to education made by leading experts in their individual fields of study. Each scholar has compiled a career-long collection of what they consider to be their finest pieces: extracts from books, journals, articles, major theoretical and practical contributions, and salient research findings.

For the first time ever the work of each contributor is presented in a single volume so readers can follow the themes and progress of their work and identify the contributions made to, and the development of, the fields themselves.

The distinguished careers of the selected experts span at least two decades and include Richard Aldrich, Stephen J. Ball, Elliot W. Eisner, John Elliott, Howard Gardner, John Gilbert, Ivor F. Goodson, David Hargreaves, David Labaree and E.C. Wragg. Each book in the series features a specially written introduction by the contributor giving an overview of their career, contextualizing their selection within the development of the field, and showing how their own thinking developed over time.

Thinking Philosophically About Education
The Selected Works of Richard Pring
Richard Pring

Language and the Joint Creation of Knowledge
The Selected Works of Neil Mercer
Neil Mercer

Educating Young Children: A Lifetime Journey into a Froebelian Approach
The Selected Works of Tina Bruce
Tina Bruce

Journeys in Narrative Inquiry
The Selected Works of D. Jean Clandinin
D. Jean Clandinin

For more titles in this series visit www.routledge.com/World-Library-of-Educationalists/book-series/WORLDLIBEDU

JOURNEYS IN NARRATIVE INQUIRY

The Selected Works of D. Jean Clandinin

D. Jean Clandinin

Routledge
Taylor & Francis Group
LONDON AND NEW YORK

First published 2020
by Routledge
2 Park Square, Milton Park, Abingdon, Oxon OX14 4RN

and by Routledge
52 Vanderbilt Avenue, New York, NY 10017

Routledge is an imprint of the Taylor & Francis Group, an informa business

British Library Cataloguing-in-Publication Data
A catalogue record for this book is available from the British Library

Library of Congress Cataloging-in-Publication Data
A catalog record for this book has been requested

ISBN: 978-0-367-22228-4 (hbk)
ISBN: 978-0-429-27389-6 (ebk)

Typeset in Bembo
by Apex CoVantage, LLC

CONTENTS

Acknowledgements *viii*

Introduction 1

SECTION I
Beginning in the midst: teacher knowledge as a matter of epistemology **21**

1 Studying personal practical knowledge 23

2 Personal practical knowledge: a study of teachers' classroom images 38

3 Developing rhythm in teaching: the narrative study of a beginning teacher's personal practical knowledge of classrooms 59

SECTION II
Journeying with narrative ideas of teacher knowledge into teacher education and professional education **77**

4 Teacher education as narrative inquiry 79

5 Narrative and story in teacher education 91

6 Creating pedagogical spaces for developing doctor professional identity 103
with Marie-Therese Cave

7 Shifting from stories to live by to stories to leave by: early career teacher attrition 113
with Lee Schaefer and Charles Aiden Downey

8 Narrative inquiry as reflective practice: tensions and possibilities 130
with Charles Aiden Downey

SECTION III
Journeying with narrative ideas of curriculum making: coming alongside teachers, children and families 147

9 Narrative understandings of lives in school 149

10 The interwoven stories of teachers, families, and children in curriculum making 160
with Simmee Chung

11 A narrative inquiry into familial and school curriculum making: attending to multiple worlds of Aboriginal youth and families 173
with Sean Lessard and Vera Caine

12 Curriculum and teacher development 191
with Jerry Rosiek

SECTION IV
Journeying with narrative ideas: considerations of the ontological, methodological, ethical, and political 209

13 Narrative inquiry: both a view of, and a methodology for, studying experience 211

14 Mapping a landscape of narrative inquiry: borderland spaces and tensions 228
with Jerry Rosiek

15 A return to methodological commitment: reflections on narrative inquiry 265
with Vera Caine and Andrew Estefan

16 Reverberations of narrative inquiry: how resonant echoes of an inquiry with early school leavers shaped further inquiries 278
with Sean Lessard and Vera Caine

17 Living relational ethics 292
with Vera Caine and Sean Lessard

18 Lingering departures: reverberations through, and in, narrative inquiry response communities 307
with Vera Caine and Sean Lessard

19 Exploring neglected narratives: understanding vulnerability in narrative inquiry 319
with Sean Lessard and Vera Caine

ACKNOWLEDGEMENTS

With a book that comes at the end of a career, as this one does, there are many people to thank. Thank you to my son, Thomas Robert Clandinin, who has taught me much about the power of imagination, curiosity, and community and the possibilities that open up in scholarship when we engage in our lives in these ways. Thank you to my husband, Michael Thomas Clandinin, who has stayed with me through it all. And to my two grandchildren, Peter and Katie, thank you for reminding me daily about why this work matters.

This work was created with many friends and colleagues. I have been fortunate to work with many undergraduate students, graduate students, and post-doctoral fellows who challenged me to keep imagining otherwise, to keep valuing relational knowing within narrative inquiry, and to keep valuing community, even when sometimes the work seemed impossible. I have also been fortunate to have mentors and colleagues who were always generous with their ideas, time, and kindness.

I have also enjoyed the support of three universities – the University of Toronto, the University of Calgary, and the University of Alberta, as well as research support from the Social Sciences and Humanities Research Council of Canada, the Alberta Government, Alberta Centre for Child, Family and Community Research, Alberta Advisory Council for Studies in Education, and internal funding from the universities where I worked.

INTRODUCTION

> Each of us constructs a life that is her own central metaphor for thinking about the world. But, of course, these lives do not look like parables or allegories. Mostly they look like ongoing improvisations, quite ordinary sequences of day-to-day events. They continue to unfold.
>
> *(Bateson, 1989, p. 241)*

As a newly minted teacher, and later as a school counsellor, in three elementary schools in an urban setting in western Canada, I grasped the immense responsibility that went with working with teachers, children, and families in order to create educative learning spaces. Perhaps my sense of responsibility was nurtured in my experience of growing up on a small subsistence farm with parents who taught me early on that we were, each of us, responsible for the land, the animals, each other, and those who lived in the farming community. I learned early about responsibility, attending to others, and knowing that I was part of the world and responsible for all who lived alongside me. When I began work in schools, I understood how crucial it was that I pay attention to the interwoven lives of teachers, children, families, and others in school. In understanding that, I believed that I could best work with others in creating educative spaces. Working towards creating educative spaces was not an abstract idea but an idea lived in practice.

I understood, at least in nascent, tacit ways, that there were many layers of complexity when families and children lived in poverty, faced racism, lived with addictions and health concerns, and experienced discrimination rooted in views of what was normal in abilities (cognitive, physical, and emotional) and ways of being in the world. And yet working with my colleagues, first as a teacher and later as a school counsellor, it seemed possible to shift oppressive school and classroom practices if we worked together and imagined how we could live differently. Making spaces to gather with other teachers was something that I did almost instinctively when I began to work in schools. I remember how we shared lunch times to make sure we had a safe space to talk about what was happening in our classrooms and in our lives. We worked together to make it possible for Fred, a child in a wheelchair, to come to our elementary school with his siblings when school board policies did not allow this. I remember, too, how we worked together to make sure that when a child and a teacher needed a break from each other because of rising emotions and moral judgements, there were non-shaming ways for a child and a teacher to take that break. I remember spending several evenings each year for a couple of years with parents of kindergarten children. A school principal asked me to work with them in order to help them to engage in educative play with their children at home. As a young mother I remember deciding it was best to be part of those sessions, not living a story as an expert child psychologist or teacher but as a mother who was also trying to cope with the complexities of being a young mother with an active child and a busy life. I remember endless cups of coffee on tired sofas in living rooms as mothers living in poverty talked with me about their lives; lives lived without adequate money, few resources, and daily experiences of discrimination and racism. And the ways forward seemed always more possible when we imagined and lived out our imaginings about what might shift the stories being lived in more educative ways.

In none of those conversations when I worked as a teacher and counsellor did we speak of knowledge, but now, in hindsight, I can see my and others' experiential knowledge was at work, shifting and changing as we each told our stories. As Mark Freeman (2010) reminds me, it is "through hindsight that we can pause, look again, and see ourselves anew, 'unconcealed' by the urgencies of the moment" (p. 15). And as I engage in the mindfulness required by hindsight, I remember wishing there were answers to these complex problems but understanding at some deep level that if we all worked together and kept open possibilities, we could make a difference in our lives; we could find ways forward, whether that entailed changing school and classroom practices and policies, setting up snack programs in classrooms for children who were hungry, or finding ways to get mothers, and sometimes fathers, into the schools alongside teachers. I knew our conversations often needed to begin outside school, where there were fewer barriers and borders than many people experienced in the place of school. I was passionate about my work and felt that change was always possible. I remember saying frequently, "We can figure that out."

I was a somewhat reluctant early teacher leaver. I worked in schools for about eight years before I left to pursue a doctoral program when that seemed a way forward in composing my life. I remember the shock when I began to take courses in my doctoral program around leadership, curriculum, and administration. While these courses were focused on schools, teachers, children, families, and administrators, I did not recognize any of the people with whom I had worked. Nor did I recognize myself, my stories of experience, in what I read. I could have, I suppose, attributed this to the exceptional people whom I knew. However, somehow, I knew that teachers were not impediments to implementers' goals; teachers were not deficit with more or less abilities – usually less ability – to implement theories and programs in their classrooms. Children and families were mostly understood in terms of risk factors and demographic and psychological characteristics. Where, I wondered, were the spaces for conversations, for coming together in collaboration to make situations better when everyone was seen in such negative, deficit terms. This was not how I had known the people whom I came alongside in schools. This was not how I had known parents and families, people who cared deeply for their children, although they sometimes struggled with inadequate resources and within oppressive social structures and policies that hindered or prevented them from expressing that care. I knew that those with whom I worked had come, sometimes slowly, to the conversations; but in those conversations, everyone's lives mattered.

I entered doctoral studies just as questions of teacher knowledge were beginning to be asked. It was an auspicious time to enter the landscape, which was in flux. Even then, I tacitly knew, as Geertz wrote, "Change, apparently, is not a parade that can be watched as it passes" (1995, p. 4). And so, as I look back, I realize that I entered that parade around teacher knowledge and began to shift it, ever so slightly, as I inserted myself into it. Attention was just beginning to be turned towards understanding teachers as active participants in curriculum making in schools and classrooms, as thinkers and decision-makers in relation to their practices, and as active constructors and co-constructors of experienced and lived curricula. These were views that seemed so much more resonant with what I knew from my work in schools.

When I learned of the work of Michael Connelly and Freema Elbaz around teacher knowledge, I had a glimmer of how I might think about ways forward. A conception of teachers as holders of knowledge rather than implementers or users of knowledge was a significant shift in how teaching was understood and one that spoke to my experiences and how I told stories of my work in schools. Rather than passive deliverers of materials to students, in the view that Michael and Freema were proposing teachers were seen as knowledgeable, not just in strategies for implementation but as holders and makers of knowledge. What interested me in what they were beginning to do was their interest in finding ways to acknowledge the experiential knowledge that teachers held and expressed in their life making. Silently, I added that children, families, and researchers also held experiential knowledge. My early work was fired by a passion to reconceptualize teachers as knowledge holders, and I recognized that I was searching for new scripts, new storylines, that would reshape how researchers, policy-makers, and teachers understood knowledge. While this was my initial passion, I began to learn about the importance of reading other scholars, sometimes from education but also from philosophy, psychology, sociology, and history, to help me think about what knowledge was and how people, all of us, came to know what we knew.

I had already searched out and read the work of some feminist and post-structuralist scholars who were reimagining what counted as knowledge. I was happy in a way that the work of many feminist scholars seemed somehow familiar to me. I had grown up speaking with what Ursula LeGuin (1989) calls the "mother tongue" (p. 151). While I had been taught "to listen to people in power, men or women speaking the father tongue", I had spent many years in my home, in my community, and in schools learning to "listen to the mother tongue, to what the powerless say, poor men, women, children" (p. 150). While I somehow understood the distinction between the mother tongue and the father tongue in the living out of lives, when I read feminist work it seemed to reach to what I knew in my body, learned growing up, and learned not only by coming alongside women who were mothers and teachers but also by living alongside children.

I find a strange lacuna as I look back on my rather late coming to ideas of feminism and feminist writers. It was not until my doctoral work that I began reading the writing of feminist scholars, poets, and fiction writers. Perhaps earlier I had been too busy with earning scholarships, studying, and holding one or more part-time jobs as I went through high school and my undergraduate work. Finding space to do the required work for university courses was usually all I could fit within my need to work to pay bills and tuition. While I had the support of my family, they could not financially support this seemingly "wild" dream I had of a university degree. Even after I obtained my undergraduate degree, it seems that I was too busy with teaching, raising a young child, and studying for a master's degree in educational psychology in a department that tended towards the behaviourist. It was during my doctoral studies that I found feminist thinking, met feminist scholars, and read as much feminist writing as I could. Virginia Woolf (1929) in *A Room of Her Own* spoke to me directly as I awakened to what having a room of my own might mean in my life. Tillie Olsen (1956) in *I Stand Here Ironing* helped me understand the social structures that shaped women's lives in poverty; Anne Oakley (1984) in *Taking It Like a Woman* called me to think about how "the personal and political merge in the struggle towards a feminist political consciousness" (p. xv). I was fascinated as I read most of these books on my own time as I do not recall being part of courses where feminist writing was much included.

One of the advantages of coming to work with Freema and Michael was that I was becoming reacquainted with the writings of John Dewey. Rereading him from my new vantage point – of someone who had worked in schools – made much more sense than when I had read him in a second-year educational foundations course in teacher education. His pragmatist understandings of experience and the ways that the past, present, and future intertwined with interactions between the personal and social allowed me to begin to find ways to talk about those conversations and educative spaces we had tried to make in schools. More recently, as I read McKenna and Pratt (2015), I realized that the ideas of pragmatist philosophers such as Jane Addams (1916) in her work at Hull House and early Indigenous knowledge holders also resonated through Dewey's work.

I became more thoughtful about the ways that each person comes to know and how their knowledge is grounded in their experiences. The more I read, the more I realized there was so much more to learn. However, even as I read, my passion for understanding more about how to think about lives in schools, particularly the lives of teachers, children, and families as their lives met in schools, did not change. And it was during my doctoral studies that I started to become awake to the diversity of lives in much broader ways, to the ways that cultural, racial, and linguistic narratives shaped diverse lives. I was still, however, passionate about wanting to understand the knowledge that was embodied in teachers' practices and expressed in their lives in school.

At one point during my doctoral studies I spent six months in an internship in the policy branch of the Ontario Ministry of Education. It was at a time when the "boat people", refugees from Laos, Cambodia, and Vietnam, came to Canada under private or government sponsorship. Fortuitously, the person who was assigned as my internship supervisor was named as the Ministry of Education point person, and I spent much of my time being involved in policy-planning and program development for the education of the refugee populations who arrived in Ontario, particularly Toronto. I did not meet any of the refugees, but watching policies and programs be developed at a distance from the lives of those the policies and programs would serve was a powerful experience for me.

At the end of my doctoral program I defended my doctoral work and was fortunate to meet Dr. Maxine Greene, who was appointed by the University of Toronto as my external examiner. I knew some months prior to the defence that she was appointed, and I began, for the first time, to read her work. The day of my oral defence, I was with her most of the day: walking across campus to the room where my oral was held; during the more than two and a half hours of my defence; talking about what I read and responding to her suggestions of what to read next; and, later in the day, listening to her public seminar for graduate students and faculty. She was a constant presence in my life after that point as she corresponded with me, encouraged me, defended me when I was overwhelmed presenting at conferences, and wrote letters to support me and my work. Her presence as a person and scholar changed my stories to live by.

Journeys with narrative ideas: a metaphor for representing a life

It matters what metaphor we each use to shape our lives. And it matters what metaphor we choose to use to represent our lives. As I learned from Lakoff and Johnson (1980), "Metaphor is pervasive in everyday life, not just in language but in thought and action. Our ordinary conceptual system, in terms of which we both think and act, is fundamentally metaphorical in nature" (p. 3). I was awake to some of the metaphors that had shaped my thinking and action over many years. As I faced the writing of this book, I struggled with choosing a metaphor to shape how I represented my life, the ways I shared the stories that lay behind my life's writing. At first, I was going to try to represent my life in a linear fashion, as "a story of how one thing led to another, and those to a third: 'and then . . . and then'" as Geertz (1995, p. 1) suggested. I did not want, as bell hooks wrote (1997), to write chronologically. While hooks chose "memories that bear upon her development as a writer" (p. xxii), I chose papers and chapters that bore upon my development as a researcher who thinks and lives with narrative ideas. While hooks wrote that her intent is "to share the spirit of that life" (p. xxii), I decided to try to do the same.

At first, I thought I could represent my life as interwoven threads within a life tapestry. Maxine Greene (1995) and Carol Gilligan (1982) both wrote of webs of relationship, and I have played with that metaphor of representation in other writing. However, as I thought about this life I am weaving in and through my teaching, my research, my writing, and my living, I came to considerations of a metaphor of journeys with narrative ideas. A metaphor of journeying with narrative ideas – that is, thinking narratively over time, place, and relationships – offered me possibilities of seeing interruptions, delays, short and long visits, detours, places to linger, and new places to visit. I journeyed with these narrative ideas into pathways, side journeys, and unmapped landscapes. Sometimes the journeys took me to unexpected places, places where I was surprised by what became visible.

Epistemological ideas about what counts as knowledge,
Ontological ideas about relational knowing and methodologies,
Ethical ideas about composing lives in relation with each other, with our worlds.
Ideas about curriculum, teacher education, research
All shaping these life journeys of mine,
I try to make them visible here.

I Beginning in the midst: teacher knowledge as a matter of epistemology

I find the process of returning to reread my early papers, papers written more than 30 years ago, using material from studies begun more than 40 years ago, a strangely calming and yet unsettling process. To return to papers I had written about teacher knowledge when I felt very much out of my depth writing about knowledge, to recollect my unease, makes me wonder if, at the time, I was enmeshed in what Dewey calls a quest for certainty. I recollect that I frequently looked to see if others were also questioning what was causing me unease. I came to see that I was in good company. Questions about the nature of knowledge were new to me, as I had been immersed in living and knew little about the philosophical questions around knowledge, but in those years in my doctoral program, I realized others were also raising questions.

I joined the research program of Michael Connelly and Freema Elbaz, caught into their ideas of conceptualizing teachers as holders and users of practical knowledge. I insisted, however, on including a personal dimension to a conception of teacher knowledge. I had been reading and was influenced by Polanyi's (1958) writing on personal knowledge, that is, that knowing is "an act of comprehension of the things known. . . . Such is the personal participation of the knower in acts of understanding" (1958, p. vii). Knowledge, within this conception, was seen as neither objective nor subjective but personal and intersubjective.

Working with Michael Connelly but with support and guidance from Freema Elbaz, Joseph Schwab, and Mark Johnson, we developed a concept in which teachers' practices were seen "as the embodiment and enactment of their personal practical knowledge (Clandinin, 1986, p. 36). We saw personal practical knowledge as experiential and more than mental cognition. Within our conceptualization, we saw personal practical knowledge as embodied in a history, in the moment, and in an act and as aimed at the event that called forth the act (Connelly & Clandinin, 1985). Personal practical knowledge, grounded in Dewey's pragmatist view of experience, is seen as tentative, subject to change, and transient rather than fixed, objective, and unchanging. Personal practical knowledge is a conception of knowledge that pushes back against teacher knowledge as only an accumulation of formal theoretical knowledge. As well, such a conception of teacher knowledge resists the idea that teachers hold only a collection of skills and strategies, understandings and perceptions. Personal practical knowledge is knowledge that is experiential, embodied, and expressed; in our conceptualization, it was expressed and lived out in terms of personal philosophy, ritual, image, narrative unity, and rhythm. In line with a Deweyan view of experience, the conceptualization of personal practical knowledge is rooted within continuity and interaction in enacted situations. It was an exciting time to be in the conversations about knowledge and, for me, especially exciting were the conversations about teacher knowledge in which teachers were seen as holding a particular kind of knowledge. I was in conversations where we were helping to name this as knowledge, with all that naming implied.

While I brought with me a passion for offering a more generative view of teachers' work in classrooms and an acknowledgement that teachers held experiential knowledge, I was fortunate I came to research in teaching and teacher education when I did. In the midst of my doctoral program a new line of research called teacher thinking (Clark & Yinger, 1977) was developing, and that seemed to create a gap into which I might fit what interested me. The shift to teacher thinking changed the focus from explaining teaching processes as focused mostly on the individual to creating spaces for considerations of teachers' active making of their personal practical knowledge. Teacher education and teaching were, during the 1970s and 1980s, rich fields of study. As Gary Fenstermacher noted in a chapter in the 1994 *Review of Research in Education*, there were three dominant lines of research in teacher knowledge: Donald Schon's, Lee Shulman's, and my work with Michael Connelly. The focus was epistemological, and I was part of developing new ideas with Michael Connelly, Freema Elbaz, and others.

I was fortunate to be in an international milieu where researchers who worked in research in teacher education, teaching, and curriculum were interested in working on a deeper understanding of teacher (and professional) knowledge. There were scholarly groups where the focus was on teacher knowledge, groups such as the International Study Association of Teacher Thinking (now the International Study Association of Teachers and Teaching), Invisible College, and later Division K of the

American Educational Research Association. I joined these groups and was part of these rich and generative conversations.

But there was another turn just beginning to happen in our work on personal practical knowledge and in the fields of education, psychology, and sociology as I was coming close to the end of my doctoral work. Our understandings of personal practical knowledge began to take a narrative turn within an interdisciplinary turn to narrative conceptions of thought. Michael Connelly and I wrote a chapter titled "Personal practical knowledge and the modes of knowing: Relevance for teaching and learning" for a *National Society for the Study of Education Yearbook* (Eisner, 1985). In that chapter, we argued

> Knowing a teaching and learning situation is a matter of the recollections from one's narratives that are called forth by the situation. These recollections are personal, in that they are derived from a person's narrative, and they are practical, in that they are aimed at meeting the demands of a particular situation. These recollections are, of course, also theoretical, both in the sense of containing conceptual content . . . and they are cultural, in the sense that individual narratives are embedded in cultural and historical narratives.
>
> *(pp. 184–185)*

Jerome Bruner's chapter "Narrative and paradigmatic modes of thought" was also published in that yearbook. In his chapter he introduced the idea that there are "two irreducible modes of cognitive functioning – or more simply two modes of thought" (p. 97). Each is a way of ordering experience; one is the paradigmatic mode and the second is the narrative mode. They differ in the uses of language and interpretation of action. The paradigmatic employs systematic categorizations and conceptualizations while the narrative mode of thought is concerned with meanings people ascribe to experiences through stories. At the same time as Bruner was offering the concept of a narrative mode of thought in psychology, the concept of personal practical knowledge was also shifting to become a narrative concept and became defined as

> a particular way of reconstructing the past and the intentions for the future to deal with the exigencies of a present situation . . . a narrative, curricular understanding of the person is an understanding that is flexible and fluid, and that therefore recognizes that people say and do different things in different circumstances and, conversely, that different circumstances bring forward different aspects of their experience to bear on the situation.
>
> *(Connelly & Clandinin, 1988, pp. 25–26)*

Within this narrative view, the contextual nature of personal practical knowledge became more pronounced. Personal practical knowledge was defined as context dependent and in constant composition as life experiences, both personal and professional, were woven together. Personal practical knowledge was moral and emotional knowledge and actively carried each person's being into interaction with classroom events. Living out personal practical knowledge intimately connected each person with the personal and professional narratives of his or her life.

By the mid-1990s we described personal practical knowledge as knowledge composed narratively in each teacher's life and in his or her practices, and it was lived out in a teacher's curriculum making practices. We wrote about personal practical knowledge as structured and embodied in images, practical principles, personal philosophies, metaphors, narrative unities, rhythms, and cycles. Personal practical knowledge is called forth in practical situations and events teachers encountered in their practice, and its justifications are often of an implicit nature.

Understanding context as a narrative landscape of personal practical knowledge

But we had not yet really focused on the contexts in which teachers lived and work. As Michael Connelly and I turned our attention to teachers' contexts in their lives – but most particularly in their schools and classrooms – we used a metaphor of a professional knowledge landscape, and we came to think of school contexts as knowledge landscapes. A knowledge landscape was composed of relationships among people, places, and things and was both an intellectual and a moral landscape. A professional knowledge landscape was narratively constructed with historical, moral, emotional, and aesthetic dimensions. The landscape metaphor allowed us to draw attention to the relational, temporal, and shifting nature of school contexts. We described the landscape as having in-classroom and out-of-classroom places, fundamentally different places

> living within the professional knowledge landscape creates epistemological dilemmas for teachers and others, such as school administrators, who also inhabit the landscape. These epistemological dilemmas are understood narratively in terms of sacred, secret, and cover stories. We described "the uneasy state of teachers' professional lives as part and parcel of moral and epistemological dilemmas associated with living in, and repeatedly crossing, back and forth between, two epistemologically different places on the landscape".
>
> *(Clandinin & Connelly, 1995, p. 5)*

As we worked with narrative ways to conceptualize the contexts in which teachers in our studies worked, we came to see some stories as having the quality of what Crites (1971) called sacred stories, stories that are often unquestioned and are shaped into institutional and social stories. Often these sacred stories shape imposed prescriptions that come from a theory-driven view of how schooling should be. These views are implicitly shared by policy-makers, practitioners, and theoreticians. We wrote of secret stories, those stories that live in teachers' classrooms, places that are mostly free from outside scrutiny. When teachers share their secret stories, they usually do so with other teachers in places that they see as safe. We wrote of cover stories lived and told by teachers in out-of-classroom places both in, and off, their professional knowledge landscapes. Cover stories are used by teachers to give an account of their practices in safe ways that allow them to keep secret their lived stories that may be in conflict with stories of school and school stories. Cover stories are designed to fit within the range of acceptable stories of school and allow teachers to sustain their secret stories.

A professional knowledge landscape is composed of school stories and stories of school, teachers' stories, and stories of teachers. Stories of school are stories told about a particular school by people such as families, school district personnel, and practitioners. These stories are told both in and outside schools. School stories are stories told by teachers within each school and are shaped when policies intersect with the histories of school landscapes and the people who live within them. Teacher stories are stories that teachers tell of themselves in which they make visible their teaching practices and their lives. Stories of teachers are stories told by others about a teacher. These stories are told both within and outside school. Conflicting and competing stories live between and within stories of school and stories of teachers. Conflicting stories are stories that collide with dominant stories of school, while competing stories live in dynamic and positive tension with dominant stories of school.

In this early conceptualization we focused on the professional knowledge landscape, paying attention to teachers' experiences within schools and within classrooms. Lee Schaefer, Aiden Downey, and I, after our work with early career teachers and early career teacher leavers, developed a more holistic view of knowledge landscapes, in which we conceptualized both professional knowledge landscapes and personal knowledge landscapes at work in understandings of personal practical knowledge. While Michael and I acknowledged that there were "off the landscape" places, Lee, Aiden, and I began to think more about personal knowledge landscapes, those knowledge contexts that shape our knowing from birth, that shape what each of us knows and who we are and are becoming. These personal knowledge landscapes are always changing as we grow, move to new places, meet new people, marry, lose parents, have children, and watch our children grow. We are always situated in a personal knowledge landscape, albeit a knowledge landscape that is continually in the making.

As Michael and I shifted our attention to teachers' identities, we saw them as stories to live by, a narrative concept of identity. Stories to live by are seen as at the nexus of personal practical knowledge and the professional knowledge landscape. Stories to live by are threaded by plotlines shaped by teachers' personal practical knowledge and the places on the personal and professional knowledge landscapes where teachers live and work. Linking personal practical knowledge to narrative concepts of contexts and identities is coherent with research that questions the separation of personal and professional identities as well as personal and professional contexts. Understanding personal practical knowledge as more holistic and coherent across a person's life and contexts is part of understanding teachers and their practice.

The ideas around what counts as knowledge and the ways knowledge is intertwined with the person and who the person is and is becoming, as well as intertwined with the contexts in which each person lives and works, were an important unfolding journey for me as I considered ideas around epistemology, ontology, and ethics. As I revisited these papers I realized that, even in this early work, I was thinking with the ideas of a relational ontology, although I often spoke of it as a dialectical idea, as that was a concept that seemed in accepted use. Ideas of a relational ontology were in nascent form but it seemed that I was already wondering about a relational methodology and relational ethics. And in these early papers, I was already awake to possible ways that the methodology I was working with had pedagogical ramifications.

At the outset of my academic journey, the first idea that I journeyed with was an epistemological one, a different conceptualization of teacher knowledge, one in which teachers held and expressed experiential embodied knowledge in their classroom practices. To represent this early work, I selected the opening chapter from my dissertation, later published as a book, a 1985 article published in *Curriculum Inquiry* (and republished as a book chapter in 2013), and a 1989 *Curriculum Inquiry* article that drew on new empirical research that I began as an assistant professor at the University of Calgary. This focus on teacher knowledge as experiential, embodied in persons, and shaped by and shaping contexts is a constant thread throughout my work. The 1989 article shifted slightly as I highlighted the centrality of social and institutional contexts in explorations of the temporal, shifting contexts in which teachers come to know. By the end of the 1990s Michael Connelly and I had collaborated on a number of empirical studies with teachers in classrooms in schools and had developed a view of teacher knowledge in which personal practical knowledge was linked to professional knowledge contexts and identities. These concepts of teacher knowledge, while they continued to be experiential, contextual, embodied in persons, and expressed in action, were now all framed using narrative terms.

II Journeying with narrative ideas of teacher knowledge into teacher education and professional education

When I completed my PhD, I was fortunate to receive a position as an assistant professor in Early Childhood Education at the University of Calgary. My position was part of a new four-year program that prepared people to become Early Childhood teachers. While I had not enjoyed my time in teacher education as a student, I was now a teacher educator. My own experiences as a student were always present as I tried to find a way to teach. The program was a new interdisciplinary one, and I was responsible for the primary methods curriculum and instruction course as well as for the placement and supervision of the students' primary grade practica. As I worked with teachers in the Calgary school districts and with other faculty members in the program, I found there was room for doing things differently from my own practicum and methods course experiences.

Working in this program and later in designing and working in a collaborative teacher education program allowed me to imagine new possibilities for teacher education. While I had been attentive to the ways teachers' personal practical knowledge significantly altered educational research, I had spent less time considering how including teachers' personal practical knowledge in teacher education might change teacher education. Teacher educators could no longer begin with theories and research but would need to encourage starting points within the lives and contexts of teachers – with their stories and life experiences. It became important to consider each teacher's experiential knowledge from his or her own schooling, his or her life outside schools, and experiences in his or her early life, all of which shape a teacher's personal practical knowledge and his or her classroom curriculum making. Working with a concept of teacher personal practical knowledge and attending to the ways that teacher knowledge is expressed in each teacher's lived and told stories of teaching were ways for me and for other teacher educators to support student teachers' professional learning.

These were the ideas I started with as a beginning teacher educator, but I turned to many muses who helped me imagine how to reconsider teacher education. One of my early muses, as I sought to reframe teacher education working with the narrative ideas of personal practical knowledge, was Vivian Paley, an early childhood teacher at the University of Chicago Lab School. Michael Connelly and I (Clandinin & Connelly, 1992) used writings from several of her books to show the power of teachers as curriculum makers in their classrooms. As a new teacher educator, I eagerly sought out her books and used them with colleagues and students to help me reimagine teacher education. Her writing helped me to think about preservice teacher education in ways that might help new teachers become curriculum makers like Vivian Paley.

I was also inspired to reconsider teacher education as I taught master's level courses to Calgary area teachers. I filled my course readings with articles and books by Noddings, Greene, Hollingsworth, Gilligan, Schon, Paley, Robert Coles, and, of course, our writings on teacher knowledge. As I responded to graduate students' weekly writing dialogue journals with these readings, they challenged me by asking questions: "If we know this about teaching, then why do we continue to do teacher education as we do? And why don't we do it differently?" Their questions and my sense of needing to teach in ways that were congruent with the ideas of personal practical knowledge worked as a call to action for me. Slowly a group of teachers including Annie Davies, Pat Hogan, and Barbara Kennard began to form with the intention of designing and living out teacher education in ways that were consistent with narrative ideas of knowledge.

Something else was at work in my early years as an academic in teacher education at the University of Calgary as my interest in feminist work continued and grew. I had started reading Hannah Arendt's (1958) work while a graduate student at the Ontario Institute for Studies in Education at the University of Toronto. Miriam Ben-Peretz, then Dean at the University of Haifa, and I, along with Madeleine Grumet and Sally Brown, planned and held a conference we named an *International Conference on Private Woman-Public Work* at the University of Haifa in June, 1988. I was spellbound as I met feminist scholars from around the world at the conference. My co-authored paper with a University of Calgary colleague, Suzanne Kurtz, was an inquiry into our search for and ultimate creation of educative spaces for ourselves and other women in the academy. In that paper, we wrote of our actions in designing and teaching a new course called "Women in Education," in arranging suppers for academic women to come together to share experiences, and in valuing our non-hierarchical ways of teaching. These early years as a woman academic and this paper and conference marked my acknowledgement of myself as a feminist scholar. I continued to read feminist work and tried to seek out feminist scholars who were also interested in research in teacher education. I remember when a newly found friend and colleague, Sandra (Sam) Hollingsworth, gifted me a copy of *Ain't I a Woman! A Book of Women's Poetry from Around the World* (I. Linthwaite, Ed., 1990). I read the book eagerly and sought more. I found Adrienne Rich's *Your Native Land, Your Life* (1986), Paula Gunn Allen's (1997) *Life is a Fatal Disease*, and May Sarton's journals Carolyn Heilbrun's (1989) *Writing a Woman's Life* spoke powerfully of the importance of questioning the scripts women are given for our lives and of abandoning metaphors that had shaped men's lives. Mary Catherine Bateson's books, especially her 1989 *Composing a Life*, also spoke of exploring

> the creative potential of interrupted and conflicted lives, where energies are not narrowly focused or permanently pointed toward a single ambition. These are not lives without commitment, but rather lives in which commitments are continually refocused and redefined. . . . The circumstances of women's lives now and in the past provide examples for new ways of thinking about the lives of both men and women.
>
> (p. 9)

I remember finding Nel Noddings (1984) book *Caring* and being struck by the possibility of how a more relational ethics might be possible. When I found Sandra Harding's (1991) *Whose Science? Whose Knowledge?*, I was challenged again in new ways to reconsider questions of context and standpoint in teacher knowledge. I returned again and again to her line "women and men cannot understand or explain the world we live in or the real choices we have . . . as long as the sciences describe and explain the world primarily from the perspectives of the lives of the dominant groups" as I wondered about research on teachers' knowledge.

As I attended academic conferences in curriculum, teaching, and teacher education, I found myself drawn to feminist scholars such as Sandra Hollingsworth, Janet Miller, Celia Oyler, and others who kept me in conversations I might otherwise have missed. The writings of feminist scholars and, more importantly, the living of feminist scholars were important in shaping who I was becoming as a scholar and researcher.

Being able to spend six years at the University of Calgary involved in teacher education allowed me to work with teachers in preservice university settings and in classroom settings. Being part of the living of teacher education was an important site for keeping open questions of teacher knowledge and for considering how teachers learn to teach and what sustains them in teaching. One of the first pieces I wrote about narrative understandings of teacher knowledge in teacher education was published after I participated in collaboratively designing a one-year experimental teacher education program with Calgary teachers, principals, student teachers, and some faculty from the University of Calgary. The 1993 book written out of this program was collaboratively written with university faculty, cooperating teachers, and student teachers.

This first experimental program in preservice teacher education informed the establishment of the Centre for Research for Teacher Education and Development at the University of Alberta. In 1990 I accepted a position at the University of Alberta to design and lead a research centre in teacher education. Other experimental programs in teacher education connected with my work in the Centre were designed to explore further possibilities. Because the Centre was interdisciplinary, questions around teacher education were expanded when I began to work with colleagues in the Department of Family Medicine at the University of Alberta. While there are a number of articles and chapters published from a 15-year collaboration, I selected a 2008 article focused on creating spaces for the storying and restorying of physicians' professional identities.

My research with Aiden Downey and Lee Schaefer was powerful in returning me to questions of teacher knowledge and epistemology, but now my attention was also more explicitly on the ontological. The 2010 *Handbook of Reflection and Reflective Inquiry* chapter with Aiden Downey and my 2014 *Teacher Education Quarterly* article with Aiden Downey and Lee Schaefer were both results of that renewed focus on ideas of narrative knowledge in teacher education.

III Journeying with narrative ideas of curriculum making: coming alongside teachers, children, and families

When I began my doctoral work, I was required to undertake an extra year of coursework and a third year of program residency because, as a master's level graduate student, I had studied psychology and was not familiar with studies in curriculum theory. I entered doctoral studies with a very narrow view of curriculum, that is, a view that curriculum was the document that contained the mandated curriculum requirements of provincial and school districts. My view was not that different from the view that many teachers hold of curriculum. However, I quickly began to question my assumptions about just what curriculum is. In my first course on the foundations of curriculum theory, the concept of curriculum as policy document came under question. I learned about other more complex views of curriculum, such as the mandated curriculum, the hidden curriculum, the null curriculum, and the planned curriculum. As I studied further with Michael Connelly and Freema Elbaz (Connelly & Elbaz, 1980) and engaged in research with teachers, I began to think of curriculum as the living out of a teachers' personal practical knowledge within a particular set of nested milieus, within various subject matters, and with particular students and their families. My doctoral work and the early work in teacher knowledge were situated in a careful study of what Michael Connelly and I saw as theories of the living curriculum. We co-authored a 1988 book titled *Teachers as Curriculum Planners: Narratives of Experience*, in which we laid out our view of curriculum making using Deweyan concepts. The book, part of our work on teacher knowledge, situated each teacher's personal practical knowledge as the starting point for understanding curriculum making. J. J. Schwab's four curriculum commonplaces, students, milieu, subject matter, and teacher, provided an important structure for the development of our idea of a living curriculum. The book bumped up against the dominant view of curriculum as a course of study prescribed through policy-making processes. In the dominant view of curriculum, curriculum is something delivered to students through various pedagogical methods. It was the dominant view that I knew something of when I began my studies. Curriculum, within the dominant view, is a kind of object.

In the view of curriculum that we were arguing for, curriculum was something made via processes over time, places, and relationships, with the teacher as central maker or planner of the living or experienced curriculum. Such a view allowed us to attend centrally to what was experienced in the classroom by the teacher and students. In our 1992 chapter in the *Handbook of Curriculum* (Jackson, 1992), Michael Connelly and I developed this conceptualization further in a chapter titled "Teacher as Curriculum Maker" Early in our chapter we stated

> Teachers and their students live out a curriculum; teachers do not transmit, implement, or teach a curriculum and objectives; nor are they and their students carried forward in their work and studies by a curriculum of textbooks and content, instructional methodologies, and intentions. An account of teachers' and students' lives over time is the curriculum, although intentionality, objectives and curriculum materials do play a part in it.
>
> *(p. 365)*

We further developed an idea of a teacher as a curriculum maker, based on our research and our Deweyan understandings of experience. In order to show our ideas narratively, we focused on two teachers, Vivian Paley and Robert Coles, as curriculum makers and, by careful textual analysis of their writings, showed how they co-composed a living curriculum with their students. In so doing, we made clear that the living or experienced curriculum that teachers made in classrooms was more correctly titled, or understood, as co-made among teachers, children, families, and others in the classroom and schools. Subject matter and milieu or context were also part of the co-making of curriculum. A concept of co-making of the living curriculum was, we argued, more authentic in attending to the ways that each child and each teacher experiences or lives a curriculum. These ideas are discussed in the 2010 chapter with Simmee Chung. We showed the ways that the lives of teachers, families, and children were interwoven in curriculum making. While we saw the important part that families played in shaping each child's curriculum, we were focused on the curriculum being made in schools.

By 2014 we had begun to shift our focus on curriculum making to the curriculum that is made not only in schools but also in familial and community places. This work had begun in the research undertaken, in part, with Chung. Working with Shaun Murphy and Janice Huber, I argued for understanding curriculum making as occurring in multiple places. Schools were one place that curriculum was being made, but curriculum was also made and experienced in home and community places. Developing a notion of curriculum making as occurring in schools but also in communities and home places allowed for a more expansive view of curriculum making that allowed considerations of the intergenerational (Young, 2005) to become more evident. In my journey with narrative ideas into curriculum theory, I could now reconnect to earlier experiences where families were important sources for shaping children's lives. Children's curriculum-making occurred in homes and community places long before children entered formal schooling. Swanson's (2019) dissertation picks up these ideas with her narrative inquiry into the lives of young children and their families before and as they enter school.

In a 2014 article with Caine and Lessard, we strengthened the connections between life making and curriculum making as we showed how familial curriculum making shaped lives in our work with Aboriginal children and youth. We argued that different places of curriculum making were akin to what Maria Lugones (1987) described as worlds. We showed the different worlds of curriculum making that children and youth experience each day as they move from their worlds of familial curriculum making to worlds of school curriculum making, a view of curriculum making that highlighted the ontological, epistemological, and ethical dimensions of curriculum making.

When Jerry Rosiek and I wrote a 2016 chapter for the *Sage Handbook of Curriculum, Pedagogy, and Assessment*, we linked the ideas of teacher as curriculum maker to teacher education and to the broader field of curriculum theory where teachers are also visible. In that chapter, written 25 years after Michael Connelly and I wrote *Teachers as Curriculum Planners*, Rosiek and I again returned to the still-contested nature of the concept of curriculum. We argued that classic and contemporary pragmatist philosophy is the most useful framework for thinking about teachers' work as curriculum makers. As we visited the literature on teachers as curriculum makers, "We see the centrality of the inclusive concept of experience – specifically the experiences of teachers and students – as the beginning and ending point of curriculum inquiry". Rosiek and I return to questions of teacher education in preparing teachers and ourselves as curriculum makers. We also return to the importance of working with teachers and others to imagine otherwise, as Greene would have it, and to ignite imaginative possibilities as Eisner would have it.

IV Journeying with narrative ideas: considerations of the ontological, methodological, ethical, and political entwined with the epistemological

In our 1990 article in the *Educational Researcher*, an article in which we introduced the term narrative inquiry into the research literature, Michael Connelly and I argued that narrative ways of thinking about phenomena are inextricably interwoven with narrative inquiry as research methodology. Narrative inquiry was, for us, more than a new qualitative research method, such as a new form of ethnography or phenomenology. Our argument then, which continues now, was for a narrative view of experience in which we understand experience as lived in the midst; as always unfolding over time, in diverse social contexts, and in place; and as co-composed in relation. I recollect that I was somewhat reluctant to enter the debates around research methodology, sensing that I was participating in difficult conversations that took me away from my main focus. I was intent on not losing sight of what we saw as our main purpose, that is, developing a narrative view of experience and of teacher experiential knowledge. However, as we found ourselves in methodological discussions about narrative inquiry, we remained steady in our understanding that relational ethics lived at the heart of narrative inquiry. We also saw the pedagogical possibilities of narrative inquiry as we explored the ideas of teachers as curriculum planners.

My work, since beginning my doctoral studies in 1978, has spanned more than 40 years. It is in the past ten years or so that I have noticed new shifts or perhaps new intentions in my scholarly work. In part, these shifts take me back to some of my earliest interests, that is, to the experiences of children, youth, and families, particularly those who live in conflict with dominant social and cultural narratives. Some of these shifted intentions are visible because of the research puzzles that called me in the last years of my work. My research puzzles are now more often focused on the lives of children, youth, and families, particularly those who are more likely to be oppressed by dominant social policies and practices. In part, these shifts are due to my long-term commitments, commitments rooted in my early life experiences.

However, these shifts are also connected with the research collaborators who have, more recently, come alongside me. Beginning with research into the experiences of youth who left school before graduating, I found myself less focused on the experiences of teachers who work in schools and more focused on people's experiences outside schools. Scholars such as Claire Desrochers, Joy-Ruth Michelson, Pam Steeves, and particularly Vera Caine and Sean Lessard, joined me in exploring puzzles around the experiences of youth who left school before graduating and who challenged me in new ways to revisit questions around belonging and lives in and out of schools. As Vera Caine, Sean Lessard, and I show in our 2013 article titled "Reverberations of narrative inquiry: How resonant echoes of an inquiry with early school leavers shaped further inquiries", the puzzles with the experiences of the youth who left school drew us to the experiences of Indigenous youth and their families. In the present, I am part of a narrative inquiry in which we are inquiring into the experiences of those who come as refugees, migrants tossed into uncertainty and upheaval by social, political, and geographical changes. For me, narrative inquiry into the experiences of refugee families resonates backwards to that doctoral student internship with the Ontario Ministry of Education. It seems my work comes full circle back to puzzles of the experiences of those who are uprooted and in search of new places in which to compose their lives. I hope I now can bring more complex understandings to the work these many years later.

My work with Lee Schaefer and Aiden Downey also took me to puzzles around the experiences of early career teachers who left teaching, as much as to the experiences of teachers who stayed in teaching. Increasingly my research is shifting to those who live in more liminal spaces outside of schools and teacher education institutions.

The work on relational ethics again drew me alongside Vera Caine and Sean Lessard and to questions about the ways the ethics of everyday lives can be thought of narratively. We share a commitment to how important it is to live our research ethics in profoundly relational ways. While ethics were always at the heart of narrative inquiry (Michael Connelly and I wrote our first article on the ethics of narrative inquiry in 1988 some 30 years ago), it was not until very recently that Vera, Sean, and I, with others, took up these questions in a focused way in our latest book, *Relational Ethics of Narrative Inquiry* (2018).

My work in these last ten years or so has allowed me enough distance to see the ways epistemological, ontological, ethical, methodological, and political commitments are woven together in narrative inquiry. I began to make those interwoven commitments visible in *Engaging in Narrative Inquiry* (2013) as well as in earlier writings such as the 2007 chapter with Jerry Rosiek in the *Handbook of Narrative Inquiry*. It was in the chapter with Jerry Rosiek that I was first able to consider questions of borderlands that narrative inquiry shared with post-structuralist, Marxist, and post-positivist stances. Jerry pushed me to take up those questions that Michael Connelly and I first addressed in our 2000 book, *Narrative Inquiry*. In a 2013 article, Vera Caine, Andrew Estefan, and I highlighted how narrative inquiry worked from different ontological assumptions, such as common university notions around owning ideas as intellectual property and writing as individuals, in order to explore the ontological and relational commitments of narrative inquirers. In that article, we showed that ownership of ideas was not our starting point; at the heart of the work was our relationships with participants and with each other. What remained particularly remarkable is the emphasis on curiosity and inquiry. What mattered most was figuring things out together. Each coming together as researchers and as researchers with participants was marked by a sense of inquiry.

In our 2018 book (*Relational Ethics in Narrative Inquiry*), our 2018 book chapter (in *Narrative and Metaphor*), and our 2018 article (in *Irish Educational Studies*), Vera Caine, Sean Lessard, and I are more visibly developing the ideas of relational ethics in narrative inquiry. As we wrote,

> A relational ontology requires that we undertake research with an understanding of relational ethics that call us to larger questions of who we are in relation with participants, but also who we are in relation with the larger world or worlds that people, including us as researchers, inhabit. This relational ontology, interwoven necessarily with a relational ethics, calls us to consider mutuality, respect, and reciprocity. But it also calls us to questions of responsibility to the person and to the worlds in which we are nested, to questions of complicity in the worlds within which we currently exist as well as to future worlds that our work leads into.
>
> *(Clandinin, Caine, & Lessard, 2018, p. 20)*

We have moved more explicitly towards showing how the relational ethics of narrative inquiry create our more generative notions of political change and action, ideas that are strengthened by reading more broadly about pragmatist philosophy.

Gathering threads

In all that I have written, both in what is included in this volume and in other writing, the Centre for Research for Teacher Education and Development at the University of Alberta is only lightly mentioned. And yet it is central to my work as a narrative inquirer. Creating and living in an academic research centre with teacher knowledge, curriculum making, teacher education, and narrative inquiry at its core has been a way for me to create a sustaining, experimental, innovative, improvisational, imaginative, and relational place to journey with narrative ideas and with others. It is a place that I was able to imagine up with others, a kind of imagining otherwise as to what a research centre might be. It has been, for me, a place to co-create, to bring together, in research conversations, people who share passions and commitments for more than 30 years, a place that provided an academic home place for me and for others. My love of, commitment to, and responsibility for each place is something learned so long ago as I grew up. The Centre is a living place for thinking narratively – a place with permeable boundaries, an interdisciplinary spirit, and possibilities for nurturing the relational ethics of responsibility and collaboration in research.

While some of my writing is solely authored and some is co-authored with my doctoral supervisor, much of my writing is collaboratively done with graduate students, former graduate students, and post-doctoral fellows. It is in working with graduate students, post-doctoral fellows, and other scholars that my ideas have shifted, changed, and been challenged. Writing for publication with graduate students is a challenge I have gratefully taken up. As I think of writing with so many people, I am reminded of the joy that comes with pushing at edges; living in liminal spaces; and living with ideas as we walked, talked, read words to each other, and shared times and places. I entered each supervisory relationship by telling students I am a hands-on supervisor who sees herself as a collaborator. I tried to work from a relational ethics with students as we worked together in coming alongside and in trying to world travel with each other. When graduate students finish and ask how they can repay me, I ask them to pay their experiences with me forward into their own work in universities, in schools, and in policy institutions. I am fortunate to see so many of them living their experiences into forward-looking stories of imagining otherwise.

References

Addams, J. (1916). *The long road of women's memory*. New York, NY: Macmillan.

Allen, P. G. (1997). *Life is a fatal disease*. Albuquerque, NM: West End Press.

Arendt, H. (1958). *The human condition*. Chicago, IL: University of Chicago Press.

Bateson, M. C. (1989). *Composing a life*. New York, NY: The Atlantic Monthly Press.

Bruner, J. (1985). Narrative and paradigmatic modes of thought. In E. Eisner (Ed.), *Learning and teaching the ways of knowing: Eighty-fourth Yearbook of the National Society for the study of education* (Part II). Chicago, IL: University of Chicago Press.

Clandinin, D. J. (1986). *Classroom practice: Teacher images in action*. Barcombe Lewes: Falmer Press.

Clandinin, D. J., & Connelly, F. M. (1992). The teacher as curriculum maker. In P. Jackson (Ed.), *Handbook of research on curriculum* (pp. 363–401). American Educational Research Association. New York, NY: Macmillan Press.

Clandinin, D. J., & Connelly, F. M. (1995). *Teachers' professional knowledge landscapes*. New York, NY: Teachers College Press.

Clark, M. C., & Yinger, R. J. (1977). Research on teacher thinking. *Curriculum Inquiry*, 7(4), 279–304.

Connelly, F. M., & Clandinin, D. J. (1985). Personal practical knowledge and the modes of knowing: Relevance to teaching and learning. In E. Eisner (Ed.), *Learning and teaching the ways of knowing: Eighty-fourth Yearbook of the National Society for the study of education* (Part II). Chicago, IL: University of Chicago Press.

Connelly, F. M., & Clandinin, D. J. (1988). *Teachers as curriculum makers: Narratives of experience*. New York, NY: Teachers College Press.
Connelly, F. M., & Elbaz, F. (1980). Conceptual bases for curriculum thought: A teacher's perspective. In A. W. Foshay (Ed.), *Considered action for curriculum improvement, ASCD Yearbook* (pp. 95–119). Alexandria, VA: ASCD.
Crites, S. (1971). The narrative quality of experience. *Journal of the American Academy of Religion, 39*(3), 291–311.
Eisner, E. (Ed.). (1985). *Learning and teaching the ways of knowing: Eighty-fourth Yearbook of the National Society for the study of education* (Part II). Chicago, IL: University of Chicago Press.
Fenstermacher, G. D. (1994). The knower and the known in teacher knowledge research. *Review of Research in Education, 20*(1), 3–56.
Freeman, M. (2010). *Hindsight: The promise and peril of looking backward*. Oxford: Oxford University Press.
Geertz, C. (1995). *After the fact: Two countries, four decades, one anthropologist*. Cambridge, MA: Harvard University Press.
Gilligan, C. (1982). *In a different voice: Psychological theory and women's development*. Cambridge, MA: Harvard University Press.
Greene, M. (1995). *Releasing the imagination: Essays on education, the arts and social change*. San Francisco, CA: Jossey Bass.
Harding, S. (1991). *Whose science? Whose knowledge? Thinking from women's lives*. Cornell, NY: Cornell University Press.
Heilbrun, C. (1989). *Writing a woman's life*. New York, NY: W. W. Norton.
hooks, B. (1997). *Wounds of passion: A writing life*. New York, NY: Henry Holt.
Jackson, P. (Ed.). (1992). *Handbook of research on curriculum*. American Educational Research Association. New York, NY: Macmillan Press.
Lakoff, G., & Johnson, M. (1980). *Metaphors we live by*. Chicago, IL: University of Chicago Press.
LeGuin, U. K. (1989). *Dancing at the end of the world: Thoughts on words, women, places*. New York, NY: Harper & Row.
Linthwaite, I. (Ed.). (1990). *Ain't I a woman: A book of women's poetry from around the world*. New York, NY: Peter Bedrick Books.
Lugones, M. (1987). Playfulness, "World"-travelling, and loving perception. *Hypatia,* 2(2): 3–19. DOI:10.1111/j.1527–2001.1987.tb01062.x.
McKenna, E., & Pratt, S. (2015). *American philosophy from Wounded Knee to the present*. London: Bloomsbury Press.
Noddings, N. (1984). *Caring: A feminine approach to ethics and moral education*. Berkeley, CA: University of California Press.
Oakley, A. (1984). *Taking it like a woman*. New York, NY: Random House.
Olsen, T. (1956). *Tell me a riddle*. New York, NY: Bantam Doubleday Dell Publishing.
Polanyi, M. (1958). *Personal knowledge: Towards a post-critical philosophy*. Chicago, IL: University of Chicago Press.
Rich, A. (1986). *Your native land, your life*. Markham, Ontario: Penguin Books.
Swanson, C. (2019). *A narrative inquiry alongside the familial curriculum making of urban Indigenous children and families*. Unpublished doctoral dissertation. Edmonton, AB: University of Alberta.
Woolf, V. (1929). *A room of one's own*. London: Hogarth Press.
Young, M. (2005). *Pimatisiwin: Walking in a good way – A narrative inquiry into language as identity*. Winnipeg, MB: Pemmican Publishing.

Selected writings

Writings selected for Section I Beginning in the midst: teacher knowledge as a matter of epistemology

Clandinin, D. J. (1985). Personal practical knowledge: A study of teachers' classroom images. *Curriculum Inquiry, 15*(4), 361–385. Reprinted in C. J. Craig (Ed.). (2013). *From teacher thinking to teachers and teaching: The evolution of a research community* (pp. 67–96). London: Emerald.

Clandinin, D. J. (1986). Introduction. Part 1: Studying personal practical knowledge. In *Classroom practice: Teacher images in action* (pp. 3–21). Barcombe Lewes: Falmer Press.

Clandinin, D. J. (1989). Developing rhythm in teaching: The narrative study of a beginning teacher's personal practical knowledge of classrooms. *Curriculum Inquiry, 19*(2), 121–141.

Writings selected for Section II Journeying with narrative ideas of teacher knowledge into teacher education and professional education

Clandinin, D. J. (1991). Narrative and story in teacher education. In T. Russell & H. Munby (Eds.), *Teachers and teaching: From classroom to reflection* (pp. 124–137). London: Falmer Press.

Clandinin, D. J. (1993). Teacher education as narrative inquiry. Chapter 1 in D. J. Clandinin, A. Davies, P. Hogan, & B. Kennard (Eds.), *Learning to teach: Teaching to learn: Stories of collaboration in teacher education* (pp 1–15). New York, NY: Teachers College Press.

Clandinin, D. J., & Cave, M. (2008). Creating pedagogical spaces for developing doctor professional identity. *Medical Education, 42*(8), 765–770.

Downey, C. A., & Clandinin, D. J. (2010). Narrative inquiry as reflective practice: Tensions and possibilities. In N. Lyons (Ed.), *Handbook of reflection and reflective inquiry: Mapping a way of knowing for professional reflective practice* (pp. 285–397). Dordrecht, Netherlands: Springer.

Schaefer, L., Downey, C. A., & Clandinin, D. J. (2014, Winter). Shifting from stories to live by to stories to leave by: Early career teacher attrition. *Teacher Education Quarterly, Winter, 41*(1), 9–27.

Writings selected for Section III Journeying with narrative ideas of curriculum making: coming alongside teachers, children and families

Clandinin, D. J. (2009). Narrative understandings of lives in school. In A. Pitt (Ed.), *Keynotes in teacher education: CATE invited addresses* (pp. 11–20). Ottawa, Ontario: Canadian Association of Teacher Education.

Clandinin, D. J., & Chung, S. (2010). The interwoven stories of teachers, families and children in curriculum making. In M. Miller Marsh & T. Turner-Vorbeck (Eds.), *(Mis)understanding families: Learning from real families in our schools* (pp. 179–195). New York, NY: Teachers College Press.

Lessard, S., Caine, V., & Clandinin, D. J. (2014). A narrative inquiry into familial and school curriculum making: Attending to multiple worlds of aboriginal youth and families. *Journal of Youth Studies, 18*(2), 197–214. doi:10.1080/13676261.2014.944121

Rosiek, J., & Clandinin, D. J. (2016). Curriculum and teacher development. In D. Wyse, L. Hayward, & J. Pandya (Eds.), *Sage handbook of curriculum, pedagogy, and assessment.* London: Sage.

Writings selected for Section IV Journeying with narrative ideas: considerations of the ontological, methodological, ethical, and political entwined with the epistemological

Caine, V., Estefan, A., & Clandinin, D. J. (2013). A return to methodological commitment: Reflections on narrative inquiry. *Scandinavian Journal of Educational Research, 57*(6), 574–586. doi:10.1080/00313831.2013.798833

Caine, V., Lessard, S., & Clandinin, D. J. (2018). Lingering departures: reverberations through, and in, narrative inquiry response communities. In M. Hanne & A. A. Kaal (Eds.), *Narrative and metaphor in education: Look both ways* (Chapter 20, pp. 278–290). Abingdon and New York, NY: Routledge.

Clandinin, D. J. (2013). Introduction and chapter one: Living, telling and retelling: Processes of narrative inquiry. In *Engaging in narrative inquiry* (pp. 9–31). London: Left Coast Press/Routledge.

Clandinin, D. J., Caine, V., & Lessard, S. (2018). Living relational ethics. Chapter 15 in *Relational ethics in narrative inquiry* (pp. 186–203). London: Routledge.

Clandinin, D. J., Lessard, S., & Caine, V. (2013). Reverberations of narrative inquiry: How resonant echoes of an inquiry with early school leavers shaped further inquiries. *Educação, Sociedade e Culturas, 36*, 7–24.

Clandinin, D. J., & Rosiek, J. (2007). Mapping a landscape of narrative inquiry: Borderland spaces and tensions. In D. J. Clandinin (Ed.), *Handbook of narrative inquiry: Mapping a methodology* (pp. 35–75). Thousand Oaks, CA: Sage.

Lessard, S., Caine, V., & Clandinin, D. J. (2018). Exploring neglected narratives: Understanding vulnerability in narrative inquiry. *Irish Educational Studies, 37*(2), 191–204. doi:10.1080/03323315.2018.1465835

SECTION I

Beginning in the midst

Teacher knowledge as a matter of epistemology

1

STUDYING PERSONAL PRACTICAL KNOWLEDGE

It is a commonplace that teachers use their experience when called upon to act spontaneously in instructional settings. It is impossible to imagine that it could be otherwise. To assume that a teacher could somehow be cut free of her[1] history and approach each situation without benefit of past experience would be absurd. Much research in teacher thinking acknowledges a teacher's past experience but this past experience has not become a research focus. At least in part, this lack can be attributed to a stance which views teachers as mere conduits of theoretical and cultural knowledge embodied in various curricula, teaching approaches and policies. The teacher is viewed as merely an agent fulfilling someone else's intentions, a transmitter of external knowledge. A teacher's experience is seen as influencing only how successful she will be in fulfilling someone else's purposes. Her experience becomes important only in understanding how she fulfils external demands. But this lack of research focus can also be attributed to a view of what constitutes valid knowledge. Knowledge is seen as theoretical and as the possession of experts. The experiential knowledge of teachers is not acknowledged. Teachers are viewed as possessing experience but not knowledge. By denying the experiential knowledge of teachers, one can reduce a teacher's experience to a series of factors in decision-making or as an influence on teacher judgment.

However, if a teacher is acknowledged as having an active, autonomous role in the classroom, and if we acknowledge the existence of experiential knowledge, the importance we attribute to understanding the influence of her past experience is enhanced. The present research adopts the view that teachers are autonomous, active agents in their classrooms. Further, the existence of teacher knowledge which is practical, experiential and shaped by a teacher's purposes and values is acknowledged (Elbaz, 1983). The general problem for this research is to develop a conceptualization of this practical knowledge teachers hold and use in their teaching. The specific task of the present study is to offer a conceptualization of a teacher's experiences as they can be seen to crystallize in the form of images. The conceptualization of image as one component of teacher's practical knowledge emerges from the analysis

Reprinted with permission. Acknowledgement: This paper was first published as Clandinin, D. J. (1986). Introduction. Part 1: Studying personal practical knowledge. In *Classroom practice: Teacher images in action* (pp. 3–21). Barcombe Lewes: Falmer Press.

and interpretation of participant observation and interview data from a study with two primary school teachers. The focus of the conceptualization will be on images as they function in the practices of teachers in classroom and school situations and in interview situations.

Reflections on my experience: the research process begins

My interest in the area grows out of my work with elementary school teachers over a six-year period. After spending a short time teaching, I completed a Master's program in Educational Psychology, with major emphasis on elementary school counselling. My intent was to return to the elementary schools as a school counsellor. The position of elementary school counsellor had been established some years earlier and was unique to the local school system. My clinical training focused on therapy with individual children and their families. I had, in addition, an internship of four months in an elementary/junior high school. My host counsellor functioned in the customary school counselling manner of meeting with individual students and making recommendations to the classroom teacher. I had a sense of unease about the appropriateness of his work for an elementary school and wondered if teachers found his help useful. As well, I sensed a negative attitude on his part towards teachers. I found this attitude difficult to deal with as I still thought of myself as a teacher and the counselling role as one of support to both teachers and students.

An incident in a counselling seminar further sharpened my concerns about what I saw counsellors doing in schools. Shortly after my return from the internship, my seminar instructor held a demonstration session with a client from his private practice. The six students in the class observed the session from behind a one-way mirror. The client, who was aware of our presence, appeared visibly upset and spoke more and more softly to our professor, her therapist. The client joined the post-mortem in the class and the students analyzed her behavior in the session using the theoretical training they had received. My observation was that she had been anxious and upset about our presence as observers as well as about the class interpretation of her behavior, which failed to take account of her perspective. Memories of the seminar incident and my sense of uncertainty about my internship experience were with me as I began my job as a counsellor in September.

The two elementary schools to which I was assigned had uniformly bad experiences with counsellors who, from the teachers' viewpoints, imposed unworkable psychological solutions. It was not a friendly climate for a new graduate armed with the same theories. However, full of enthusiasm and sure I could make a difference, I began to apply my textbook theories to teachers and to their classrooms. My success was minimal. I learned instead to spend considerable time in classrooms observing children and their instruction and talking with teachers about their purposes and intentions. Upon reflection, I found that teachers had fairly well worked out, although not articulated, ideas regarding their purposes and intentions in the classroom. They had, for the most part, notions about themselves as teachers; notions about what worked for them instructionally; notions about children, including specific children and children in general; ideas about their school milieu and themselves in relation to that milieu as well as notions about the instructional content that would allow them to fulfil their purposes.

When teachers referred a child to me, they wanted me to make a difference but they were indifferent as to what theory or test I used. It made little sense to suggest what I saw as a solution to a particular child's problem without taking into account the notions that each teacher held and used in relation to that child. Applying a solution based on theory or test results that did not take into account the larger context in which the child functioned did not seem appropriate. I spent time talking with the teacher and observing the child in class in order to gain a more complete understanding of the child's school situation. Based on those understandings and possibly some individual sessions with the child, I formulated some tentative notions about how the teacher could work with the child to make a difference. The teacher and I, often with input and suggestions from the child's parents, worked out at that point what seemed to be the best approach to take in working with a particular child.

Reflecting now, I can see that I was developing a new and more adaptive role for myself as a counsellor working with teachers. Certainly, at the time, I was unable to articulate what I was doing. Not only was I conscious of a discrepancy between my training and what I was doing, but I was aware of a discrepancy between what other counsellors in the system were doing and what I was doing. For example, at a regular elementary school counsellors' meeting when another counsellor described how The Magic Circle program was being instituted in the primary classrooms of his schools, I was able to recognize my work as different but was unable to explain the differences. The Director of Counselling recognized a difference in my work from that of the other counsellors and, in my third year in the schools, invited me to sit on a policy formulation committee when he proposed a shift from 'crisis' counselling to work with teachers. At the meetings, however, I was unable to articulate clearly my work in the schools. In the discussions I was, however, able to point out where I saw his proposed shift as different from my work.

Notwithstanding the difficulty of explaining myself, I was satisfied with the quality of my work in schools. Even though I was conscious of running in opposition to my training and to the overall notion of what elementary school counsellors did, I was receiving positive reactions and reinforcement from the situation for what I was doing and for the direction I was taking. While there were several indicators that I was making a difference, the most meaningful to me at the time was that teachers who had originally been reluctant to have my involvement had begun to express actively their enthusiasm towards my involvement in their programs.

At one point I was described as a change agent by a teacher in one of my schools. My notion of a change agent was that of someone who implemented theories and as far as I could see, I was implementing no theories. At the time I rejected the notion. And yet, in reflecting, I can see how I might be described as a change agent. Through my work with teachers, both individually and in groups, changes were being made. But it was not through the application of theories to teachers, but rather through working out policy changes, programs and ideas with teachers, always with an awareness of the notions teachers already had and used in their planning and teaching.

Although I had strong feelings about the importance of working with teachers in this way, I lacked any way of articulating my experience. Elbaz's work (1983), a case study of one teacher, provided a way to think about my previous experiences as a problem in teacher knowledge. Her conception of practical knowledge seemed consistent with my own intuitive and, at that point, unreflected upon notions of teacher knowledge. Her notion of image as a component of teacher knowledge gave me a starting point from which to think about my work with teachers. My work had focused on teachers as they worked with individual students. The students' teachers, parents or the principal had asked for my involvement with them. Usually the incidents with these students were fairly vivid for myself and for their teachers. Because my work with many of the teachers spanned several years, their actions with these students often guided their actions with students they perceived as similar in subsequent years. For example, after a Grade 4 teacher had worked with me for a year with a particular student, Julia, she asked me for help with a new child the next year by saying, 'I think she's a lot like Julia and I've been trying some of the things we did with Julia. Would you come in and see what I've done and meet her?' 'Julia' served not only as a way for her to talk to me about the student but as guide to her in her work with the new student. The notion of image gave me an exciting entry point into rethinking how those past experiences could have guided the teacher.

Again using the notion of image as a component of teacher knowledge, I had a way of talking about the importance of understanding how a teacher thought about her colleagues and children, both generally and in particular. I now had an insight into describing many situations like the following one, that I had not been able to understand previously. A kindergarten teacher, Elaine, with whom I worked for a number of years, made specific recommendations each year for the Grade 1 classroom placement of each of her students. I observed her in this process for two years. She made the choices quickly and without benefit of outside information. At the time, when I questioned her on the reasons for her decisions, her comments were of the sort 'she seems right for him' or 'they'll be good for each other'. The notion of image gave me a way to think about what she was doing, something I had not been able to do, other than in an uncertain way. I now had a concept for understanding the possible bases for her intuitive decisions.

The concept of image seemed relevant to another situation that has always seemed much different from the one above involving Elaine, but equally puzzling to me. When a primary consultant's position in our board became available, I recommended to a primary teacher, Marianne, that she apply for the position. She was a successful, dynamic teacher who had worked with me on several professional development ventures. Her response to my suggestion was, 'I can't do that. I'm only a Grade 1 teacher.' I was puzzled as to why she didn't see herself as fitting the job description. Once again the notion of image gave me a way of thinking about a previously uncertain situation. With a concept of image I could now view her as having an image of herself as a Grade 1 teacher, not as someone who worked with teachers. It made it possible for me to understand why she had difficulty seeing herself in the job description.

This work with teachers provides an entry point into my research on teacher knowledge. The terms and concepts of practical knowledge have allowed me to reflect on my experience in such a way that the preliminary dimensions of the research problem have become clear. Furthermore, the more informal, reflective analysis of my own experience has allowed the development of a 'natural' or more spontaneous concept of image as a way of understanding how teachers use their past experience in instructional situations.

The significance of the study

In my work with teachers I experienced a personal dissatisfaction with the way teachers are viewed. The prevailing view and organization of the educational enterprise give little credit to their knowledge. My role as a school counsellor was illustrative of the prevailing stance. I was placed in a highly prescriptive role *vis-à-vis* teachers. Because I had advanced training in Educational Psychology, I was assumed to have theories that could be applied to classroom situations. There was, perhaps, some understanding within the educational hierarchy that the teachers might, on the basis of past experience, adapt or modify a theoretical prescription. If they did change the prescription, it was usually taken to indicate a lack of expertise in applying it. But the position I filled in the educational system is only one of many which are in a prescriptive relationship to teachers. Experts in the disciplines and in subject matter areas prescribe solutions drawn from theory to classroom situations. Teachers are, at best, viewed as adjusters or adapters of externally imposed knowledge (Connelly and Ben-Peretz, 1980; Sarason, 1982). The stance adopted in my earlier work with teachers and in the present research is of teachers as thinking, deliberative agents, oriented towards action. Teachers are seen as assuming a position of autonomy over instructional acts.

Teachers are commonly acknowledged as having had experience but they are credited with little knowledge gained from that experience. The omission is due in part to the fact that we have not had ways of thinking about this practical knowledge and in part because we fail to recognize more practically oriented knowledge. The importance of conceptualizing practical knowledge derives from two avenues of thought. One relates to the widely acknowledged disillusion with much curriculum implementation work (Fullan and Pomfret, 1977). In part, the lack of success of curriculum implementation efforts derives from the use of a perspective which minimizes the teacher as an active, autonomous agent *and* a holder and user of practical knowledge. It is not the case that researchers and implementors deny the reality of teacher independence and initiative. Rather, these teacher characteristics tend to be either overlooked or, when recognized treated as an impediment in the implementation process. When a more adequate view of the teacher is adopted, i.e. a view that acknowledges the teacher as an active knowing agent, the importance of coming to understand teachers' practical knowledge is heightened. By a more adequate understanding of teachers' practical knowledge we may be able to provide more adequately for ways of thinking about school change.

The second avenue of thought relates to the fact that teachers as professionals are not seen as possessing a body of knowledge (Lortie, 1975). Consequently, teaching is not recognized as having the status and prestige of other professions, even within the teaching profession. The general stance is that teachers do not possess a body of knowledge unique to their profession. What knowledge they are supposed to have is thought to be in a discipline or subject matter area such as science or reading and not in the profession of teaching. In the research community, this view is slowly shifting as a growing number of researchers (Elbaz, 1983; Connelly, 1980; Schön, 1983) begin to conceptualize this practical knowledge of teachers.

The impetus for this study is a dissatisfaction with the way teachers are viewed and their role conceived in the educational enterprise. This dissatisfaction and my personal struggles to work with teachers in a way that allowed me to value their experiential knowledge lie behind this study.

Key terms in research on teacher thinking

Because much work has been done in the area of teacher thinking, it is important to consider it as a backdrop to the present study. The intent in this section is to place the present research in the context of ongoing research in the area of teacher thinking, not to offer a comprehensive review of research in the area. Excellent reviews examining teacher thinking have been completed (Burns, 1982; Clark and Yinger, 1977; Larocque and Oberg, 1980).

The key terms of the present research are research perspective, role of the agent, view of the teacher, teacher's experience and teacher's personal practical knowledge. These five terms will be used to structure an account of research on teacher thinking and to place the present research within this context.

1 The research perspective

Research on teacher thinking can be distinguished roughly into two classes: research adopting a theoretical researcher's perspective and research adopting a teacher's practitioner perspective. In the former class, the teacher tends to be seen as playing out more or less well a particular theory, policy, planned curriculum or researcher's view of how teachers think about their classroom work. Consequently teacher thought is divided into such practical categories as planning, interaction, reflection and evaluation. These categories tend to be predetermined and embodied in surveys, questionnaires, observation instruments and coding schemes. Because the theoretical perspective is set prior to data collection, teachers are seen to fit more or less well within the framework.

Morine's (1976) work is illustrative. She collected written plans for two experimenter-prescribed lessons taught by teachers to groups of their own students. She then analyzed these plans according to the following seven predetermined characteristics: 1) specificity of written plans, 2) general format of plans, 3) statement of goals, 4) source of goal statements, 5) attention to pupil background and preparation, 6) identification of evaluation procedures, and 7) indication of possible alternative procedures. Her conclusions were that teachers tended to be fairly specific (characteristic 1) and use an outline form in their plans (characteristic 2), but paid little attention to behavioral goals (characteristics 3 and 4), diagnosis of student needs (characteristic 5), evaluation procedures (characteristic 6), and alternative courses of action (characteristic 7). This account of teacher planning is given in Morine's research terms for it was to Morine's perspective that the teachers responded. In their planning, teachers may well have been doing much that was not captured by the imposed research framework.

Other research on teacher thinking adopts a teacher practitioner perspective. In research of this kind an attempt is made to understand teachers from their own perspective. The work of Bussis, Chittenden and Amarel (1976) is illustrative. They examined what they term 'teachers' understandings' using in-depth open-ended interviews to probe the constructs which teachers bring to their work and the relationships among these constructs. The teachers gave their accounts in their own terms, not in terms imposed by the researchers. The research intent was to understand how particular individual practitioners understood their work. Others (Clark and Yinger, 1980; Finch, 1981; Hayes, 1980; Janesick, 1982) have also adopted a teacher practitioner perspective in their research.

But studies which *claim* to adopt a teacher's perspective may, in their methodology, still be conducted from the researcher's theoretical perspective. Mireau's (1980) case study of one teacher is, at first glance, a study which adopts a teacher practitioner perspective. Mireau, using a variety of methodological techniques, did an intensive study of one teacher working in his classroom. While the study purported to give an account from the teacher's perspective, what it does is give an account of the teacher from a wide variety of theoretical terms imposed by the methodologies. This study highlights the point that when the literature in the area of teacher thinking is reviewed, there are studies which claim to have a teacher practitioner perspective, but which, when the methodology and knowledge claims are examined more closely, are conducted in theoretical terms prescribed by the researcher. In Mireau's case the superficial appearance of a teacher perspective study results from the adoption of a case study methodology and from the eclectic use of a variety of theories to classify and explain the teacher's work.

The research perspective adopted in teacher thinking studies has significance for the resulting knowledge claims. Knowledge derived from research adopting a theoretical researcher perspective is knowledge of the universal: of what things are and how they work in general. Hence Morine, noted above, can claim that teachers' written plans, in general, exhibit the characteristics noted. In studies adopting a teacher practitioner perspective, the knowledge claimed is knowledge of the individual case: of what things are and how they work in particular instances. Consequently, Bussis *et al.* (1976) can claim knowledge of individual teachers in their work. The adoption of the latter perspective does not, of course, rule out the possibility of generating universal constructs, such as image or ritual, which are differentially expressed in individual cases.

The present research draws on work which adopts the perspective of the teacher practitioner. Teachers are assumed to hold, use and develop personal practical knowledge. The intent is to understand the personal practical knowledge of two teachers from their perspectives and, in consequence, to elaborate a teacher-based conception of image. The research claims made are, consequently, not about teachers in general but, rather, about particular teachers and their imagery. The construct of image is, of course, treated as a universal conception applicable to the study of teacher practitioners and others.

2 The role of the researcher

Studies on teacher thinking can also be distinguished into two classes based on the role adopted by the researcher: an agent-free role or an agent-central role. The researcher is viewed, in any philosophical account of enquiry, as a commonplace (Herron, 1971). In research characterized by the adoption of an agent-free role, the researcher may not appear as an agent but, when the research is examined closely, the researcher's role becomes apparent.

I posit two classes of research based on the role of the researcher. However, it may be more appropriate to view the role of the researcher as on a hierarchy of possible relationships with the phenomenon that make the researcher as agent more or less central to the research. For example, in field-based classroom studies, the researcher may videotape the teacher at work (Marland, 1977), may observe the teacher using an observation scale (Hildyard, 1982) or may engage in participant observation with the teacher (Janesick, 1977). As one moves from the first to the third study, the researcher can be seen to acknowledge more openly his role as central to the research process. To explore fully the role of researchers as agents in teacher thinking research would in itself constitute a study. Such is not my purpose here. The role adopted by the researcher may be a consequence of his predilections or a consequence of the methodology selected for the study. In either case, however, the methodology is intimately connected with the researcher role.

The agent-free role is characterised by a neutral, objective stance *vis-à-vis* teacher participants; by methods for retaining anonymity such as surveys and questionnaires; by statistical procedures for removing error variance; and by methods for removing researcher bias. This role conceptually separates the researcher from teacher participants. Yamamoto's (1969) study of teacher images of the ideal pupil is illustrative. Yamamoto tested sixty student teachers with three instruments to determine what kind of concepts teachers held of the ideal pupil. He administered the following three statistically reliable instruments to each participating teacher: an ideal pupil checklist, a self-esteem scale and a dogmatism scale. Techniques such as random order of administration of instruments and statistical techniques to remove researcher bias were included as part of the methodology. The accounts of teacher participants are given as statistical comparisons of instrument ratings. Yamamoto's role as researcher appears both neutral and objective in the enquiry.

The agent-central role is characterized by a caring, subjective stance *vis-à-vis* teacher participants and by methods which highlight the values and purposes of both researcher and teachers in the study. Elbaz's (1983) case study is illustrative of this stance. She studied one teacher over a period of two years using an open-ended interview methodology. She began the enquiry with the eventual purpose of conceptualizing a teacher's practical knowledge. Elbaz acknowledged the centrality of Sarah, the participating teacher, but she also acknowledged her own values and purposes as central to the enquiry. Her own purposes and values determined the course of the interviews and in that way she shaped what Sarah offered. The constructs of practical knowledge emerged from Elbaz's interpretation of the interview data. Her role as agent was central to the enquiry.

In the present research the researcher assumes an agent-central role. As researcher, I entered fully into the teacher's classroom and school situation and participated in a wide range of the teacher's activities. My participation in the classroom, in the interviews and in the interpretive process was minded by my personal practical knowledge and shaped by my purposes. The research process was dependent not on minimizing my role as agent but, rather, on acknowledging the centrality of my role and viewing the knowledge claims made as dependent upon the shared meaning created by researcher and teacher participants.

3 The view of the teacher in the research

The research perspective and the role adopted by the researcher necessarily condition how the teacher is viewed in the research process. When a theoretical researcher perspective is adopted, teachers are viewed as more or less representative of the theoretical stance. The nature of individual theories is such that when a theoretical perspective is adopted, only a partial view of the subject, in this case the teacher in her classroom, emerges (Schwab, 1971; Connelly, 1972). Any particular theory is only one of several possible starting points that could be used to give an account of a teacher. When the account is given in terms of the particular theory, it is at best a partial account of the teacher. Much is left unexplained.

Thus, in the research literature, teachers are seen as exemplifying one or another characteristic (Hunt, 1976). For example, depending on the theoretical starting point chosen, teachers have been investigated in terms of the sensitivity of their judgment to the reliability of information received (Shavelson, Cadwell and Izu, 1977); in terms of their interactive decision-making (Clark and Peterson, 1976); and in terms of the types of decisions made in planning situations (Joyce and Hartoonian, 1964). In Morine's (1976) study noted above, teachers were presented in the researcher's terms and, from that perspective, the account of the teachers was limited to the terms of theory, i.e., as reflecting a researcher's theory of how teachers plan. Nothing is revealed about the uniqueness of the individual teacher's planning. In short, the theory is deficient as a complete account of teachers' planning.

Beyond this, however, and of more concern to my study, is the consequence these partial, theoretically determined accounts have for teachers and how they are seen. They, too, are seen as deficient and come to view themselves as deficient when participating in theoretical situations. Fox's (1972) account of biology teachers' deference to biological sciences researchers in curriculum planning settings is illustrative. Gilligan (1982) makes a similar point about how women have been viewed in her analysis of Freud's conclusion that women showed 'less sense of justice than men' following his observation of a sex difference in what is considered 'ethically normal'. Gilligan states that, 'thus a problem in theory became cast as a problem in women's development' (Gilligan, 1982, p. 7) and women, as a consequence, have seen themselves *and* have been seen as deficient in moral development.

The habit of converting a deficiency in theory into a deficiency in the phenomenon is readily seen in how teachers are treated in the school change and implementation literature. The prevailing stance in implementation research views teachers as facilitators of curriculum developers' intentions. When programs fail, teachers are often viewed as the weak link in transmitting the innovation. Research then focuses on one or another of a teacher's characteristics to specify more accurately where the breakdown occurred. When an aspect of, for example, decision-making skills is specified, teachers are given in-service training to bolster their deficient skills. This process feeds a negative, fragmented view of teachers and encourages further research to specify more precisely other teacher deficits noted in still other theories.

When a teacher practitioner perspective is adopted, teachers are viewed as persons and their actions are seen to have meaning in their situations. Teachers are accepted as persons creating their own meaning. For example, Janesick (1982), in her case study of a teacher, adopted this view of the teacher. She described a teacher's perspective as 'a reflective, socially derived interpretation of that which the teacher encounters that then serves as a basis for the actions he or she constructs. It is a combination of beliefs and behavior continually modified by social interaction' (p. 162). Janesick's work gives an account of a teacher as a person as he confronts the reality of his classroom. In part, her account of the teacher is an account of how the teacher views and makes sense of his world.

The present research adopts a stance similar to Janesick's in terms of the view of the teacher. Teachers are viewed as persons in interaction with their milieu. However, the account of the teachers in my study is not only an attempt to see the world through the eyes of the teachers. In part, I attempt to offer such an account, but I also offer a conceptualization of teachers' personal practical knowledge in which teacher practices are expressions of the images the teachers hold. From the point of view of my two participating teachers, the conceptualization is an interpretation of their perspective. It is a statement of *their* perspective. From the point of view of the conceptualization, each teacher's imagery is the material basis for the idea of image resulting from the research.

4 The role of experience in teacher thought

The present study focuses on conceptualizing the experiential knowledge of teachers. Experience is a key term and consequently it is important to examine the concept of experience in research on teacher thinking; to examine briefly the literature on image from the perspective of experience and to place the present study within this context. Let us turn first to the research on teacher thinking.

The experience teachers bring to their work is commonly acknowledged in teacher thinking research and the role assigned to experience is often an explanatory one. Teachers are said to do or think something in some particular way because of their 'experience'. Experience becomes in these instances almost a magical way to account for certain actions. Yinger's work (1977) is illustrative. He studied a grade 1–2 teacher over a five-month period and explained the teacher's routines by appealing to experience. He summarized that 'much of this teacher's planning behavior could be portrayed as the selection, organization, and sequencing of routines developed as a result of experience' (Clark and Yinger, 1977, p. 284). Four types of teaching routines were described in his study: activity routines, instructional routines, management routines, and executive planning routines. Functionally, routines were characterized as 'methods used to reduce the complexity and increase the predictability of classroom activities, thus increasing flexibility and effectiveness' (p. 284). Just what was involved in experience is not made explicit.

Experience, used in a similar explanatory way, is seen by some researchers to penetrate all judgment and decision-making. Clark and Yinger (1977) summarize the importance of work on teachers' implicit theories by writing, 'Because much of the judgment and decision making that teachers exercise follows from their interpretation of their experience, it is important to study how teachers make sense of their world' (p. 295). Research which follows this line focuses on characterizing teachers' conceptual bases as personal perspectives, implicit theories, conceptual systems or belief systems. Experience is assumed to enter into these conceptual bases. However, even in research of this kind, experience is used as a way of explaining the conceptual bases.

In the present research, the intent is to search into the personal experiences of two teachers in order to understand experience as it crystallizes in the form of images and thus forms part of the teachers' personal practical knowledge. The literature of imagination, imagery and image has been explored to locate connections between image and experience.

Scruton (1974) distinguishes between images as a phenomenon in imagination and images as a phenomenon in memory *and* their corresponding links to experience. In imagination, 'what is pictured has not in fact been experienced' (p. 104). In memory, images picture 'something that has already been seen or heard etc.' (p. 104).

How image and experience are linked has been a source of controversy in both the psychological (Nicholas, 1974) and philosophical (Boulding, 1956; Scruton, 1974; Warnock, 1976) literature. Controversy has surrounded the notion of an image as a 'private mental picture formed like a copy of a sense-impression, only slightly more faded' (Scruton, 1974, p. 92). This notion of the link between experience and image has been largely replaced by a concept of image as a 'dynamic symbolic system capable of organizing and transforming perceptual information' (Paivio, 1974, p. 51). According to this literature, 'image' is viewed as functioning in a dynamic process rather than as a passive recorder of experience. Furthermore, memory of experiences recorded in images is seen to involve reconstructive or generative processes and is, consequently, selective and incomplete.

A similar view of the link between experience and image is adopted in therapeutic literature (Assagioli, 1965; Vaughan, 1979). Here 'image' is seen as a central concept in accounting for the flow of thought as a person interacts with an essentially diverse environment. In this view, images are seen as the mediator between the unconscious and conscious levels of being. What is known at the unconscious level finds expression in a person's thought and action through a person's images. Images are thus seen as the source of inspiration, ideas, insight and meaning.

The present research draws on research that views all teacher thought as imbued with experience. However, the intent is to develop a concept of image to give an account of the teacher's experience within personal practical knowledge rather than to use experience as a mere explanatory device. The literature of imagination, imagery and image provides a rich source of distinctions for how image might be linked to experience in teacher thinking studies. It is within the context of both the philosophical and psychological positions described above, in which the concept of image is seen to link experience and image in dynamic and constructive ways, that the present research is placed.

5 The conceptualization of teacher knowledge

Research on teacher thinking which deals with knowledge and teachers can be distinguished into two types: research on what we know about teachers and research on what teachers know. For example, Lortie's (1975) study is a kind of research focused on knowledge *about* teachers. He offered a sociological description of teachers in which he described the backgrounds, education, teaching histories and attitudes towards teaching of teachers in general and, through his study, offered insight into teachers and teaching in general. This kind of study is not dealt with in this book.

Studies of the latter type, that is research on what teachers know can also be distinguished into at least four kinds. One kind of study focuses on what teachers know of theory. For example, such a study provides an account of all of the pieces of knowledge such as knowledge of philosophy, sociology and psychology that teachers in general or even a teacher in particular might be shown to hold. Such accounts might result from an evaluation of teacher education or professional development programs. Clandinin, Wahlstrom and Schermann's (1979) study of early childhood teachers is illustrative of such work. Teachers identified various philosophical, sociological and psychological theories which they knew from teacher education and/or professional development programs and, based on the responses, an account of early childhood teachers' knowledge of theory was given.

A second kind of study which looks at what teachers know focuses on what teachers know in practice. Butt's (1982) research is illustrative of this kind of study. He offered a catalogue of components of knowledge teachers, in general, could be seen to hold. He noted knowledge of such things as timetables, curriculum guides and teaching strategies.

A third kind of study which focuses on what teacher know examines the kind of knowledge teachers hold. Young's (1981) study is illustrative of such work. He gave an account of teacher epistemologies in terms of existing philosophical categories and offered an account of teacher knowledge in theoretical terms. For instance, based on interview data, teachers were classified as having a scientistic or other view of knowledge.

Research on practical knowledge is a fourth kind of study focused on what teachers know. Elbaz (1983), in her work, does some of what each of the other kinds of studies do *but* she does something else as well. She does, for example, in her account of the content of Sarah's practical knowledge, offer an account of some of the theoretical and practical components of Sarah's knowledge. In this way, the work does something similar to the studies of Clandinin, et al and Butt noted above. Elbaz also offers a meta-level analysis of the kinds of knowledge teachers hold. But, in this, the work differs from work such as Young's noted above. While Young made use of categories derived from existing philosophical categories, Elbaz's work on practical knowledge is an attempt to define the form of practical knowledge in its own terms rather than in terms derived from theory.

Elbaz does something else which marks the study as a study of a different kind. She develops the notion of practical knowledge not as knowledge which is just content nor knowledge which is just structure but knowledge which is, in Johnson's (1984) words, 'a contextually relative exercise of capacities for imaginatively ordering our experience' (p. 467). Elbaz's work on practical knowledge opens the way for looking at knowledge as experiential, embodied and based on the narrative of experience.

The present research builds upon Elbaz's (1983) account of practical knowledge. Elbaz offered the constructs of image, practical principle and rule to give an account of the structure of practical knowledge; the construct of orientation is offered to define how practical knowledge is held. Elbaz defined image as 'a brief, descriptive and sometimes metaphoric statement' (p. 254). As the concept of image emerged from her research, it appeared to take on the character of a linguistic tool or, in Lakoff and Johnson's (1980) terms, the character of a public metaphor. The construct of image does not take into account the private experience invested in an image which is part of the construct of image offered in the present research. Elbaz's concepts of practical knowledge emerged from interview situations in which the teacher reflected on her teaching. The interview situation in the present study is viewed as one in which the teacher is communicating about her practice in theoretical terms. Communication in the interview situation is seen as an expression of a teacher's personal practical knowledge and is, in the present study, one of the situations in which personal practical knowledge is expressed and is therefore subject to enquiry. A teacher's classroom practices, such as her routines and rhythms, are also seen as expressions of a teacher's personal practical knowledge.

The task of the present study is to offer a conceptualization of image as a central construct for understanding teacher's personal practical knowledge and for linking such knowledge to past experience and to ongoing practical expressions. These expressions, in classrooms, other school settings and in interviews, are the starting points of the enquiry. The present study reaches both into the teacher's practices *and* into the teacher's personal and professional experiences to offer a conceptualization of image.

Design of the study

The research intent is to develop a conceptualization of image as a component of teacher personal practical knowledge. The purposes and perspectives of this study necessarily condition its design. The conception of personal practical knowledge is of knowledge as experiential, value-laden, purposeful and oriented to practice. Personal practical knowledge is viewed as tentative, subject to change and transient, rather than something fixed, objective and unchanging. It is through phenomenological, dialectic methodologies that the conception of personal practical knowledge advanced in this book has been developed.

Personal practical knowledge as a concept embodies a dialectical view of theory and practice. In the dialectical view (McKeon, 1952), theory and practice are viewed as inseparable; practice is seen as theory in action. In this view, theory is assumed to change and modify according to the shifting exigencies of the practical world. The essential task of the dialectical is to resolve oppositions in theory, oppositions in practice and oppositions between theory and practice. Elbaz assumes a dialectical relationship between theory and practice in her conception of practical knowledge where she has 'shown how the world of practice continually shapes the teacher's knowledge and, conversely, how the teacher herself structures the practical situation in accordance with her knowledge and her purposes.'

The present research is conceptualized dialectically both in the methodologies adopted in the relationships established with the two teachers *and* in the conception of personal practical knowledge offered. Qualitative methodologies have been chosen. In part, justification of the methodologies comes from the dialectical relationships that characterize the interdependence between the researcher and the researched. I cannot, as researcher, enter into a teacher's classroom as a neutral observer and try to give an account of her reality. In order to understand her, I enter into the research process as a person with my own personal practical knowledge. The research process is a dialectical one characterized by Dwyer (1979) as 'a particular form of social action that creates dialectical confrontations and produces intersubjective meaning' (p. 211). The meaning created in the process of working together in the classroom, of offering interpretations and of talking together is a shared meaning. Neither teacher nor researcher emerges unchanged.

Intensive dialectical relationships with the two teachers were established over more than a year of participant observation and interviews. Two teachers in their classroom reality, coping with their students, parents, other staff, principal, consultants and program demands are the focus of the study. In order to be able to offer an understanding of the teacher's personal practical knowledge, an understanding of how the teacher works in her classroom milieu is necessary.

Accounts of developing interpretations were offered to the teachers over the study period. These are written from the perspective of my personal practical knowledge, minded by my reading in theoretical literature. The interpretations of teacher's personal practical knowledge advanced in the book are not accounts of the teachers' actions from the perspective of a theoretical framework. Rather, the theoretical literature enriches my personal practical knowledge, and it is from the perspective of my personal practical knowledge that I develop constructs to give accounts of my intimate, detailed understanding of the two teachers in the study.

The construct of image which I develop in this study is an interpretation, in Polanyi's (1958) terms, derived from my personal practical knowledge rich with my own images and enriched with diverse theoretical readings *and* a detailed understanding of two classroom teachers.

Organization of the study

The study is presented in three main parts. The first, which includes this introduction, is an account of the methodology used in the study and of preliminary work that led to a tentative conceptualization of image. The second is a series of interpretive accounts and characterizations which give a rendition of the two teachers' personal practical knowledge presented in terms of their imagery. Woven into these interpretative accounts is a description of the methodology of the study and of the links to the theoretical literature used in the interpretive process. The final part of the book has three chapters. The first offers a conceptualization of image as a component of personal practical knowledge. The second is an account of the subject matter practices in language arts of the two participating teachers. The third is a reflective look back on the research process and ahead to the educational possibilities of the conceptualization offered.

Note

1 Concerning pronouns in this study, exclusive use of either masculine or feminine pronouns in referring to the teacher would seem to generate either inaccuracies (the majority

of elementary school teachers are women) or unintended political messages. Both forms will be used.

References

Assagioli, R. (1965) *Psychosynthesis*, Harmondsworth, Penguin Books.

Boulding, K. (1956) *The Image*, Ann Arbor, MI, University of Michigan Press.

Burns, R. (1982) 'Conceptualizing the process of teaching: A review of the literature', Paper prepared for the IEA General Assembly Meeting, Toronto, Canada.

Bussis, A.M., Chittenden, E.A. and Amarel, M. (1976) *Beyond Surface Curriculum*, Boulder, CO, Westview Press.

Butt, R. (1982) 'Making sense of classroom reality', Paper presented at the Annual Meeting of the Canadian Society for the Study of Education, Ottawa, June.

Clandinin, D.J., Wahlstrom, M.W., and Schermann, A. (1979), 'The young child in Ontario', Unpublished Research Report prepared for the Commission of Inquiry into the Education of the Young Child, Toronto.

Clark, C. and Peterson, P. (1976) 'Teacher stimulated recall of interactive decisions', Paper presented at the Annual Meeting of the American Educational Research Association, San Francisco, CA.

Clark, C.M. and Yinger, R.J. (1977) 'Research on teacher thinking', *Curriculum Inquiry*, 7, 4, pp. 279–304.

Clark, C.M. and Yinger, R.J. (1980) 'The hidden world of teaching: Implications of research on teacher planning', Paper presented at the Annual Meeting of the American Educational Research Association, Boston, MA, April.

Connelly, F.M. (1972) 'The functions of curriculum development', *Interchange*, 3, 2–3, pp. 161–77.

Connelly, F.M. (1980) 'A conceptualization of the interface between teachers' practical knowledge and theoretical knowledge in effecting board policy', Proposal submitted to the National Institute of Education Grants for Research on Knowledge Use and School Improvement, May.

Connelly, F.M. and Ben-Peretz, M. (1980) 'Teachers' roles in the using and doing of research and curriculum development', *Journal of Curriculum Studies*, 12, pp. 95–107.

Dwyer, K. (1979) 'The dialogic of ethnology', *Dialectical Anthropology*, 4, pp. 205–24.

Elbaz, F.L. (1983) *Teacher Thinking: A Study of Practical Knowledge*, London, Croom Helm.

Finch, M.E. (1981) *Behind the Teacher's Desk: A Study of the Teacher and the Change Process*, Unpublished doctoral dissertation, Washington University.

Fox, S. (1972) 'A practical image of "the practical"', *Curriculum Theory Network*, 10, pp. 45–57.

Fullan, M. and Pomfret, A. (1977) 'Research on curriculum and instruction', *Review of Educational Research*, 47, 2, pp. 335–97.

Gilligan, C. (1982) *In a Different Voice*, Cambridge, MA, Harvard University Press.

Hayes, H. (1980) *Teacher Orientation: An Interview Study of Teachers of English*, Doctoral dissertation, University of Toronto.

Herron, M.D. (1971) 'The nature of scientific enquiry', *School Review*, 79, pp. 171–212.

Hildyard, A. (1982) 'Preliminary findings from the Ontario English-speaking classroom environment study: Teaching for learning', Paper presented at the meeting of the Canadian Society for the Study of Education, Ottawa, June.

Hunt, D. (1976) 'Teachers are psychologists, too: On the application of psychology to education', *Canadian Psychological Review*, 17, 3, pp. 210–18.

Janesick, V. (1977) *An Ethnographic Study of a Teacher's Classroom Perspective*, Doctoral dissertation, Michigan State University.

Janesick, V. (1982) 'Of snakes and circles: Making sense of classroom group processes through a case study'. *Curriculum Inquiry*, 12, 2, pp. 161–90.

Johnson, M. (1984) 'Review of teacher thinking: A study of practical knowledge', *Curriculum Inquiry*, 14, 4, pp. 465–8.

Joyce, B. and Harootunian, B. (1964) 'Teaching as problem solving', *Journal of Teacher Education*, 15, 4, pp. 420–7.

Lakoff, G. and Johnson, M. (1980) *Metaphors We Live By*, Chicago, IL, University of Chicago Press.

Larocque, L. and Oberg, A.A. (1980) 'Implications of research on teacher decision-making for future research, teacher education, and curriculum making', Paper presented at the Annual Meeting of the Canadian Association for Curriculum Studies, Montreal, June.

Lortie, D.C. (1975) *Schoolteacher: A Sociological Study*, Chicago, IL, University of Chicago Press.

Marland, P.W. (1977) *A Study of Teachers' Interactive Thoughts*, Doctoral dissertation, University of Alberta.

McKeon, R. (1952) 'Philosophy and action', *Ethics*, 62, 2, pp. 79–100.

Mireau, L. (1980) *Teacher Expectancy Effects and Student Attributes*, Doctoral dissertation, University of Alberta.

Morine, G. (1976) 'A study of teacher planning' (BTES Technical Report 76-3-1), Far West Laboratory for Educational Research and Development, San Francisco, CA.

Nicholas, M. (Ed.) (1974) *Images, Perception and Knowledge*, Dordrecht, Holland, D. Reidel Publishing Company.

Paivio, A. (1974) 'Images, propositions, and knowledge', in Nicholas, M. (Ed.), *Images, Perception and Knowledge*, Dordrecht, Holland, D. Reidel Publishing Company.

Polanyi, M. (1958) *Personal Knowledge*, Chicago, IL, University of Chicago Press.

Sarason, S.B. (1982) *The Culture of the School and the Problem of Change*, Boston, MA, Allyn and Bacon.

Schön, D. (1983) *The Reflective Practitioner*, New York, Basic Books.

Schwab, J.J. (1971) 'The practical: Arts of the eclectic', *School Review*, 79, pp. 493–542.

Scruton, R. (1974) *Art and Imagination*, London, Routledge and Kegan Paul.

Shavelson, R., Cadwell, J., and Izu, T. (1977) 'Teachers' sensitivity to the reliability of information in making pedagogical decisions', *American Educational Research Journal*, 14, 2, pp. 83–97.

Vaughan, F.E. (1979) *Awakening Intuition*, Garden City, NY, Anchor Press.

Warnock, M. (1976) *Imagination*, London, Faber and Faber.

Yamamoto, K. (1969) 'Images of the ideal pupil held by teachers in preparation', *California Journal of Education Research*, 20, pp. 221–33.

Yinger, R.J. (1977) *A Study of Teacher Planning: Description and Theory Development Using Ethnographic and Information Processing Methods*, Doctoral dissertation, Michigan State University.

Young, R.E. (1981) 'The epistemic discourse of teachers: An ethnographic study', *Anthropology and Education Quarterly*, 12, 2, pp. 122–44.

2

PERSONAL PRACTICAL KNOWLEDGE

A study of teachers' classroom images

Theoretical perspective and key terms[1]

The theoretical perspective of the research derives from the notion of personal practical knowledge with its concern for the development of a person-centered language and perspective for accounting for school practices. According to the perspective, actions are both the expression and origin of the personal knowledge of the actor. Thus, action is imbued with knowledge and knowledge with passion. Action and knowledge are united in the actor and the account of both is of *an* actor.

The phrase "personal practical knowledge" has been discussed in detail elsewhere (Connelly and Clandinin, 1984, 1985). The following is a brief summary of what is intended by the phrase. What is meant by "personal" as defining knowledge is that the knowledge so defined participates in, and is imbued with, all that goes to make up a person. It is knowledge which has arisen from circumstances, actions and undergoings which themselves had affective content for the person in question. This use of "personal" draws attention to the individual local factor which helps to constitute the character, the past, and the future of any individual. By personal as defining knowledge, is meant that knowledge which can be discovered in both the actions of the person and, under some circumstances, by discourse or conversation.

By "knowledge" in the phrase "personal practical knowledge" is meant that body of convictions, conscious or unconscious, which have arisen from experience, intimate, social, and traditional, and which are expressed in a person's actions. The actions in question are all those acts that make up the practice of teaching including its planning and evaluation. "Personal practical knowledge" is knowledge which is imbued with all the experiences that make up a person's being. Its meaning is derived from, and understood in terms of, a person's experiential history, both professional and personal.

There are at least four kinds of studies which focus on what teachers know (Clandinin, in press). One kind of study focuses on what teachers know of theory. For example, such studies provide accounts of all of the pieces of knowledge such as knowledge of philosophy, sociology, and psychology that teachers in general, or even

Reprinted with permission. Acknowledgement: Clandinin, D. J. (1985). Personal practical knowledge: A study of teachers' classroom images. *Curriculum Inquiry, 15*(4), 361–385.

a teacher in particular, might be shown to hold. A second kind looks at what teachers know in practice. Such research offers a catalogue of components of knowledge which teachers, in general, could be seen to hold. A third kind examines teacher epistemologies in terms of existing philosophical categories. Accounts of teacher knowledge in theoretical terms are thus given. Research on personal practical knowledge constitutes a fourth kind of study focused on what teachers know. The notion of personal practical knowledge is not of knowledge which is just content nor knowledge which is just structure. It is, rather, knowledge which is "a contextually relative exercise of capacities for imaginatively ordering our experience" (Johnson, 1984, p. 467).

It is assumed that knowledge so defined is not found in lists of the contents of teacher education textbooks, workshop outlines, or teacher task analysis. These matters, of course, all have their part but such lists, with their categories of concepts, theories, facts, tasks, properties, and skills, do not define a teacher's personal practical knowledge. These lists of objective and definable content are leavened by one's personal and practical experience, subsumed, as Polanyi would say, in one's "subsidiary awareness" (Polanyi, 1958, p. 88). It is this personal and existential matrix that makes up what a teacher "knows" about teaching. Where, then, is this knowledge found? Personal practical knowledge and, in particular, images are found in a person acting. Accordingly, the study of teachers' personal practical knowledge begins in the study of practice. Personal practical knowledge is revealed through interpretations of observed practices over time and is given biographical, personal meaning through reconstructions of the teacher's narratives of experience. Personal practical knowledge is, therefore, found in practice. It is knowledge which is experiential, embodied and based on the narrative of experience.

Image

This article offers a conceptualization of teacher "image."[2] "Image" as a component of personal practical knowledge and as based on the narrative unity (Clandinin and Connelly, 1984; Connelly and Clandinin, 1985) of an individual's life is seen as a central construct for understanding teachers' knowledge. It is important that the notion of image as part of personal practical knowledge not be confused with the notion of image as a "concept" and as a propositional knowledge term. If a critic claimed this definition for my work, it could then be easily argued that the term "image" adds little of substance since standard views on the concept of image and of related events, concepts, and propositions treat the same thing, namely, a form of conceptual knowledge. And this criticism might be true if, after all, my interest was with propositions and concepts about practice. But this is not my interest. Lakoff and Johnson's (1980) work in philosophy follows similar interests to my own in research on teaching. They have developed an alternative account in which human experience and understanding, rather than objective truth, plays the central role. It is, as they say, "an experiential approach . . . to questions of our everyday experience" (p. *x*). Johnson further argues that it is "our images and deep metaphorical structures, as well as our concepts and propositions that constitute our practical knowledge" (Johnson, 1984, p. 467).

My interest is in the imaginative processes by which meaningful and useful patterns are generated in practice. Propositional knowledge in this domain refers only to concepts of, and their relations to, practice. But practice involves more than this. It involves the calling forth of images from a history, from a narrative of experience, so that the "image" is then available to guide us in making sense of future situations. Images are within experience and are not only in the logically defined words which specify their conceptual status. Accordingly, for my work, images are embodied and enacted. Their embodiment entails emotionality, morality, and aesthetics and it is these affective, personally felt and believed, meanings which engender enactments.

Curricular significance of the study

The curricular importance of conceptualizing personal practical knowledge derives from at least two avenues of thought. One relates to the widespread disenchantment with much thinking about curriculum implementation work (Fullan and Pomfret, 1977). In part, the implementation of curriculum innovations did not produce intended changes in classrooms because implementers inadequately accounted for teachers. Connelly and Ben-Peretz (1980) describe three roles teachers have been required to play in implementation. In all three roles, teachers are expected to facilitate someone else's intentions. This failure to understand the teacher as an active holder and user of personal practical knowledge helps explain the limited success of curriculum implementation. When the more vital teacher view is adopted, the importance of understanding teachers' personal practical knowledge is heightened and we are led to more adequate ideas of school reform.

The second reason for the study of personal practical knowledge relates to the popular belief that teachers as professionals do not possess a body of knowledge (Lortie, 1975). Consequently, teaching does not have the status of other professions. What knowledge teachers are thought to have is of a subject matter such as science or reading, not professional knowledge. By recognizing and conceptualizing teachers' personal practical knowledge, one way of enhancing their professional status is secured.

Methodology

The conception of personal practical knowledge is of knowledge as experiential, value-laden, purposeful, and oriented to practice. Personal practical knowledge is viewed as tentative, subject to change and transient, rather than something fixed, objective, and unchanging. These characteristics led to the use of dialectical research methods since it was felt that both the ongoing study and its results would be best pursued with a reflexive outlook between participant and researcher and between action and idea.

Personal practical knowledge as a concept embodies a dialectical view of theory and practice. In the dialectical view (McKeon, 1952), theory and practice are viewed as inseparable; practice is seen as theory in action. In this view theory is assumed to change and modify according to the shifting exigencies of the practical world. The essential task of the dialectical is to resolve oppositions in theory, oppositions in practice, and oppositions between theory and practice. Elbaz (1983), whose work is a forerunner of my own (Clandinin, 1983), can, for example, be seen to assume a dialectical relationship between theory and practice in her conception of practical knowledge where she has shown how the world of practice continually shapes the teacher's knowledge and, conversely, how the teacher herself structures the practical situation in accordance with her knowledge and her purposes. The present research is conceptualized dialectically both in the methodologies adopted in the relationships established with the two teachers *and* in the conception of personal practical knowledge offered.

The foregoing considerations gave rise to the use of qualitative methodologies in the study of image. In part, justification of the methodologies comes from the dialectical relationship that characterizes the interdependence of researcher and researched. As researcher, I cannot enter into a teacher's classroom as a neutral observer and try to give an account of her reality. Instead, I enter into the research process as a person with my own personal practical knowledge. My knowledge of teaching interacts with that of my participants. Inevitably, the data collected reflects my own participation in the classroom and my own personal practical knowledge colors the interpretations offered. The research process is, accordingly, an interactive, dialectical one characterized by Dwyer (1979) as "a particular form of social action that creates dialectical confrontations and produces intersubjective meaning" (p. 211). The meaning created in the process of working together in the classroom, of offering interpretations and of talking together, is a shared one. Neither teacher nor researcher emerges unchanged. In terms of narrative it is appropriate to view this process as the negotiation of two people's narrative unities.

The notion of narrative unity is borrowed from Maclntyre (1981) and is defined as a continuum within a person's experience which renders life experiences meaningful for the unity they achieve for the person. What we mean by unity is the union in a particular person in a particular place and time of all that he has been and undergone in the past and in the past of the tradition which helped to shape him. The notion of narrative unity is not merely a description of a person's history but a meaning-giving account, an interpretation, of one's history. We can see within the history of an individual a number of narrative unities. The notion of narrative unity allows us the possibility of imagining the living out of a narrative as well as the revision of ongoing narrative unities and the creation of new ones.

Intensive dialectical relationships with the two teachers were established over more than a year of participant observation and interviews. The study focused on these teachers in their classroom reality – coping with students, parents, other staff, the principal, and consultants and with program demands, for to understand the teachers' personal practical knowledge, one needs to understand how they work in their classroom milieu.

Two primary teachers, Aileen and Stephanie, participated in the study.[3] Aileen is an Early Childhood Education teacher with 12 years' experience in kindergarten to Grade 3 classes. During the research period, she taught Junior and Senior kindergarten in a traditional elementary school and was the only teacher on the staff using what she calls a "play-based" approach to teaching. Aileen became interested in participating in the study when she was pursuing a graduate degree. Stephanie is an elementary school teacher with 12 years' experience in two inner-city schools. During the research period she taught a split Grade 1 and 2 class in the first year and a Grade 1 class in the second. Stephanie agreed to participate in the study when her school was approached to participate in a large scale research project (Connelly and Clandinin, 1984).

Participant observation methodology was used in both classrooms. I worked in Stephanie's classroom for three half-days per week from April, 1981 to June, 1981 and from September, 1981 to February, 1982, and in Aileen's classroom for the equivalent of one full week in February and March, 1982.

In each classroom I took an active role as a teacher assistant and colleague. I became more deeply involved in Stephanie's class and took a more central role in planning sessions, in discussions of student progress, and in taking responsibility for class projects. (This paper focuses primarily on Stephanie. For a full account of work with both teachers, see Clandinin, 1985).

My involvement with students precluded note-taking during school visits. After leaving the school, usually the same day, events were reconstructed in anthropological style field notes. Dictaphone notes were made and entered into a Dec-10 mainframe computer using a Digital word processor. The principal topics on which notes were made were student activities, discussions with the teacher, observations of the teacher's activities, projects completed, the physical appearance of the classroom, and my own activities. My notes attempted to give a complete account, recording as much detail as could be remembered.

Two unstructured, open-ended interviews were held with each teacher: March and June, 1980 with Aileen and June, 1981 and January, 1982 with Stephanie. The second of each of the interviews were focused, in part, by the teachers' reactions to the narrative accounts discussed below. These interviews were taped and later transcribed and computer-entered. Transcripts were shared with the teachers to give them an opportunity to correct and modify the interview data.

Field note and interview data were initially divided into content units, coded by brief descriptive phrases. This initial interpretive process was enriched by a "theoretical memo" process (Glaser and Strauss, 1967), in which preliminary interpretations and comments on segments of the data were written as I analysed field note and interview data. After initial analysis, the data, which now included raw data, descriptive phrases, and theoretical memos, were re-read in order to identify practices which seemed "minded"[4] by what I speculated were images.

Preliminary narrative accounts were prepared and shared with teachers. These accounts took the form of long letters from me to each participant. The accounts not only provided feedback on my interpretation of classroom activities and interviews but also advanced tentative notions of image grounded in my interpretation of events. The accounts were designed to capture the personal practical knowledge of each teacher by detailing her images and their expression in minded practices in both classroom and interviews. These accounts also described my participation in the classroom and offered tentative ideas on the concept of image for consideration by the teachers.

The teachers responded to the narrative accounts in the second of the above-noted interviews (June, 1980 with Aileen and January, 1982 with Stephanie). Their responses provided insight into their imagery as it was embodied in their practice. These responses, combined with the ongoing participant observation work, led to the preparation of a second narrative account and a brief discussion with each participating teacher in November, 1982.

The essential outline of the notion of image presented in this paper was developed in these four narrative accounts (two per teacher) and has, therefore, been discussed with each teacher. In this way, the reflexive dialectical methods that characterized the practical classroom research are replayed at the ideational level.

Thus, reflexivity is apparent at several levels in the study. There is, at one level, ongoing reflexivity between researcher and teacher participating in classroom practices. At another level, reflexivity marks the relationship between the interview and classroom participant observation data as transcript and field note material are read, given meaning, and re-read with new insights. Reflexivity also marks the relationship between the narrative accounts and the interview discussions that focus on the account. We can see, therefore, that as the methodology of the study is worked through, reflexive dialectical relationships are a recurring mark. There is a dialectical relationship between the concrete and the experiential on the one hand *and* the concrete and theoretical on the other as the methodology unfolds.

In sum, the key idea in this study is of image as an experiential construct. It is a term which reflexively links the person to her practice at one level and, at another level, offers the potential of making links between participant observation data on individual teachers with ideas about teachers in general. I came to understand Aileen and Stephanie's classroom practices in terms of their past experience as it could be seen to crystallize in the form of their imagery and as their imagery was embodied in their practice. Although the interpretations offered in the study are of two individual, distinctive persons, the structure of how and of what I can give an account is the same. I give accounts, in general, of practices, experiences, images, and relationships while acknowledging the particular practices, experiences, images, and relationships of each individual. I talk about Stephanie and Aileen as individuals and also about teachers in general as persons whose experience is reconstructed in the form of images which are expressed in practice. In this way image relates individual participant observation data to teachers in general. Methodologically, then, image is both a practical and a theoretical term. It is a term designed to embody the dialectic of practice and of inquiry.

Stephanie's image of the "classroom as home"

We now turn to a conceptualization of the nature of image through an examination of what I call Stephanie's "classroom as home" image. Through the analysis, the dimensions of the construct of image become apparent.

As noted in the account of the methodology of the study, the notion of image developed through a cyclical sequence of participation observation, interview, and interpretation. My understanding of what I have termed Stephanie's image of classroom as home developed through such a process. The following account, abstracted from the July, 1982 narrative account written to Stephanie, provides a context for understanding the development of the particular image and the concept of image. The excerpt has been altered very slightly because of the changed audience. For example, in the first sentence, "our June, 1981 interview" is altered to read "the June, 1981 interview" and "you" is altered to read "Stephanie."

The emerging image of classroom as home

In the June, 1981 interview Stephanie explained working in the classroom as being something like "running a house." This statement was tentatively identified as an expression of an image which I labeled the "classroom as home" image. After the interview, I began to read the field notes in order to see how I might interpret the way Stephanie's classroom practices could be minded by such an image. I had problems offering an adequate interpretation in the first narrative account. In the January, 1982 interview,[5] Stephanie responded to my interpretation in the following ways:

Transcript segment 1

T. Right, that I refer to our class as our home as our house . . .
I. Yes, yes, and . . .
T. Yes, yes I think so.
I. Okay . . .
T. Yes especially with young children, and even older children, I mean. I don't even know how, I think I say things that slip out, as Freudian slips and I don't even

know why, but you know deep down there's something back there, you picked up everything . . .

(S.W., 2, 61)

Transcript segment 2

T. Yes, I don't know, now don't ask me, now you're going back and want the Freudian reasoning for that but I don't know why it even comes out except that I, the closeness and, and, and . . . I don't know. I don't see how you can, you can segregate, you know that's the big thing there which education always tried to do and it was there in all different parts of the bureaucracy I guess and it's separate, and this is what causes so many problems I think caused a lot of our problems, and the sixties came out of that, people were saying no. . . .

I. Uhhuh

T. no, you know, we want a more together life and not have this type of, of a segregation as it was . . . to our, to our lifestyle . . .

(S.W., 2, 62)

Transcript segment 3

T. You know but that idea of the home well it's a home. I mean, it's or a way, my idea of how a home should be, maybe that was a wrong word to use, maybe or a community, I should have just called it . . .

I. Uhhuh

T. but sure every little area . . .

I. A home is the way you like to think of, of this as being?

T. Of a home being, like when I say home this would be my idea, is a group of people interacting together and cooperating together . . .

I. Uhhuh

T. so that's, that was why I used that term or you could even say mini-community, I think would even be better in that sense cause we're all coming from different backgrounds but yah, I mean, I spend as much time here as I do in my own home and you, you know it should feel, I mean, I feel that you should feel comfortable here, you know which I do . . . cause you know you want to just get out as soon as that bell goes, you've had it, its been a rough day or week, fine but I mean I think you have to have a feeling for a place because if not, I think it shows, it shows in your work, it shows how you work with the children, it shows in the children themselves, how they relate to each other you know . . .

I. Uhhuh

T. and I, I've always been that way, and so this really I guess starts right back from my early years as the big thing was to get that sense of environment to me was very important. I didn't care that they learned one and one is two if they were at each other's throats daily cause you've got to live here, you know, and I just personally, I, I couldn't stand . . . being the . . . you know . . . you know being there to stop fights and whatever, to live and work in that kind of atmosphere . . .

I. Uhhuh

T. so environment and atmosphere have always been very important to me because we're living here, it's a living, learning experience, a living area, it's not a dead room, this room comes alive as soon as we all come in here, you know . . . it, it

> breathes again and lives again and that's how I see it and that's how I hope, really homes should have, should be, you know, interacting together.
>
> *(S.W., 2, 64–65)*

I realized as Stephanie spoke, in the interview, that I had not completely captured either the depth or the significance of the image as a part of her personal practical knowledge. The image as it now appeared seemed more powerful and important than merely an analogous comparison between running or managing a home and managing a classroom.

In the interview Stephanie indicated the classroom was "a home." Her classroom was her "idea of how a home should be," "a group of people interacting and cooperating together. . . ." She felt it "should feel comfortable there" and that "you have to have a feeling for the place because if not, I think it shows, it shows in your work, it shows in how you work with the children, it shows in the children themselves, how they relate to each other."

The image of "classroom as home" as it was expressed in the interviews and in the classroom subsumed various elements of the content of her personal practical knowledge. Knowledge of the instructional process; knowledge of herself as a teacher and person; and knowledge of appropriate subject matter for primary school were all captured by the image. The following three narrative fragments were seen as the embodiment and enactment of Stephanie's "classroom as home" image.

1 At the end of September, the class was being restructured to reduce the class size. Fifteen of the children were being sent to a new classroom. Stephanie wanted to make the last day a special one. She created a party setting much as one would in one's home when friends leave or move away. The following field notes record the event.

> Stephanie told me that because it would be the children's last day in the classroom, as a whole class, she wanted to do something special. She had brought her popcorn maker in and we were going to make popcorn. She also brought in her camera and wanted to take pictures. Stephanie and I discussed the best way to serve the popcorn. Stephanie initially suggested we let the students pass the popcorn as they worked at making it. However, as it turned out, this plan did not work as the students all wanted to gather around and watch the popcorn be made. Stephanie then suggested we just serve them family style by handing the bins around as they were seated on the carpet. Family-style was Stephanie's way of describing it.
>
> *(Field Notes, September 25, 1982)*

2 A second series of events involving a unit on planting was also an expression of the "classroom as home" image. Stephanie had, very early in our work together, asked me to put together a unit on planting. As we worked on the unit and later in the summer and fall, she tried out her planting and growing skills at school and then took her newly acquired skills and knowledge home to put them to use. The following field note segments are a partial account of the events.

> Stephanie found that Al, a Grade 5 teacher, does a lot of planting and growing in his classroom and she had been asking him a lot of questions about how to

set things up. He gave her a geranium and said he would teach her how to make cuttings. Stephanie was quite amazed that the geranium she had, had grown from a cutting. Stephanie is also delighted because an avocado she has been trying to grow has finally started to grow. This is the first time Stephanie has been able to do this.

(Field notes, May 8, 1981)

She commented that she was "very happy about how the beans were growing," and she was "excited about what we had been planting." She had collected many more pots; she wanted to transplant some of the plants from the school to her garden; and she wondered about starting tomato plants. She said they had cleaned both their front and back yards and had taken out a tremendous amount of garbage. She wanted to have space to plant things. She filled an old bathtub on her front lawn for the first time in two years with geraniums. What we had done at school had really made her excited to get things done at home.

(Field notes, May 20, 1981)

Later in October

I forgot to mention earlier in the morning, before school started, her friend came over to the school with two pumpkins from their garden. We put the pumpkins under the language experience chart. Stephanie had left the earth on the pumpkins because she wanted to let the students know she had grown them.

(Field notes, October 26, 1981)

3 Stephanie's practices around the Hallowe'en celebration were an expression of Stephanie's image of "classroom as home." Her preparations for the event seemed to me to be reminiscent of how I get ready for a celebration in my own home. The box of Hallowe'en decorations, the displays to create atmosphere, and the culmination of the week of festivities in a party are presented in the following field note segments.

I arrived at the school at 8:30. I went right down to Stephanie's class. She was in the room, the door was open. I was immediately struck by how much had happened in the room over the weekend. The farm display at the back was set up, the pictures off the back wall were down, there were criss-crossed clotheslines hanging from the ceiling with Hallowe'en displays, the Hallowe'en words were up in the display and the front board displays were all arranged.

(Field notes, October 26, 1981)

She showed me some Hallowe'en pictures she wanted me to laminate that morning. She also wanted me to mark and file the work. When we were going through the Hallowe'en box digging out the pictures for laminating, she found some sample Hallowe'en books and decided she wanted to have the children make those. She needed one more pumpkin cut out and laminated. The pumpkin needed to have the word "mask" printed on it. The preparation of the Hallowe'en pictures seemed to be her first priority.

(Field notes, October 26, 1981)

After recess time I worked with the children on the baking of the pumpkin seeds. I came back down to the classroom about twenty-five to twelve and told Stephanie

> she should be on her way out to get more party supplies. Stephanie told me she didn't think there would be time for a story. When I arrived back in the classroom, several children were hanging balloons, Wallace's table was being covered with a black tablecloth made of crepe paper, Gail and another student were sorting apples for bobbing and there was much party activity going on. I tried hastening Stephanie out of the classroom by telling her she had to get back to take the pumpkin seeds out of the oven. She said she would do that on her way out of the school. She wanted all the books and boxes left stacked in the centre of the children's tables so the napkins could be handed around and so the children would have room at the tables. I told her I would have the children do that.
>
> *(Field notes, October 30, 1981)*

The importance of the home center; the importance of baking and cooking; the amount of personal money spent in the classroom and the beautiful displays she used to create a warm homey atmosphere, also were expressions of the image of the "classroom as home."

The preceding section, taken from a narrative account, provides a sense of how my understanding of what I call Stephanie's image of classroom as home emerged through the research process. In the remainder of the article, I outline the dimensions of the classroom as home image. I explore first how the "classroom as home" image links Stephanie's personal life with her professional teaching life.

The image as a link between Stephanie's educational and personal life

What I refer to as Stephanie's image of the "classroom as home" highlights the experiential link between a teacher's educational and personal private life. This image captures, in its origin and function, aspects of both spheres of Stephanie's life. Stephanie, in talking about her teaching, speaks of her classroom as a home, "You know about that idea of the home. Well it's a home. I mean . . . my idea of how a home should be" (S.W., 2, 64).[6] In this verbal expression of the image, both personal private and educational aspects of her life are captured; the image draws together both the home and classroom. An examination of how the image provides this link between Stephanie's personal private and educational life through its origins in her experience is presented first.

Origins of the image of "classroom as home"

The image has its origin in Stephanie's personal private life. She holds a view of herself as a child and as a student who was "always different" and who marched to "another beat" (S.W., 2, 38). She described her own school experiences as a "packaging" experience and felt that those who did not fit the package were "scattered by the side" by the educational system (S.W., 2, 13). She describes herself as one of the ones who didn't fit the package and was "left out" (S.W., 2, 13).

A sense emerged from the transcripts that she had experienced a home such as the home she wants to reconstruct in her classroom. It is a place where "people cooperate and interact together" (S.W., 2, 66). No clear sense of where or in what manner she participated in such a home emerged. She describes the emotional and social attributes of the imagined home as a place where people can interact and cooperate but where each person has his or her own space and where each is "free to march to their own drummer" (S.W., 2, 38). Two other aspects of the "home" were apparent: a home is to be full of treasured things and it is to be a "living area" (S.W., 2, 66). The "classroom as home" image is, thus, rooted in her personal school and home experiences. But the image also has its roots in her professional experience. In Teacher's College, she again felt out of step – out of step with the way student teachers were being taught, that is, as "mini-models where you had to model the style of the teacher" (S.W., 2, 56) and with what and how they were to teach. She saw herself as someone who reacted to this felt-pressure for conformity and "so," she says, "I came liberal" (S.W., 1, 45). The significance of this personal interpretation of her experience is that she felt a continuity of experience as her experience of public schooling was replayed as she entered professional life.

Not until Stephanie had her own class did she begin to feel "in step." She underwent what she called "a metamorphosis" (S.W., 2, 40) after she began teaching. In her classroom she was able to create a space in which she felt "in step." She spent then, as she continues to do now, long hours creating an environment in which she and her students could feel comfortable and cared for, in short, a home environment.

In its origin then, the image is rooted in four areas of Stephanie's experience: in her professional experience, "so this really I guess starts right back from my early years as the big thing was to get that sense of environment" (S.W., 2, 65); in her professional training, "that's the big thing there which education always tried to do and it was there in all different parts of the bureaucracy" (S.W., 2, 62); in her own school experience, "and I think it did a lot of harm in those years" (S.W., 2, 62); and in her private life, "like when I say home this would be my idea – a group of people interacting together and cooperating together" (S.W., 2, 62). These professional and personal origins are linked in Stephanie's classroom practices by the image of the "classroom as home."

This brief narrative account of Stephanie's personal and professional biography, as reconstructed in her personal knowledge of her classroom as a home, sets the stage for the reader to see how the personal and professional are linked both in Stephanie's personal and professional life. The following two instances illustrate how the image links her personal and professional life in practice.

The planting unit

The image was expressed in a number of classroom events recorded in my field notes. One instance detailed above in the narrative account, was the work on the planting unit. When Stephanie first asked me to work on the unit, I did not understand it as anything more than a science unit in the program. At the time I saw it more or less as a random choice and thought it could have been any other unit. However, I now see Stephanie's request as minded, in part, by the "classroom as home" image. The link between her personal private life and her educational life is especially important in providing an understanding of how the image functions within her personal practical knowledge.

To many people and particularly to Stephanie, a home should have a garden or at least have growing things as part of it. Her emphasis on a "living" (S.W., 2, 66) component of the home image suggests that importance, as does her choice of her personal home, an old house she is renovating in an inner city neighborhood. To be able to grow things is important to Stephanie. Her interest in the planting and growing activities serves functions in both her personal and professional life.

On one side, the planting activities contribute to the "home in the classroom." The bean plants, the garden, the avocado, and the geranium, discussed briefly in the excerpt from the interpretive account, contributed to the home-like classroom environment. On the other side, the planting activities at school were a way for her to try out something for her personal life. With the success of our activities at school, Stephanie took her newfound skills home. As noted earlier in the narrative account, she planted her front yard bathtub with geraniums and, in her backyard, grew a garden complete with vegetables and pumpkins for Hallowe'en. The classroom "home" became a testing ground for her personal home.

Thus we see how the unity of the personal and professional in Stephanie's personal practical knowledge is expressed in both the personal and professional spheres of her life. Further, we see how the personal and the professional interact reflexively within the image of "classroom as home." The effect on both home and school of the image expressed in action is dramatic. Elements in both are transformed. On the school side, school subject matter is selected and organized in a particular way; the classroom atmosphere is changed; inner-city students are given new experiences; Stephanie sees herself as a resource to other teachers interested in planting; and she seeks out staff members who are interested in similar activities. On the personal side, her home life is enriched as new hobbies develop and the physical appearance of her personal environment is enhanced. This, in turn will, I speculate, affect such matters as her relationship with friends as she shows off her garden, and her interaction with neighbors as she works in her garden.

The celebration of cultural holidays

The image is dramatically expressed in Stephanie's rhythm[7] of the school year. Stephanie responds in her practice to the cycle of major celebrations in mainstream Canadian society, events such as Hallowe'en, Christmas, and Easter, events celebrated by many people in their homes with family traditions and rituals.

Stephanie's image of the "classroom as home" is given meaning by her particular rhythms of teaching. Just as there are rhythms in our North American Christian home life[8] tied to cultural givens such as the work week and cultural holidays such as Christmas, Thanksgiving, and Easter, there are similar rhythms in Stephanie's classroom life. Rhythms serve to modulate an individual teacher's imagery and to moderate, smooth out, and make harmonious personal and social action. Stephanie's rhythm is one in which she expresses the rhythms of her culture at the same time as she accommodates the cultural holidays of others. The result is a harmonious living out of the school year in such a way that her own personal and cultural rhythms and those of her students find expression in her classroom.

The ways in which Stephanie approaches each celebration are expressions in part, of the "classroom as home" image. For example, in the narrative account noted above, we saw how at Hallowe'en she transformed the classroom. She devoted her weekend to decorating it; she made Hallowe'en activities a priority for both her own and my activities; and she rejected what I wanted to do, i.e., read a story, in favor of making the room more home-like by setting up tables with tablecloths and napkins. The focus for the celebration moved from her private home to the classroom home.

Her classroom practices are ones of living out and knowing the classroom rhythmically and as a home. Because she knows the classroom in these ways, the celebration of Hallowe'en in the classroom is a way for Stephanie to make the children feel "at home" and to permit them to participate in her culturally influenced rhythms of the classroom.

These two expressions of the image – the planting unit and the celebration of cultural holidays – illustrate how the "classroom as home" image links Stephanie's personal private and professional life. As the image was expressed in action, new forms of expression were added. Stephanie's home, both in the classroom and in her personal home, became places where plants flourished. Stephanie's classroom became a place where her personal cultural holidays and those of her students could be celebrated.

Temporality and the image of "classroom as home"

The expression of the image both in verbal communication and in classroom practices is always in the present. Its origins are in the past. As the image finds new forms of expression in practice, however, it reaches into the past and reorders both professional and personal private experiences. For example, one expression of the "classroom as home" image was in the baking and cooking activities Stephanie suggested I do with the children in the classroom. These activities constituted a new expression of the image. As a result of this expression of the image we might imagine Stephanie came to see earlier baking activities with students, for example, making potato latkes which she had done for the school Festival of Lights (Field notes, December 16, 1981), as important in creating a home atmosphere. Similarly, we might imagine that previous baking-related experiences in her personal private life were important in creating Stephanie's personal home.

Experiential images, therefore, have an historical character, both in their origin and in their reconstruction of past experiences, to meet the demands of a particular situation. But experiential images also have a future character. The image of home points the way to future expressions in both Stephanie's personal and professional life. For example, Stephanie told me in a conversation "that once you have taught kindergarten or been in the primary, any grade level within the primary is not too much of a challenge" (Field notes, September 10, 1981). If Stephanie were to teach in another grade or in another subject area such as English as a Second Language (an area into which she would like to move), the "classroom as home" image would find expression in new settings. In future situations in both her personal and professional life, the image would still be expressed in her practices. It would be marked by an emphasis on environment, her interactions with others, and the importance of creating a space where each participant would be free to "march to his or her own drummer."

In this temporal (past, present, and future) aspect of the image, insight is gained into how image as a knowledge component is related to the phenomenal world and to future knowledge. New situations are experienced from the perspective of the image as a part of personal practical knowledge. Teaching at a different level or in a different program area are interpreted from Stephanie's perspective of the "classroom as home" image. New situations in her personal life, such as planning for another holiday celebration, can also be interpreted as being experienced from the perspective of the image. New knowledge can be added as previous experience is reordered and shaped by expressions of the image. Hence, Stephanie gains knowledge of herself as a person able to successfully grow plants as a result of the expression of the "classroom as home" image in her school planting practices.

Emotional and moral dimensions of the image of "classroom as home"

To understand the image of home as a link between Stephanie's personal private life and her educational life is an important step in understanding her teaching practice as an expression of her personal practical knowledge. Image as a form of personal practical knowledge is an embodied, experiential meaning complex and we understand Stephanie's image of home as a crystallization of her experience, experience in which emotions and morality are elements. Without an understanding of the moral and the emotional, this account remains lifeless and lacks the fire that characterizes her teaching.

The emotional dimension

The image of "classroom as home" is strongly held. As the image was expressed in our second interview, Stephanie tried to reject it . . . "you know, about that idea of the home. Well it's a home. I mean, . . . my idea of how a home should be. Maybe that was a wrong word to use, maybe a community, I should have just called it . . ." (S.W., 2, 64). But after briefly exploring the possibility of rejecting it, she returned to affirm the image of "classroom as home," as pointing to crucial ways in which she knows her teaching.

The words used to convey her meaning were ones which conveyed the image's emotional dimension. She talked about "the closeness" (S.W., 2, 62); the relational aspects, "interacting" and "cooperating" (S.W., 2, 64); and "the living" aspects of being with others (S.W., 2, 65). In her verbal expression of it, there seemed little doubt there was an emotional coloring to the image.

This coloring derives from the experiences that gave rise to the image. The experiences were emotional ones and this emotion is carried forward as part of the image. Dewey (1934, p. 42) describes emotion as "the moving and cementing force" in an experience. Emotion, says Dewey, "selects what is congruous and dyes what is selected with its color, thereby giving qualitative unity to materials externally disparate and dissimilar." The experiences in which Stephanie's image of "classroom as home" are rooted, make real Dewey's view of emotion in experience. Emotion was evident in Stephanie's verbal expression of the experiences of her home, school, professional training, and teaching. She described her school experiences with words loaded with emotion, such as "bitter" (S.W., 2, 17), "terrible" (S.W., 2, 17), and as "desperately unhappy" (S.W., 2, 38). The "metamorphosis" (S.W., 2, 40) she underwent in her early years of teaching was described as allowing her "to get the confidence" (S.W., 2, 41) to "give of herself" (S.W., 2, 40).

The emotion within each of these early experiences is recollected by Stephanie and we sense how emotion has been, and continues to be, a "moving" and "cementing" force in the image of "classroom as home," an image central to her teaching. It is, perhaps, easiest to understand the emotional strength of the image when we consider its moral dimension. The two are so closely connected in experience that it is difficult to talk about one without the other. Stephanie does not "know" abstractly that a teaching act is good or bad; she *feels* it as such. It is their combination, their unity in the image, that contributes to the image as a "moving force" in practice.

The moral dimension

In Stephanie's verbal expression of the image, a sense of its moral coloring emerged. The image is not neutral; a classroom *should* be like a home and both classroom and home *should* have certain features. There is, then, in her verbal expression of the image a "should" and a "should not" character. A sense of the possibility of "better" or "worse" action emerges. For Stephanie the better action allowed her "to live here" (S.W., 2, 65) and "to treat people as individuals and humans" (S.W., 2, 63).

In its practical expression, a sense of the moral dimension of the image also emerged. For example, the party Stephanie held in her classroom to mark the departure of some of her students in September, 1981, noted above in the narrative account, is an expression of her "classroom as home" image. The party was an exceptional gesture, such as one might make to mark the departure of friends from one's home. In the expression of the image, there was a better and a worse way to acknowledge the students' departure. Stephanie could have chosen to act differently. We might, for example, imagine alternative expressions of the "classroom as home" image in this instance. But not to mark their departure by an expression appropriate to that of persons leaving her home would not have been the "right" thing for Stephanie to do.

The moral character of the image provides Stephanie with a judgmental standard for her practices. This standard is unique to Stephanie. When practices are discordant, the moral coloring of the image highlights the discordancy. In my work with Stephanie, this was most clearly evident when I took action, or attempted to take action, which conflicted with an expression of her imagery in practice. For example, I suggested that we have the children take home the growing bean plants when I felt the unit was complete. Stephanie resisted my suggestion as she felt the plants were continuing to add to the "classroom as home" environment (I.A.2). In its practical expression, environment was an important element of the image. A certain kind of environment "should" be created in the expression of the image. My interference created a discordant note and Stephanie acted to stop my plan.

As is the case with the emotional, the moral coloring of the image emerges from the experiences in which it has its origin and from her judgment of the experiences as "good" or "bad." Accordingly, the moral character of the "classroom as home" image emerges, in part, from Stephanie's judgment of her school experience as a "packaging experience" (S.W., 2, 13) in which she was hurt. The image takes on the moral shadings of her judgment of the experience as bad, and from this experience she derives a standard of judgment of her own practices. Similarly, her experiences of herself as a child who was marching to a different drummer; who failed to fit into the standard mold; and who eventually came to see herself as "slow" and not able to "see things properly in a perspective" (S.W., 2, 38) all contribute to the moral coloring of the "classroom as home" image. These experiences were negative and her judgment of them contributes to her standards of judgment for her practices.

In my final narrative account of Stephanie, I characterized her within a governing framework of relationships. The relationship theme illustrates how the moral coloring of Stephanie's "classroom as home" image emerges from its origins in her experiences of relationships with others and in her judgment of herself within those relationships. The experiences appear to be ones in which the particularly critical moral issue of hurting is involved. My account of Stephanie's experience parallels Gilligan's account of women's moral development. "It is," says Gilligan, "in their care and concern for others that women have both judged themselves and been judged." (1982, p. 165). The relationship context helps both to explain the moral vividness of the image, and how this image serves as a guide to Stephanie in her relations with students.

Gilligan highlights the importance of understanding women within a framework of relationships. To understand Stephanie's image of "classroom as home," the relationship aspects of the originating experiences and the resulting moral coloring of the image must be confronted. I noted above Stephanie's struggle in her early teaching experiences to see herself as a worthwhile person after her experiences in both school and professional training in which she saw herself as being hurt. Through what Stephanie termed her "metamorphosis" she came to see herself as a person worthy of care and as someone whom she considered it "moral" not to hurt. Her earlier experiences were seen by her as negative, and while she doesn't judge herself as wrong within her relationships, she now has a standard for judging herself in her relationships with others both in school and outside of it.

In sum, the image of "classroom as home" became a nucleus around which significant elements of her experience, complete with moral coloring, were attracted and shaped. The moral character of the "classroom as home" image derives from significant elements of her home, school, professional training, and teaching experiences. In the coalescence of Stephanie's experiences into the image, all life experiences, not only those from her personal private life nor only those from her educational professional life were attracted and drawn together to form her personal practical knowledge. Thus we see how the moral coloring of the image is grounded in her experiences and ultimately in how she judges herself within her relationships.

The concept of image summarized

The concept of image is frequently used in the social science literature. However, my use of the concept is as a form of personal practical knowledge and the term assumes its meaning within the framework of personal practical knowledge. I do not view it as a therapeutic tool as, for example, it is used in the psychological literature (Assagioli, 1965; Progoff, 1975), nor as a standard for instructional purposes in the way Howard (1982) develops the notion for music instruction. Rather, image, in this research, is a kind of knowledge, embodied in a person and connected with the individual's past, present, and future. Image draws both the present and future into a personally meaningful nexus of experience focused on the immediate situation which called it forth. It reaches into the past, gathering up experiential threads meaningfully connected to the present. And it reaches intentionally into the future and creates new meaningfully connected threads as situations are experienced, and new situations anticipated from the perspective of the image. Image is the glue that melds together a person's diverse experiences, both personal and professional. An image has emotional and moral dimensions and I have shown how these characteristics mark out the knowing contained in the expression of image in classroom and interview practices. In accordance with this view, action, and the personal knowledge embodied in it, is imbued with meaning-giving emotionality and morality. The concept of image, as developed in this study, emerges from the imaginative processes by which meaningful and useful patterns are generated in minded practice. Minded practice involves the emergence of images out of experience so images are then available as guides for the person to make sense of future situations.

In subsequent pages I turn to a general consideration of the origin and expression of images.

The origin of image in experience

The central idea of the research is that teachers' classroom images grow out of their experience, both private and professional. They are a kind of coalescence of experience, with moral, emotional, and personal overtones reflecting the quality of the experiences in which they are based. Just as each image is specific to a particular teacher, the experiences in which the image is rooted, and the way it is related to that experience, are also specific to the teacher.

Some experiences have a "watershed" character and form vivid detailed visual images.[9] Aileen's image of a particular child's face is illustrative. She now views her experience with this particular child as a turning point in her teaching, frequently calling his face to mind when confronted with other children's problems. The image has a copy-sense impression. This child's face and Aileen's relationship to the child form the core experience around which the image has developed. Stephanie's image of her high school math experience is similarly rooted in one watershed experience. In her case, however, while the image is vividly emotional, it contains less visual detail.

Other images, equally powerful, are less directly linked to specific events in the teachers' lives. These images are formed from a coalescence of many diverse experiences over a long period of time. Their formation occurs in processes similar to those described by Dewey in his notion of the "continuity of experience" (1938) and by MacIntyre in his notion of the "narrative unity of life" (1981).

Some of the images linked to experience in this narrative sense assume a metaphorical quality. Aileen's image of "language is the key" is illustrative. For Aileen, language is the central cognitive, substantive, and social theme around which her classroom is organized. This is seen in her play-based kindergarten program, justified by her in terms of children's language development; in her graduate level study in a combined Early Childhood and Language Education program; and in her tendency to equate children's cognitive development with their language development. Her phrase "language is the key" expresses metaphorically her deep sense of the importance of language in her teaching. Images of this kind take on the quality of Lakoff and Johnson's "experiential metaphors" (1980).

Other images exhibit the same quality as "language is the key" but retain more of the specifics associated with images connected to watershed experiences. Stephanie's image of "the classroom as home" is illustrative. Unlike Aileen, who often asserts that "language is the key," Stephanie only infrequently refers to the classroom as a home. Yet in the organization of classroom activities; in the interpersonal relationships she establishes with students; in the daily opening and closing class routines; and in her curriculum planning around annual cycles of school events, Stephanie is clearly living out her image of "classroom as home." The specificity of this image is seen in the organization of her own home life and in her cultural traditions. Images with this metaphoric quality have a "real analogy" sense like that described by Black (1962).

This study has not, of course, exhausted either the possible *kinds* of experiential images nor their various possible experiential origins. Such an understanding will emerge from the results of long term studies of images of more teachers than the two in this work. Furthermore, unraveling the historical antecedents to particular teacher images is a task that depends on the aspects of classroom experience in which one is interested. Gendlin (1962) puts the matter well when he reminds us of the many meanings an experience may have for a person. "Any experienced meaning," he writes, "will be differentiate into countless experienced meanings, each of which, because it is a meaning, will again be differentiable into countless meanings. Apart from this specification, it is always multiple. Experiencing is multiple, nonnumerical." (Gendlin, 1962, p. 152). We may imagine, therefore, that the search for understanding of the experiential origins of images is rich in possibilities.

The expression of images

In earlier sections, we saw how the "classroom as home" image was expressed in Stephanie's classroom and in her home. In this section, I distinguish between the verbal expression of images and their expression in classroom practices. Logically, either form of expression may occur without the other. A teacher may, in her explanations of her teaching, express herself with images which may not be expressed in her classroom practices. Likewise, a teacher's classroom practices may be expressions of images that are not verbally expressed.[10]

Perhaps because of the widespread and common use of interview methodologies for the study of classrooms, teachers' speech *about* themselves has often been equated with their practice. If there is a spoken report of a practice, there is a tendency to say that there is such a practice. But my study of teacher images in classroom and in interview practices leads me to view this matter more akin to that of Einstein when he wrote, "The words or the language do not seem to play any role in my mechanism of thought. The physical entities which seem to serve as elements in thoughts are certain signs and more or less clear images which can be voluntarily reproduced and combined" (Einstein in Hadamard, 1945, p. 142).

Einstein was speaking of a different situation and of images with different content but the translation of images into words seems remarkably like Stephanie's translation of the "classroom as home" image, with its disparate elements, into words in our interview. Stephanie struggled to give an adequate verbal expression. She tried one, rejected it, and settled on the classroom being a home. She chose to use a metaphor to capture the image. In her choice of metaphor she chose one with a public meaning. We often say a place is homelike or homey when we want to convey a notion of warmth or coziness. The verbal expression then, at one level, is a public one.

Hunt comes close to what I intend in his notion of "teachers as their own best theorists" (Hunt, 1976). A teachers' verbal expression of an image is essentially her theory, her explanation to others, of her practices. This, in general, is the relationship between the two modes of image expression that emerged in this study.

The verbal expression of images

Some of the teachers' images were frequently expressed verbally, for example, Aileen's images of "language is the key" and of "myself as an island." Whenever discussion turned to the purposes of instruction or to her professional place within the school, she used these images to explain herself.

Other images were not expressed verbally as, for example, Stephanie's image of herself as "maker." She did, however, readily agree to the interpretation of her practice, which showed how she taught language arts through the making of books, pictures, and models. What I have called Stephanie's image of "making" is part of the image of "classroom as home," which is more deeply embedded in her life. Occasionally, Stephanie referred to the "classroom as a home" in her conversations and she occasionally discussed classroom management with the children in terms of what was proper to the running of a home.

Overall, the verbal expression of an image tends to function metaphorically in situations where the teacher is explaining herself to another. These verbal expressions of images represent "personal theories" of oneself. In this sense, verbally expressed images allow teachers to generalize on their experience and to offer theoretical accounts of what they do.

Expression of images in practice

Because a teacher's world is essentially one of action, they are not often called upon to verbally explain themselves and to put terms on their actions. Talking about what they do is not a necessary part of their practice. However, an interesting (and unanticipated) benefit of this study was the value teachers placed on the reflective opportunity to read and discuss interpretations of their work.

Since the central focus of the research was to understand practice, all of the images described were built up out of field notes made in classrooms. It was from reflection on practice that this study's concept of image grew. The images are essentially images of practice. In the two instances where my first insight into the images came verbally, i.e., Aileen's "language is the key" and "myself as an island" images, I sought confirmation and expression of its meaning in classroom events.

The account of Stephanie's "maker" image, an image expressed only in practice, grew up out of repeated observations and was tested through discussions of the narrative accounts with Stephanie. At most, the verbal showed up in practice in Stephanie's student directions such as "show me" rather than "tell me." One of the implications of this method of studying images is that they are not merely mental constructs to be expressed; they are embodied in action. When we see practice, we see embodied images (Johnson, 1983).

Conclusion

There is a dialectic between the two purposes of the study: the practical understanding of the two teachers *and* the theoretical notions of personal practical knowledge, particularly image, as a language and perspective for inquiry. The theoretical ideas are based on the classroom data and, in turn, enrich our understanding of the teachers.

The conceptualization of image developed in this study contributes to a theoretical understanding of the nature of personal knowledge that differs from that usually thought of when we consider the problem of knowledge, a point well made by Polanyi (1958). Personal practical knowledge is an emotional and moral knowledge. It actively carries our being into interaction with classroom events. Personal practical knowledge is, furthermore, intimately connected with the personal and professional narratives of our lives. It is not something which has an independent and objective standing apart from our personal histories. Readers have seen how the image of "classroom as home" originates in both the personal and professional spheres of Stephanie's life; binds the two together in a narrative unity; and are reflected back upon each as the image is expressed in Stephanie's home and school activities. Finally, it is evident from the discussion of the verbal and practical expressions of images that personal practical knowledge need not be clearly articulated and logically definable in order to exert a powerful influence in teachers' lives.

This research has at least two practical consequences. One is that with the concept of personal practical knowledge as a language and perspective for viewing school practices, we assume a stance which credits and values teachers' knowledge. A second is the formation of a different notion about the improvement of schools, a notion that builds on the personal practical knowledge of teachers by working with them rather than on or against them.

Acknowledgement

This work was supported by research grants from the Social Sciences and Humanities Research Council of Canada (Grant #410-80-0688-Xl) and the United States National Institute of Education (Grant #NIE-G-81–0020).

Notes

1 I am indebted to Professor Joseph Schwab for his detailed comments and assistance in developing this introductory section.
2 Professors Elliot Eisner and Mark Johnson have aided my thinking on image. The one has encouraged my development of the study of imagination as a novel way of thinking about the practice of teaching and the other has encouraged me to reflect on the philosophical significance of an experiential conception of knowledge.
3 To protect the privacy of participants, pseudonyms are used throughout the paper.
4 The use of the term minded was triggered by Jenning's (1982) notion of minded action in his discussion of religious ritual. In our work on personal practical knowledge (Connelly and Clandinin, 1984), we view teachers' practices as the embodiment and enactment of their personal practical knowledge. In my work on images, I understood Stephanie's and Aileen's practices as the embodiment and enactment of their personal practical knowledge of which their imagery was a part. The concept of minded practice is used to capture this understanding.
5 The interview transcripts have been edited slightly to improve their readability.
6 Bracketed material refers to coded field note, interview, and narrative account material.
7 Rhythm is used in the commonplace sense of something recurring repetitively, perhaps cyclically, and which has an aesthetic quality as performed. Rhythms as part of personal practical knowledge serve to modulate an individual teacher's imagery and the narrative unities of which the imagery is a part (Clandinin and Connelly, 1984).
8 What we mean by the rhythms in our North American Christian home life are the patterns of events tied to Sunday designated as the Sabbath with shops and school closures, Monday designated as the first day of the work week, school and business closures for Christmas, Easter Sunday, Good Friday and so on.
9 The concept of a watershed experience is credited in my thinking to Professor James Britton who, in a personal discussion of image, described one of his images of what he termed a watershed experience in World War II. He described the image in vivid detail and credited the experience with being a profound influence in his personal knowledge.
10 Verbal is used in the conceptual sense of having to do with words, whether written or spoken, as opposed to ideas and actions.

References

Assagioli, R. *Psychosynthesis.* Middlesex: Harmondsworth, 1965.

Black, M. *Models and metaphors.* Ithaca: Cornell University Press, 1962.

Clandinin, D. J. *A conceptualization of image as a component of teacher personal practical knowledge.* Unpublished doctoral dissertation, University of Toronto, 1983.

Clandinin, D. J. *Classroom practices: Teacher images in action.* Barcombe Lewes: Falmer Press, 1985.

Clandinin, D. J. "Terms for inquiry into teacher thinking: The place of practical knowledge and the Elbaz case." *Journal of Curriculum Theorizing*, in press.

Clandinin, D. J., and Connelly, F. M. "Teachers personal practical knowledge: Calendars, cycles, habits and rhythms." Paper presented at the *Curriculum in the Making Conference*, University of Haifa, March, 1984.

Connelly, F. M., and Ben-Peretz, M. "Teachers' roles in the using and doing of research and curriculum development." *Journal of Curriculum Studies*, 12 (1980): 95–107.

Connelly, F. M., and Clandinin, D. J. "Teachers' personal practical knowledge." In *Teacher thinking: A new perspective on (persistent problems in) education*, edited by R. Halkaes and J. K. Olson. Heirewig, Holland: Swets Publishing Service, 1984.

Connelly, F. M., and Clandinin, D. J. "Personal practical knowledge and the modes of knowing: Relevance for teaching and learning." In *Learning and teaching the ways of knowing*, edited by E. Eisner, NSSE Yearbook. Chicago: University of Chicago Press, 1985, pp. 174–198.

Connelly, F. M., and Dienes, B. "The teacher's role in curriculum planning: A case study." In *Studies in curriculum decision-making*, edited by K. Leithwood. Toronto: OISE Press, 1982, pp. 183–198.

Dewey, J. *Art as experience*. New York: Capricorn Books, 1934.

Dewey, J. *Experience and education*. New York: Collier Books, 1938.

Dwyer, K. "The dialogic of ethnology." *Dialectical Anthropology*, 4 (1979): 205–224.

Elbaz, F. *Teacher thinking: A study of practical knowledge*. London: Croom Helm, 1983.

Fullan, M., and Pomfret, A. "Research on curriculum and instruction." *Review of Educational Research*, 47, 2 (1977): 335–397.

Gendlin, E. T. *Experiencing and the creation of meaning*. New York: The Free Press of Gelcoe, 1962.

Gilligan, C. *In a different voice*. Cambridge, MA: Harvard University Press, 1982.

Glaser, B. G., and Strauss, A. L. *The discovery of grounded theory: Strategies for qualitative research*. Chicago: Aldine Publishing Company, 1967.

Hadamard, J. *The psychology of invention in the mathematical field*. Princeton, NJ: Princeton University Press, 1945.

Howard, V. A. *Artistry: The work of artists*. Indianapolis: Hackett Publishing Company, 1982.

Hunt, D. "Teachers are psychologists, too: On the application of Psychology to Education." *Canadian Psychology Review*, 17, 3 (1976): 210–218.

Jennings, T. W. "On ritual knowledge." *Journal of Religion*, 62, 2 (1982): 111–127.

Johnson, M. Personal communication, 1983.

Johnson, M. "Review of Elbaz, Freema, Teacher thinking: A study of practical knowledge." *Curriculum Inquiry*, 14, 4 (1984): 465–468.

Lakoff, C., and Johnson, M. *Metaphors we live by*. Chicago: The University of Chicago Press, 1980.

Lortie, D. C. *Schoolteacher: A sociological study*. Chicago: University of Chicago Press, 1975.

Macintyre, A. *After virtue: A study in moral theory*. London: Gerald Duckworth & Co. Ltd., 1981.

Mckeon, R. "Philosophy and action." *Ethics*, 62, 2 (1952): 79–100.

Polanyi, M. *Personal knowledge*. Chicago: The University of Chicago Press, 1958.

Progoff, I. *At a journal workshop*. New York: Dialogue House Library, 1975.

3

DEVELOPING RHYTHM IN TEACHING

The narrative study of a beginning teacher's personal practical knowledge of classrooms[1]

Introduction

In this article I offer a way of understanding how novice teachers develop a personal and practical knowledge of teaching. While there is widespread consensus that the first years of teaching are particularly important, researchers traditionally have understood beginning teachers' experience as a survival stage (Katz 1972; Ryan 1986), a period of struggle that must be gone through in order to learn to be in control of a classroom and before one can get on with becoming an effective teacher. Few researchers and teacher educators have looked beyond the commonplace account of the lack of skills of novice teachers to explore the transition from novice to experienced teacher.

My work is based on the assumption that experienced teachers hold a certain kind of knowledge, knowledge that is practical, experiential, and shaped by a teacher's purposes and values (Elbaz 1983; Clandinin 1986a). The present study is aimed at understanding how this knowledge develops. It is not a study of what teachers should know about classrooms nor of what they should be able to do in classrooms. I focus on a novice teacher's experience and offer an account of the development of his practical knowledge during his first year of teaching. My concern is with both personal and practical knowledge, knowledge that reflects the individual's prior experience and acknowledges the contextual nature of that teacher's knowledge. It is a kind of knowledge carved out of, and shaped by, situations. The study, therefore, explores the experiential basis of teachers' personal knowledge as it is made practical within the context of the first year teaching situation.

My perspective on understanding the beginning teaching experience is a narrative one (Connelly and Clandinin 1985) in which the interest is to understand novice teachers' constructions of classroom reality. We do this experientially and biographically by understanding these constructions as, in part, reconstructions of novice teachers' life narratives. To date, our research has focused on the development of a language and way of understanding the personal practical knowledge of

Reprinted with permission. Acknowledgement: Clandinin, D. J. (1989). Developing rhythm in teaching: The narrative study of a beginning teacher's personal practical knowledge of classrooms. *Curriculum Inquiry*, *19*(2), 121–141.

experienced teachers[2] with no attention to the practical knowledge of novice teachers. Studies have focused on teacher images (Clandinin 1986a), rules and principles (Elbaz 1983), personal philosophy (Kroma 1983; Connelly and Clandinin, 1984), and on teacher and student experience of classroom cycles and rhythms (Clandinin and Connelly 1986) of experienced teachers. With the exception of the work on cycles and rhythms, these studies have not explored the cultural/professional context within which personal knowledge is embedded. In short, in Johnson's terms (1987), we have, for the most part, stressed personal practical knowledge's "embodied" character while taking for granted its "embeddedness." However, paying attention to the cultural and professional context within which personal knowledge is embedded seems particularly important when we want to understand how novice teachers develop practical knowledge.

In earlier work, we became interested in the ways in which experienced teachers know the structure of time in schools. The cyclical organization of time is a particularly striking feature of the professional context of teaching. We saw experienced teachers as holding a rhythmic knowledge of teaching around the cyclic temporal structure of classrooms and schools. We saw schooling, as much as any other organized form of social life (Zerubavel 1979, 1981), as exhibiting a periodic cyclic temporal order. Time in schools is organized cyclically into school cycles such as yearly, daily, between holiday, reporting, and Monday to Friday cycles. These cycles are embedded one within the other and are marked by characteristic features such as a certain duration. Each part of the cycle, beginning, middle, or end, has certain characteristic features.

In our work with experienced teachers, these cycles are experienced not merely as objectively imposed cycles but as having meaning; that is, they are experienced rhythmically. In the narrative of experienced teachers, there is an annual reconstruction of experience and it is through this cyclic repetition of school life that teachers come to "know" their classrooms rhythmically. This knowledge, recollected as they teach, allows them to cope with variations as they reconstruct a story already lived out that is appropriate to the situations they confront.[3] This living out of the narrative is modulated rhythmically. They know the down times will be followed by up times; they know that cyclic disruptions are temporary; they know that the end of a cycle whether it is day's end, week's end, or year's end is characterized by special features and that activities will be experienced differently at these times.

While we understood from this work how experienced teachers "knew" the cyclical nature of school time, that is, in their rhythmic knowledge of their teaching, we wondered how beginning teachers would experience the cyclic nature of school time *and* how they would develop this rhythmic knowledge. While we understood that there is a possibility that in teacher education programs, prospective teachers are taught a knowledge of rhythm in somewhat the same way skills are taught, we saw this as a knowledge of rhythms, or more appropriately, a knowledge of school cycles. We saw this knowledge as different from, although possibly compatible with, a rhythmic knowledge of teaching that develops experientially from working in classrooms. This set the context for the inquiry into the experience of novice teachers.

I have recently begun work with novice teachers in order to offer accounts of their experiences. In this article, I describe my work with Stewart,[4] a beginning kindergarten teacher. In this exploration of Stewart's experience, I focus on the development of his personal practical knowledge, particularly on one image[5] that forms part of his personal practical knowledge. The article by no means represents a complete account of Stewart's personal practical knowledge nor even of our overall collaboration. Materials from our work together are used to illustrate the notion of developing rhythm in his personal practical knowledge of teaching.

Stewart, the teacher in the study

Stewart is a first year kindergarten teacher in a large urban board in a Western Canadian province. Like many beginning teachers, he is on a temporary contract. From September to December he had a temporary placement in a school where he taught a morning and an afternoon kindergarten class. During these first four months, he was part of a kindergarten team of four teachers. All four teachers team planned together. Stewart and another teacher on temporary contract team taught their two classes; that is, they shared their work with the two classes of children. After the Christmas break (from January to June), Stewart took over the morning kindergarten class of another teacher who went on leave. In this new school, he was the only kindergarten teacher on staff and he held a half-time appointment.

Prior to Christmas, while he taught full-time, Stewart continued part-time work in a department store. After Christmas, he assumed much heavier time commitments in the department store in order to supplement what had now become a half-time teaching salary.

Stewart had two experiences in teacher education. Some years ago he completed the necessary requirements to become a high school science teacher. He chose not to teach then and went to work in a department store where he began to assume some managerial and organizational responsibilities. After several years of doing this, he returned to university to complete the requirements to become a kindergarten teacher. During his time at the university, Stewart was a student in my Early Childhood Education class. While at the university, he did considerable volunteer teaching in a kindergarten class at a neighboring school. He also completed one practicum experience in a kindergarten classroom.

Method

The method used for offering an account of a teacher's personal practical knowledge is a narrative one with a particular focus on personal experience (Connelly and Clandinin 1986). A narrative method has as its principal feature the reconstruction of classroom meaning in terms of unities and rhythms in the lives of classroom participants. A narrative method involves a number of data sources including biographical data, journal material, interview transcripts, and field note material from which narrative reconstructions of classroom practice are written.

My work with Stewart stretched over his first year teaching. During that time, he kept a daily journal that recorded what seemed to him to be his most significant classroom experiences. These were shared with me on a weekly basis. There were frequent informal conversations throughout the year and there were three semistructured interviews (October, November, March) in which the journals, and Stewart's ongoing experience, were discussed. These interviews were tape recorded and Stewart received a copy of the interview transcript prior to the conduct of the next interview. One preliminary narrative account was prepared and shared with Stewart. This account took the form of a long letter from me to Stewart. The account not only provided feedback on my interpretation of classroom activities and interviews, but also advanced tentative notions of images and Stewart's developing rhythmic knowledge of school cycles.

It is important to note that Stewart's records are not meant to portray the exceptional as, for example, in the way expert teacher research focuses on exceptional teachers. Rather, in this work I am attempting to find the meaning contained in the everyday experience of novice teachers. What the article attempts to do is capture a commonplace that we have often experienced but about which we have not researched and written. The research intent is to probe beneath the commonplace of a novice teacher's experience to understand the implications of that learning experience for teacher education. My work with Stewart adopts a reflective attitude and a willingness to probe the real, everyday, commonplace events of the day-to-day business of learning to teach. This probing of the beginning teaching experience allows us an opportunity to uncover "the layers of those elementary structures of everyday life which provide the foundation of social experience, language and social action and thus of the complex historical world of human life" (Schutz and Luckmann 1973, p. xxi). The work, thus, is an attempt to uncover the "elementary structures" of Stewart's everyday life that provide a foundation of teaching. Schutz goes on to say that:

> The sciences that would interpret and explain human action and thought must begin with a description of the foundational structures of what is prescientific, the reality which seems self-evident to men remaining within the natural attitude. This reality is the everyday life-world. The everyday life-world is the region of reality in which man can engage himself and which he can change while he operates in it by means of his animate organism.
>
> *(Schutz and Luckmann 1973, p. 3)*

The work with Stewart is a study of a novice teacher's commonplace or everyday-life-world and how he comes to know it during his first year of teaching. The study in this way offers insight into the process of learning how to teach.

The emerging image of teaching as relating to children

I now turn to a description of what I came to call Stewart's image of "teaching as relating to children."

Clues to the image were first apparent in reading Stewart's journal entries and interview transcripts. One such clue was his insistence that he only wanted to teach at the kindergarten level rather than in the elementary grades where he felt the prescribed curriculum would interfere in his work with children. I wrote about it in the narrative account in the following way.

> This experience seems to be in behind your dogged insistence of only teaching kindergarten despite opportunities for full-time teaching at higher grades. "I don't want a Grade 6 class any more than I want a Grade 1 Class. You've chastised me about getting in first and then wheeling and dealing for a kindergarten, but I live and teach for today-I can't imagine sitting in one of their daily time quota sessions-you *have* to have so many minutes for this-so many for that – here; take this and teach it, will you? It's good for the kids. Okay kids, turn to page 21-do numbers 1 through 6 then shut off your minds for the duration of the day"!
>
> *(Narrative Account, February, 1986)*

In my tentative interpretation, this seemed to point towards an image in which his insistence on being a kindergarten teacher was grounded. Stewart was adamant that he did not want to deal with curriculum guides that were prescribed at each grade level, even if that jeopardized his opportunity to find a teaching position. I speculated that this insistence on teaching kindergarten was an expression of an image, an image I came to call "teaching as relating to children." That Stewart held such an image became apparent over the course of our work together. The following section, excerpted in part from the narrative account, gives some sense of what I came to see as the image.

> One of the images seems to be of teaching as relating to children. While you haven't expressed it in quite those words, it seems to come out in words like ". . . the joy – it's there in the kids. And the grief and tension vaporized when they came to me and the magic welled up in me and those kids let go – to me. To me!" (9/3/85); ". . . I want to be with them when those lights go 'flash' in their minds" (9/3/85); and in your comment that the highlights of your program "for me is when I am with the kids . . . my joy comes from the interactions. The only way I safeguard that joy is being totally prepared prep-wise and plan-wise."
>
> *(Narrative Account, February, 1987)*

When Stewart responded to the narrative account, he talked again of "the joy" (April, 1987) that he found in teaching through relating to "kids." His teaching occurred when he was "working *for* the little ones" (9/16/85). He could teach because "I know I empathize with them a lot (I can even think like a child at times!" (9/16/85).

The image of "teaching as relating to children" as it was expressed in the interviews and in his journal accounts of classroom practices, subsumed various elements of the content of his personal practical knowledge. Knowledge of the instructional process, knowledge of himself as a teacher and a person, and knowledge of appropriate subject matter were all captured by the image. The following descriptions of three of Stewart's practices in September of the year were seen as the embodiment and enactment of Stewart's "teaching as relating to children" image.

The first practice describes a day when Stewart's team partner was absent. Stewart had insisted on only completing part of the planned program rather than, as he saw it, sacrificing the teaching relationship with the children. He wrote:

> I maintain that everyone's job is primarily to remain calm and in control – if tiny parts of the program suffer, that's too bad-it's more important to maintain the child-adult relationship than it is to maintain the day plan that says "we will finish the little witch book at this time."
>
> *(10/23/85)*

While we might have imagined that a beginning teacher would have wanted to cover planned content, for Stewart it was important that teaching continue. For Stewart that meant he had to continue to relate to children and that took priority over content except as he was able to continue to cover the content and maintain the teaching relationship.

Other practices in which the image found expression were around ensuring adequate time for centers. The importance of this practice was captured by his comment:

> The rest of day was pretty good. My team partner thought it hectic and at one point said, "Let's end centre time now – I've had it with centres for this morning!" I like centres the best because you can one-to-one it more.
>
> *(9/26/85)*

Stewart persisted in keeping the center time going, arguing that centers gave him more time for relating to individual children. His more experienced team partner wanted to go on with a whole group activity but Stewart wanted to continue to work in a situation that allowed for individual teacher-student relationship.

A third practice in which this image found expression was his search for an evaluation and record-keeping process that "still lets me interact with my kids" (10/16/85). Stewart found it difficult to use class time to fill out check lists, to write detailed observations for children's behavior, or to write anecdotal records, practices frequently engaged in by kindergarten teachers while the children are in the classroom. He felt that using class time for such activities took him away from his time to relate with children. At several points in the journal and interviews, Stewart details his search for such a system that would not take him away from his work with children.

The preceding section provides a sense of how my understanding of what I call Stewart's image of teaching as relating to children emerged. As I worked with Stewart, the image seemed to function as an experience-based structure of Stewart's personal practical knowledge. As the image found expression in his practices, several dimensions of the image became apparent. The dimensions of emotionality and morality seemed particularly striking qualities of his knowledge. Stewart's image of teaching as relating to children is not a neutral image. The image is deeply held and the words he used to convey his meaning give a sense of this emotionality. He used the words "emotional commitment" (10/24/85), "sharing something real" (9/23/85), and "joy" (10/24/85) when he expressed the image verbally. The emotionality is illustrated in his verbal expression of the image in statements such as "when I *feel* being natural is more important" (9/23/85). The emotionality is clearly tied to a moral dimension of the image. For Stewart, there are better and worse ways of relating to children. In his verbal expression of the image, we get a sense of the ways in which the image provides him with a judgmental standard for his practices. This was evident in such verbal expressions as "Nothing bugs me more than realizing I've said something that's gone ten miles over their heads – just as nothing really turns me on like that wide-eyed appreciation when my words do click in" (9/16/85). This moral standard flows out of Stewart's image of teaching as relating to children. While we often teach such principles as "teach to the level of the child" in teacher education, it is without the moral sense that Stewart holds. It is the moral coloring of the image that provides the moral standard for Stewart. When practices are discordant, the moral coloring of the image highlights the discord. He describes how the image finds expression in his work with children, and how the moral dimension of the image provides a guide.

> They like to "fool" around and have fun but they are not disrespectful to me or to others. Only time will tell . . . but on days like today, when they're higher than kites and yet still willing to give me the power to help them learn, I *feel* like I'm doing something right.
>
> *(11/21/85)*

Another practice that Stewart judged as a "better" practice was one when the moral dimension of the image of relationship also provided the judgmental standard. He wrote about the experience of a trip to the firehall as follows.

> Pretty soon someone started our song – just singing as they skipped along – and I picked it up and it went along the group like a campfire tune. Great stuff! Joy from kids.
>
> *(10/17/85)*

This experience was judged successful using the moral standard provided by the image of teaching as relating to children.

The image of teaching as relating to children emerged from both the personal-private and educational-professional spheres of Stewart's life. Part of the image could be explained as propositional knowledge learned from educational lectures on the place of the child in education and on communication skills important to working with children. However, part of it also comes from his ongoing experience of the life world, from his narrative of experience.

Stewart talked about the experiential origin of the image in this way.

> I don't know why I'm teaching other than a queer twist of fate put me in contact with a bunch of 4½–5 year olds one summer and I really responded positively to them. It was so good for me that I've come this far on that experience and want still more.
>
> *(9/6/85)*

The image also emerges from his professional training when he worked as a volunteer while he was a student. He saw his job as a volunteer to be one of keeping the little things out of the teacher's way so she could teach through relating to children. This allowed the teacher to teach. He wrote about it this way:

> When I volunteered, I always thought my strong point was making the class atmosphere "work" for the teacher by making sure the little things didn't become stumbling blocks.
>
> *(9/16/85)*

The image finds expression in both his personal and professional experience. For example, he describes how the image functions in his personal life in the following journal story.

> My friend/boss at the store was helping me get over some of the rough edges of my first few days and he said that it didn't really matter if others were more experienced than I; I was still the best teacher and he knew it without even meeting them . . . he said it isn't your experience or your brains, it's how you use what you do have and he reminded me of a time when he'd come to my place to check on my furnace and we'd been interrupted by four of my neighbourhood kids who wanted to know if Big Stewart could come out to play!
>
> *(9/13/85)*

In this story, Stewart tells us how he sees himself in relation to the children in his community. This too is an expression of the image. The image functions in his professional practices in similar ways. The relationship with children is central in the classroom as evidenced by the following two journal entries.

> I just feel good working *for* the little ones and I know I empathize with them a lot (I can even think like a child at times)!
>
> *(9/6/85)*

In a later journal entry, he describes an experience with a child where he questioned his own insistence on telling children not to damage books. He is concerned that he has created a situation in which his relationship with the children may be at risk.

> I should be more careful with them – I don't want them to be so afraid of me that something so material as a book can cause them grief like that. There's nothing worth that – that makes me feel as bad as he does.
>
> *(10/24/85)*

It is the emotional and moral dimensions of the image that bind the experiential sides together. In the first experience with young children, Stewart talks about it as "so good" for him and it is this sense of goodness that serves as a guide to him in structuring other situations. It is this sense of relating to children with its emotional and moral sides that serve as standards to his practice and that are expressed in his comments such as "there's nothing worth that."

The image so far described as part of Stewart's personal practical knowledge can be seen to have social origins in his personal and professional experiences. The image in its expression, in his practices both in and out of school, had important moral and emotional dimensions. This image was an important part of Stewart's personal knowledge when he began to teach and began to work in the particular context that defines schools. In this article, the particular social context I have focused on is the rigid cyclic temporal social structure of schooling. As Stewart began to work in this context, I anticipated a change as the image began to be expressed in practice.

We turn our attention now to an exploration of what new personal knowledge structures emerged to deal with this new social experience. Stewart had, of course, experienced basic temporal cycles but as he began teaching, he experienced, as a teacher, a new and particular form of temporality seen in the school cycles.

Image in tension with school cycles

Early in the yearly (September to June) school cycle, the image found expression in practices such as Stewart's practice of allowing the children and their parents to come into the school as soon as they arrived at school, even if that was earlier than the regular school starting time. Stewart saw this practice as allowing him time to talk to the parents prior to class time and thus freeing him to use class time for full involvement with the children.

Another practice was using the time prior to the arrival of the children in the mornings and in the afternoons for preparing his centers and ensuring he was ready so details that could be worked out ahead of class time would not, as Stewart saw it, interfere with his work in class with the children. He talked about this practice in the following way.

> I am there at 7:30 and, you know, I like to be totally ready to go at 9 or quarter to 9 when the kids are there and I really like to have all my time during centre time for my interactions with the kids so I don't like to, for instance, the paint bottles, I hate, during centre time, having to go fill up the paint box. That should be done long before that, you know, and if the water is filthy, the last time you want to clean that water table is during centre time because you are stealing your own time and that really makes me mad so I come in very early

and I usually stay about a half hour later just to make sure that everything is out of my way.

(Interview No. 1)

Still another practice was his concern that center time and sharing time be kept intact at all costs for, as he saw it, that was when he had the most opportunity for one-to-one interaction with children. The following interview transcript gives a sense of this.

like sharing, one of my most important times to me, when you get to have the kids talking to you about what they did .

(Interview No. 2)

The following journal entry also highlights the expression of the image in practice when Stewart refuses to deal with other staff when he is teaching. He is describing what happened when the principal and the kindergarten supervisor made an unexpected visit during class time.

I naturally did what I usually do when someone walks in, I just go on with my kids and say, "Look around. I'll be right with you" – we went to gym.

(10/8/85)

These three practices, which can be seen as early expressions of the image of relationship, are used illustratively. Early in the term, however, Stewart began to be aware of the cyclic nature of schooling. Each of these practices was called into question by various school cycles.

By mid-September, the first practice was in conflict with the school's daily cycle of allowing children into the school at 8:43 a.m. and 1:13 p.m. Stewart wrote about the tension this way.

I think I'm heading for another run-in with the principal . . . he wants me to throw my kids and moms[6] outside if they come into the school before 8:43 or before 1:13. I really don't mind if my kids come in early . . . that's the time I'd rather talk to moms (not during my precious class time!) . . . It requires the child's first teacher to be the heavy phony (one minute you're throwing them out; the next you have a rosy plastic smile on your face and you're saying – Hi there – Welcome).

(9/18/85)

The second practice of arriving early so all preparation is done prior to school opening came into tension with several school cycles such as his team partner's daily cycle of school arrival and departure and the weekly cycle of planning meetings with the other two kindergarten teachers.

The following two journal entries highlight this tension. The first journal entry captures the tension between the expression of the image in his practice and the daily cycle of his team partner.

Friday I ended the day at 4:30 and it was extremely hard *not* to say something when my partner and aide split at 4:00 p.m. After a big unit, there's a lot of clean up to do and there's a lot of set up to do for the next unit on Monday – plus I insist on clean paint stations and clean water centre, play dough and tables . . . Today I began at 7:30 as usual and the set up for the new unit took a rush job to get done by 8:45. My partner came in at 8:30 and my aide at 8:35.

(10/15/85)

The following journal entry highlights tension between the cycle of planning meetings and the expression of the image in Stewart's practice.

> You have maybe 15–20 minutes to prep your morning and suddenly someone wants to chat with you or needs you for some pointless triviality . . . and then . . . you meet the moms and all the new bunch coming in and, without your approval, your morning descends on you . . . the morning still barely limps to its given finale. And . . . isn't there a planning meeting at that time. . . and you rush back to class and you want just 5 minutes to suck back and re-load (simply to get the p.m. name tags out!) . . . when BOOM – your afternoon descends on you!
>
> *(9/5/85)*

The journal entry highlights the impact of school cycles on Stewart's practice of being completely "with" the children during class time.

The following journal entry highlights the tension Stewart experiences between the expression of the image in keeping center times as long as possible and what he sees as his teaching team's pressure to cover various subject matter skills with the whole group of children.

> One thing I still can't get a handle on is my day plan is so full I can't fit it all in – yet when I look at the paper, it seems that I should be doing more. I've tried twice to do a pre-math graphing chart with them – I just seem to lose time in little driblets and I have to master my time control better – either simplify more or become more aware of time's importance. I hate getting caught in centre time but I hate equally disturbing a fluid set of centres.
>
> *(9/17/85)*

In this entry, he poses the tension as a dilemma and it is apparent he has not yet developed a rhythmic knowledge of his classroom teaching.

His felt sense of tension as his expressions of the image result in conflict with the cyclic nature of schooling is captured in his comment:

> I should make the program on the kids . . . I make it in terms of what blocks have to be filled because I don't get any other time. I can determine what happens in the blocks of time that I have but . . .
>
> *(Interview No. 1)*

The tension Stewart feels and his sense of school cycles as objectively imposed on experience are both expressed in the comment.

The tension Stewart experiences as his image of teaching as relating to children, part of his personal practical knowledge, conflicts with the cyclic ordering of school time draws our attention to teacher dilemmas (Lampert 1985). A dilemma for Lampert is a conflict between equally desirable teaching actions. These dilemmas are not merely programmatic dilemmas that have a kind of propositional character and solution or resolution about them. They are experiential dilemmas. People are torn through their felt values, their emotionality and morality, to go one way in the face of a social structure that makes it difficult to do so.

In the following section, we see several dilemmas confronted by Stewart as his image conflicts with the imposed social structure of cyclic school time. We also see some of the ways in which he copes with these dilemmas as he develops a rhythmic knowledge of teaching.

Rhythm in personal practical knowledge

In earlier articles, we speculated that it is in the first years of teaching that a teacher develops his or her rhythmic sense of knowing the classroom and of knowing teaching. For beginning teachers, we speculated that school cycles would appear as unexpected, intrusive, imposed structures. School time would, in general, appear fragmented and would serve to disrupt their teaching. But we speculated that even within the first year of teaching, there would be a transformation of beginning teachers' understanding of cycles as meaningless, fragmented, and objective impositions to events having personal meaning in the way they "know" their teaching. Teachers would, we thought, come to know this through the narrative of their lived experience of teaching. Something much like this occurred with Stewart. There was a decreased sense of balance when Stewart's practices, expressions of his images, conflicted with school cycles and resulted in personal dilemmas. This faltering at the unexpected, these dilemmas, and the ensuing reconstruction of the narrative to regain balance is at the heart of the process of growth from novice to experienced teacher with a rhythmic understanding of teaching. Dewey put it this way:

> Life itself consists of phases in which the organism falls out of step with the march of surrounding things and then recovers unison with it . . . Here in turn are balance and harmony attained through rhythm . . . [which] comes about . . . because of tension.
>
> *(1943, p. 14)*

The tension between the expression of Stewart's personal knowledge in practice *and* the school cycles resulted in the development of some sense of rhythm in Stewart's teaching. In his teaching, he was responding to school cycles, always trying to regain balance. As the year progressed, he began to develop a rhythmic knowledge of teaching. There were fewer dilemmas as he learned to know the cyclic ordering of school time. A rhythmic knowledge of the experience of teaching that allowed Stewart to "feel" balance began to develop. In reading the journal entries, field notes, and interview transcripts, several examples of the development of a rhythmic knowledge of teaching became apparent.

When Stewart began to teach in September, he had particular difficulty with the cyclic organization of the school gymnasium and library time. He found it hard to accommodate what he saw as the important cycle of his kindergarten program to the larger school cycle in which it was embedded.

> We're running into grief on scheduling – it's the usual thing of having to fit a supposedly unscheduled ECS class into a scheduled school system – gym and library! I've accepted the time slots available (should I say, given?) for my class but I've kept my routine covering the times that I'm not scheduled in the gym. I'll have some exercise or movement every day even if I'm not allowed in the gym everyday – ditto on library.
>
> *(9/11/85)*

By March, this no longer seems problematic to Stewart as he accepts the school cycles as more meaningful.

We see him developing a rhythm that allows him to fit his day plans into his unit plan. He talks about it in the following way.

> I know in my unit plan that I'm going to do that somewhere in this unit but the day plan is a waste of time. It doesn't even really key me into who my parent volunteer is because I have that right beside my desk on that large calendar and things like telling me when assembly is, well, I get an announcement in the morning when that is. Thursday is always library day . . . you know, I think my main emphasis is on my unit plans. If I'm sure of what I want to do, then I feel good about my day.
>
> *(Interview No. 3)*

Stewart seems to have developed a rhythmic way of knowing this aspect of his teaching. While early in the year, Stewart had felt he needed to keep detailed daily plans as part of what he saw as the school's daily cycle, he had little understanding of their value. He kept records of all other classroom activities organized around cycles but many of them seemed meaningless. As the year progressed, no longer did the library cycle, the parent volunteer cycle, or the cycle of daily planning seem meaningless. Rather, he comments,

> if you have a craft centre and you have down there on your day plan you are going to make a nurse's hat, like we did today, and a doctor's hat, there is no point in writing that down four or five days in a row. You've got four kids that are going through a centre.
>
> *(Interview No. 3)*

He offers an account of knowing his classroom by saying, "Our day plans are different because we have unit plans, we have week plans, we have sequence plans, I guess" (Interview No. 3). In this description, Stewart is drawing attention to his own rhythmic knowledge of various planning cycles.

Stewart also develops a rhythmic knowledge of his teaching in which he knows how to find time to interact with children while they are in class. He talks about his knowing in this way.

> I feel a great deal of security when I'm organized and I'm ready to face my day and I know that with this unit (one he has taught before in student teaching), this is what's going to happen. When I pull that Easter thing out, I've done it before. That's a security blanket for me because I know when I go to do the eggs and . . . sewing around the edge of the eggs, I know what to do . . . Like you can just go to that unit, you can get everything ready, you are all prepped, you're feeling great about your day and the kids are going to fit in.
>
> *(Interview No. 3)*

But with his developing rhythmic sense of knowing teaching, Stewart raises concerns that the way he has come to know teaching is not one that allows for a comfortable expression of at least the one image we have discussed in this article. Prior to Christmas break and while he was still working in a team situation, Stewart talked about the "team planned" program.

> We're constantly fighting this battle-too many activities – too many ideas – too much and not time to do it right whatever it might be . . . we're choosing

> the activities first and then the objectives rather than trying to find an activity that might come close to displaying the objectives we think necessary . . . why can't we pick a few useful activities and really do them the right way.
>
> *(12/4/85)*

Stewart expands on this in an interview.

> There are so many ideas, we stuff them all in and nothing gets done properly. The same with our daily program . . . I am sure we have a better time sharing when we first come in, when I talk to the kids about the Ewok show last night or you know something like that. To them it's their only chance to talk. That's wrong. I know it's wrong and I feel it is wrong and I think it's wrong too.
>
> *(Interview No. 2)*

However, when he finds himself in his own classroom, he expresses concern about the way he has come to know teaching as he deals with the cyclic nature of schools. His concern is that he "knows" the unit and its activities and does them without needing to reflect on what the children need. He says, "I don't have to sit there and think about my kids" (Interview No. 3) and yet focusing on individuals' experience is an important expression of his image in practice.

Late in the year, he is still developing a rhythmic knowledge of the cycle of unit planning. He expresses concern that the cycle of units or themes still seems objective and imposed. In the following sequence of journal entries, we get a sense of Stewart's developing rhythmic knowledge of planning.

Early in the year, he expressed concern about beginning a new unit.

> Began our Halloween unit today – every centre has some subtle change to it and I wish I could find a better way to introduce these changes. Usually time leaves me 5 minutes to list the differences and I know some of my kids can't cope without a bit of demonstrating to ease them into it. I feel angry at myself for not allowing more time . . . .
>
> *(10/21/85)*

A bit later, as he is working on another unit, he expresses concern that it is time to move on to another unit, Pioneers, before he and the children are finished working on the present unit, Fairy Tales. He writes,

> Our fairy tale unit has been pretty good and our kids are just getting the idea of what can happen if you let your imagination go . . . now we have to pop the big let down on them and try to crystallize the concept of a different "long, long ago!" Kids are eager for anything but it seems a shame to have to press on into something we're not so sure of. We had slotted two weeks for fairy tales but we lost three days to parent-teacher interviews and holidays so we really robbed ourselves.
>
> *(11/15/85)*

In this journal, he is expressing concern that the cycle lacks meaning for him as he works with the children. In other entries, words such as "imposed three weeks of Pioneers" (12/4/85) and "trying to stick to the Pioneer unit in order to start [the] Christmas [unit] on time" (12/4/85) capture the sense of an objective cycle rather than a meaningful rhythmic knowing.

This same sense of imposition of an objective cycle of units is still being expressed much later in the year when he is teaching alone. He describes a new unit on community. He comments here on an experience of making a Co-op shopping center in his classroom.

> And I wanted the kids to have that Co-op shopping centre, so I painted it all white. I shouldn't have done that. I should have made them do it because then they have a sense of having done it themselves, from the start. They've created this store themselves and it is their store. . . I wanted them to have it right away and I didn't want to take the time to have them do it. . . Even if we only had a week or two weeks to do the theme in, two or three of those first days should have been for building with them.
>
> *(Interview No. 3)*

Within that first year of teaching, Stewart was still struggling to allow for an expression of the image within the cyclically imposed time constraints of schooling.

Dilemmas resulted from the expressions of Stewart's image of "teaching as relating to children" as they came into tension with various school cycles. These dilemmas created situations in which we could see growth and change in Stewart's personal practical knowledge. Through the reconstruction of his experience, Stewart began to develop a rhythmic knowledge of teaching, but it was through that process of reconstruction of experience that a further dilemma became apparent. For while Stewart came to deal with the imposed school cycles through using previously prepared and taught curriculum materials and units, he had to confront the dilemma that he no longer looked first to the children as in his first practical expressions of the image of "teaching as relating to children." As Stewart sensed the tension around his dilemma, he began to question the ways in which he "knows" teaching. We might imagine that for Stewart in his next year of teaching this tension will result in further reconstruction of experience and new expressions of his personal practical knowledge. In the tension and the resulting reconstruction of experience, personal practical knowledge is shaped and developed.

In the final section, we turn our attention to the entailments of this work for the education of beginning teachers.

Entailments for the education of beginning teachers

In this article, I have given a brief account of the experience of one novice teacher, Stewart, from a narrative perspective. In presenting the account, I have probed beneath the obvious and commonplace experience of a first year teacher to reveal, in part, his knowledge structures, aspects of his personal practical knowledge. The knowledge structure explored in this article, an image of teaching as relating to children, was seen to be nonpropositional in character, have an experiential origin, and to have emotional and moral dimensions. I then explored the dilemmas that were created when Stewart's image, in its practical expressions, conflicted with the cyclic ordering of school time, which is a powerful part of the school context. As Stewart worked through these dilemmas, we could see a reconstruction of his experience that allowed us to see a process of growth and change in Stewart's rhythmic knowledge of teaching.

In this account of a novice teacher's experience, it is clear that learning to teach involves much more than learning and applying skills. Learning to teach involves the narrative reconstruction of a teacher's experience as personal practical knowledge is shaped through its expression in practical situations.

In the final section of the article, I deal with what I have come to see as the entailments of this work for the education of novice teachers. The first has to do with what constitutes appropriate experience for a novice teacher to reflect on during the experience of learning to teach in his or her first year of teaching. The second deals with the situation in which a first year teacher typically finds him or herself, that is, alone and, as Stewart was, without someone who would even acknowledge the uncertainty of teaching except in the research relationship.

In an earlier article (Clandinin and Connelly 1986), we commented that to understand rhythm in the narrative of teaching is to understand something of the way in which a person conforms to the cyclic, temporal structure of schooling and of social life and becomes what we call a "teacher" while at the same time stamping his or her own particular cultural and personal mark on the teaching process via the rhythms he or she develops. It is the first years of teaching that seem particularly important for, once in place, the rhythmic knowing of a classroom becomes a shaping force on the ways in which teachers experience their classrooms.

When we understand rhythm as part of teachers' personal practical knowledge which is embodied, biographical, historical, cultural, and *in* their teaching practice, it becomes difficult to detach education from life, for education and knowing education are part of life. This point leads to the first educational entailment of my work with Stewart.

A full accounting of the understanding a given teacher brings into and develops in the classroom requires an opportunity for inquiry into the whole of a teacher's life. The appropriate experience for reflection becomes all experience that led up to and contributed to the teaching experience; that is, it becomes an exploration of a teacher's personal practical knowledge. Reflection on a teacher's personal practical knowledge is a "dialectical exploration of the principal structures by means of which that person 'has a world' or experiences situations in a meaningful way" (Johnson 1987).

Stewart, however, began to teach in a situation that he perceived did not value reflection as a way of helping teachers come to know their teaching situation. He commented on professional development in the following way.

> They call it professional development but I, I guess that's what it is, it is the professional side of the business, it's not your personal, it's not your emotional side, it's not the way that I'm feeling about my kids right now that they are interested in. It's . . . they're interested in whether I have the skills.
>
> *(Interview No. 3)*

In this statement, Stewart is commenting on the focus of support he was given as a novice teacher. The focus was on the professional side but, even there, it was only on what Stewart terms "skills." As he saw it, his opportunities for reflection were as part of the research experience and were not a part of his ongoing experience of teaching in the school and classroom.[7]

A second entailment follows from the first. As Stewart tells his story of his experience of beginning teaching, he found himself alone. He commented, "You need somebody to talk to. When you desperately need it, then it is not there" (Interview No. 3) and "I don't get a lot of support right now at all and you get really bad days. . . I get support from the kids. . . that's the only one I can think of (Interview No. 1).

Stewart frequently found himself looking to his students for feedback and support as he came to know his teaching. The following comment captures this feeling.

> What do you do in the week, like last week you can't find, when you say to Carrie (a student) at the end of the week, I think I need a hug and she comes and gives you a hug and you realize that you really did need that hug. . . . Where do you find it when you really need it?
>
> *(Interview No. 3)*

Even those individuals who found themselves in positions to support novice teachers such as Stewart, found it difficult to acknowledge the tension as the novice develops a rhythmic knowledge of teaching. One of Stewart's journal entries highlights this sense. Stewart was talking about a session with the school's vice principal.

> I also talked about my weaknesses in the observations-as program-basis area and he immediately told me not to reveal "weaknesses". . . I said that didn't matter – if he was evaluating me to provide detailed comment on my strengths and weaknesses, it was ridiculous for *me* to *hide* the fact and miss the help.
>
> *(11/18/85)*

In this journal entry, Stewart highlights his feeling of isolation from meaningful support as he learned to teach. Stewart's work in the research project allowed him opportunities for ongoing reflection as part of his experience as a novice teacher. The opportunity to reflect on the uncertainty of learning to live within the particular cultural, historical, and cyclic situation of each classroom is one way of providing significant support. This sense of having the certainty of support in the professional uncertainty of becoming a teacher is important (Floden and Clark 1987). Programs of teacher education must find ways to support beginning teachers during the first critical years of teaching. It is clear that the form in which this support is offered must be characterized by features that allow for the reflective reconstruction of the novice's narrative of experience.

Acknowledgement

This work was supported by a research grant from the Alberta Advisory Committee for Educational Studies.

Notes

1 Editor's Note: This article is a further contribution to the special series on Personal Practical Knowledge.

2 The term personal practical knowledge (Connelly and Diennes 1982; Clandinin 1985) marks the boundaries of our inquiry into teaching. The term "knowledge" points to our underlying epistemological interest and associates us with those interested in problems of knowledge and knowing in the curriculum. The term "practical" qualifies this epistemological interest by aligning us with writers such as Schön (1983) whose interest is in the epistemology of practical thinking. The term "personal" qualifies our interest in how specific individuals know their classroom situation. Accordingly, the term "personal practical knowledge" defines our interest in understanding teaching acts in terms of personalized concrete accounts of people knowing.

3 I use Crites' (1971) notion of how experience is collected and reconstructed to form stories useful for coping with life situations and for creating possible scenarios for the future.

4 The beginning teacher's name has been changed to protect his anonymity.
5 Image in this work (Clandinin 1985, 1986a) is defined as part of a person's personal practical knowledge embodied in the person and connected with the individual's past, present, and future. Image draws both the present and future into a personally meaningful nexus of experience focused on the immediate situation that called it forth. It reaches into the past, gathering up experiential threads meaningfully connected to the present, and it reaches intentionally into the future and creates new meaningfully connected threads as situations are experienced and new situations anticipated from the perspective of the image. Image is the glue that melds together a person's diverse experiences, both personal and professional. An image has emotional and moral dimensions and these dimensions mark out the knowing contained in the expression of image in classroom and interview practices. Action, and the personal knowledge embodied in it, is imbued with meaning-giving emotionality and morality. In earlier work, I have written about an image of "classroom as home" which is part of Stephanie's, a primary school teacher's, personal practical knowledge. As the image is expressed in her practices, it becomes a shaping force in the way she knows her teaching and learning situation. For a more detailed account of the nature of image, see Clandinin (1985, 1986).
6 In most kindergarten programs, it is common for parents, usually mothers, or caregivers, to walk children to school. This is not because they want particularly to visit the school but, rather, to ease the children's transition between home and school and for various safety reasons.
7 The collaborative nature of narrative research has educational benefits for both researcher and teacher participants. Reflection ensues through participation in the research process. The research process offers potential for allowing us, classroom teachers as researchers and researchers as classroom teachers, to reflect upon the narrative that define our personal practical knowledge as it is embodied in our classroom practices. See Clandinin (1986b), for a more detailed account of the collaborative nature of narrative research.

References

Clandinin, D. J. "Personal practical knowledge: A study of teachers' classroom images." *Curriculum Inquiry*, 15, 4 (1985): 361–385.

Clandinin, D. J. *Classroom practice: Teacher images in action*. London: The Falmer Press, 1986a.

Clandinin, D. J. "Classroom research: Teaching and change." *Journal of Curriculum Studies*, 19, 2 (1986b): 195–200.

Clandinin, D. J. and Connelly, F. M. "Rhythms in teaching: The narrative study of teachers' personal practical knowledge of classrooms." *Teaching and Teacher Education*, 2, 4 (1986): 377–387.

Connelly, F. M. and Clandinin, D. J. "Personal practical knowledge at Bay Street School: Ritual, personal philosophy and image." In Halkes, R. and Olson, J. (Eds.), *Teacher thinking: A new perspective on persisting problems in education*. Lisse: Swets in Zeitlinger, 1984.

Connelly, F. M. and Clandinin, D. J. "Personal practical knowledge and the modes of knowing: Relevance for teaching and learning." In Eisner, E. (Ed.), *Learning and teaching the ways of knowing*. Eighty-forth yearbook of the National Society for the Study of Education. Chicago: University of Chicago Press, 1985.

Connelly, F. M. and Clandinin, D. J. "On narrative method, personal philosophy and narrative unities in the study of teaching." *Journal of Research in Science Teaching*, 23, 3 (1986): 15–32.

Connelly, F. M. and Diennes, B. "Teacher decision-making and teacher choice in curriculum planning: A case study of teachers' uses of theory." In Leithwood, K. (Ed.), *Studies in curriculum decision-making*. Toronto: OISE, 1982.

Crites, S. "The narrative quality of experience." *Journal of the American Academy of Religion*, 39, 3 (1971): 291–311.
Dewey, J. *Art as experience*. New York: Capricorn Books, 1934.
Elbaz, F. *Teacher thinking: A study of practical knowledge*. London: Croom Helm, 1983.
Floden, R. and Clark, C. *Preparing teachers for uncertainty*. Unpublished manuscript, 1987.
Johnson, M. "Review of classroom practice: Teacher images in action." *Curriculum Inquiry*, 17, 4 (1987): 465–469.
Katz, L. "Developmental stages of preschool teachers." *The Elementary School Journal*, 23((1972): 50–54.
Kroma, S. *Personal practical knowledge of language in teaching: An ethnographic study*. Unpublished doctoral dissertation, University of Toronto, Toronto, Ontario, 1983.
Lampert, M. "How do teachers manage to teach?" *Harvard Educational Review*, 55, 2 (1985): 178–194.
Ryan, K. *Induction of new teachers*. Bloomington, IN: Phi Delta Kappa Educational Foundation, 1986.
Schön, D. A. *The reflective practitioner: How professionals think in action*. New York: Basic Books, Inc., 1983.
Schutz, A. and Luckmann, T. *The structures of the life-world*. Evanston, IL: Northwestern University Press, 1973.
Zerubavel, E. *Patterns of time in hospital life: A sociological perspective*. Chicago: University of Chicago Press, 1979.
Zerubavel, E. *Hidden rhythms: Schedules and calendars in social life*. Chicago: University of Chicago Press, 1981.

SECTION II

Journeying with narrative ideas of teacher knowledge into teacher education and professional education

4

TEACHER EDUCATION AS NARRATIVE INQUIRY

In elementary school classrooms, in seminar rooms of graduate school, in walks and talks with good friends, in writing projects, and in our journals, my colleagues and I began to be aware of the ways in which we, as teachers, were writing our lives (Heilbrun, 1988) as we worked in our classrooms. As we listened to each other's stories and told our own, we learned to make sense of our teaching practices as expressions of our personal practical knowledge (Clandinin, 1986; Connelly & Clandinin, 1988), the experiential knowledge that was embodied in us as persons and was enacted in our classroom practices and in our lives. It was knowing that came out of our pasts and found expression in the present situations in which we found ourselves. For many of us it was an acknowledgment that had been missing as we lived out our lives in the prescriptive environments of schools where our stories as teachers had not been valued and the kind of knowledge we possessed had not been given voice.

With the realization that we were writing our own lives as knowing people came a sense of the need to give voice to our experiences and to find places where we could begin to figure out what it was that each of us knew as teachers. We began to tell stories of our experiences as children, as teachers, as students, as women, as men, and as people in our Western society. We came to see, as we reconstructed our lives, the ways in which they were storied ones. We came to make sense of what we were doing both as living our stories in an ongoing experiential text and as telling our stories in words as we reflected on life and explained ourselves to others.

As we acknowledged these new ways of talking about our knowledge and our lives, we looked back over our stories and journals to find the narrative threads of our individual lives. We saw the ways in which we had been shaped by our culture, our gender, our institutions, and our profession, but we also saw that each of us had learned to write her life in unique ways that came from her personal experience of the world.

Reprinted with permission from Teachers College Press. Acknowledgement; Clandinin, D. J. (1993). Teacher education as narrative inquiry. Chapter 1 in D. J. Clandinin, A. Davies, P. Hogan, & B. Kennard (Eds.), *Learning to teach: Teaching to learn: Stories of collaboration in teacher education* (pp 1–15). New York, NY: Teachers College Press.

We began to know our own stories better by hearing others' stories. As we listened to others' stories, we not only heard echoes of our own stories, but saw new shades of meaning in them. We learned to value each time we wrote in our journals, responded to another's journal, told one of our stories, and listened to another's story. Through these experiences we gained new possibilities for writing our lives differently.

As we read the work of researchers and practitioners and talked about their ideas and how they helped us make sense of our lives, we also saw new possibilities for changed practices. Each was an educative experience. We knew as we listened and as we spoke and wrote our stories, to value the knowing that we had come to see in our work and in ourselves.

This new sense of ourselves as knowing people emerged over time as we developed a language and ways of working with each other. We learned to make spaces for each other in which to hear our voices, to know that in our voices were our ways of making sense of ourselves and of our work. Words such as Britzman's (1990) helped us to find ways of talking about what we were figuring out.

> Voice is meaning that resides in the individual and enables that individual to participate in a community. . . . The struggle for voice begins when a person attempts to communicate meaning to someone else. Finding the words, speaking for oneself, and feeling heard by others are all a part of this process. . . . Voice suggests relationships: the individual's relationship to the meaning of her/his experience and hence, to language, and the individual's relationship to the other, since understanding is a social process.
>
> *(p. 14)*

Britzman's words about what it means to have a voice gave us a sense that we could find ways of talking about our knowing that were part of how we lived our lives. We began to tell stories of other experiences to which we had not given voice, stories of many experiences that formed the texts of our lives. The distinctions placed between who we were as professionals and who we were as persons blurred as we talked about our lives and the ways in which we worked with children and each other in schools and classrooms, in our homes, and among our families.

As we wrote about our work and the knowing found in our work and in our lives, we began to wonder about the ways in which teacher education was constructed and lived out. We began with wondering about graduate programs in education, staff and professional development, and the ways in which such programs were constructed. The language and the strategies of these programs emerged from talk of one vision, one way of knowing, of skills that could be coached. This language seemed disconnected from the meaningful experiences of our lives. We began to write and talk about other ways of continuing to have educative experiences, other ways of making connections to our lives and our work and to the people with whom we worked each day. As we wondered about the experiences our institutions constructed for us, we began to talk of preservice teacher education. We found the language of teacher education an uncomfortable one with its talk of standards, percentages, skills, strategies, exit and entrance criteria. We had come to feel uncomfortable with this language because we had learned to talk about our own teaching in terms of personal and practical knowing, emotionality, moral dilemmas, and ethics of caring. Noddings (1986) helped us to express some of what we felt about the language of teacher education when she wrote that "we approach our goal by living with those whom we teach in a caring community, through modeling, dialogue, practice and confirmation. Again, we see how unfamiliar this language has become" (p. 502).

Noddings's words helped us begin to question the feelings we had when we found ourselves trying to live out our lives bounded by the structures of teacher education. We felt constrained by unfamiliar boundaries, boundaries that we had begun to break out of when we thought about our lives as teachers of children. The ideas of expert-novice, prescriptions for "right" practice, and generic rules that could be applied in any situation felt as uncomfortable in teacher education as they had in how we were beginning to speak of our teaching. And yet our talk of friendship, ethics of caring, and what Elbow (1986) calls the believing game seemed to have no place in discussions of teacher education. We found no place for making sense of teacher education as part of our ongoing narratives of experience (Connelly & Clandinin, 1990) or for seeing teachers as holders of personal practical knowledge. When we wanted to talk about student teachers as learning to live and tell their stories in practice, of personal knowledge being made practical, we became lost in the gaps and silences of the institutional stories of teacher education.

Quietly and cautiously, we had begun to question the lived story of teacher education, a story rooted in long institutional narratives of university-professional relationships. In the pages that follow we tell of our wondering about teacher education. We describe the ways in which we tried to construct and live out a new story of teacher education, through a collaborative experimental program.

Planning the project: beginning the inquiry

The story of this inquiry into restructuring or restorying the lived and told stories of teacher education has, as all narratives of experience do, multiple possible beginnings. I could begin to tell this story, or more appropriately these stories, in many ways depending on the temporal, personal, or institutional frame I placed around the story. I could begin, for example, with each of the participants' narratives of experience situated within particular institutional, cultural, and social stories. If I took that as my starting point, I would trace the narrative threads that led each participant to the program. I might, for example, begin with a telling of my story that highlighted an image of community rooted in my experiences as a child in a rural community in Alberta. I was raised to be in tune with the rhythmic changes of the seasons, nurtured by parents, family, and community members whose very survival depended on being responsive to nature and other community members. But that is only one of the possible narrative threads that led me to this new program in teacher education. There are many such threads, some more telling than others.

The story could begin with such a telling for any participant in the program. I might, for example, begin with Pat Hogan's story with its narrative roots in a search for place within a community, with establishing a community both in which to feel she belonged and that sought to move forward some mission that gave place to others. There are many such possible narrative beginnings. The characters in this story were 28 student teachers, 28 cooperating teachers, five university teachers, other team partners, school administrators, and countless children and parents. I could begin this story with any of their stories, with each participant's story told in many ways.

There are other possible narrative beginnings. Another beginning could be, for example, the discussions of my research on teaching seminars on different conceptions of teaching fostered by the work of John Dewey, Philip Jackson, Elliot Eisner, Joseph Schwab, Madeleine Grumet, Bob Yinger, Eleanor Duckworth, Donald

Schön, David Hawkins, Michael Connelly, Deborah Britzman, and Vivian Paley. This telling of the story would begin with the questions raised by seminar participants about why our institutions "did" teacher education as they did if scholars held different conceptions of teaching, of curriculum, of teacher education.

I could also begin with each cooperating teacher's story of student teaching, of teacher education, of methods classes, of working with student teachers in other years. Those, too, would be possible beginnings to the story of the inquiry.

I could also begin by telling of the connections among the participants. Many joined the program because they had friends in the program. They wanted to share a further adventure, to participate with colleagues and to engage in a collaborative inquiry into teacher education. They wanted to learn to live and tell their stories of teaching, of curriculum, and, perhaps, of their lives differently through working in more connected ways with valued colleagues. In this telling, I would begin with stories of collaboration, of caring, of participants playing the believing game, trying to see things from another person's perspective. I would raise questions about how the story of teacher education would look different if university teachers and cooperating teachers took seriously and tried to live out the ideas talked about in courses on teaching and curriculum.

The story could also begin with the students who participated and how they sought out the program, hearing that their friends were coming. They, too, had heard stories of "the dreaded practicum year" that was both the best year of the program and the worst. They wanted to be part of living a different story of teacher education. Becoming participants in the program with us allowed them that possibility.

All are possible beginning points and, depending on which one I select, I would give a different telling of the story. In any telling, however, I would want to note some common marks. I would emphasize that the inquiry was marked by a search for voice, a search for place. In the inquiry all participants tried to take each other seriously. They tried to listen closely to their own voices, the voices of other participants, and the voices of theory as they struggled with a new story. All participants tried to come to new understandings of the ways in which their stories had been lived out within social, cultural, and institutional stories that had both shaped their knowing and continued to shape the new stories they were trying to live and tell. The inquiry was marked with deep emotions. Colleagues in different small groups and large groups laughed and cried together as they came to understand what it means to teach and to be a teacher. It was an inquiry marked by the moral issues of what it means to engage in educative experiences with children, with teachers, and with other people. The story told of the inquiry is one in which the participants cared deeply about what was happening and have, as a consequence, learned a great deal about other possible stories to live and tell in teacher education.

But I have here sketched out the barest of possible beginning points for these stories. As the stories are told in the pages that follow, I hope the richness of each particular story will allow others to imagine different ways I might have told the story.

A temporal telling of the story

When called on to explain the Alternative Program to others, I have found myself constrained by the customary narrative form of beginning, middle, and end. I first outline the inquiry's purposes and name the participants. I describe the activities in which participants engaged and the outcomes of the program. I will do some of that here so readers get some sense of the development of the program and of our inquiry.

The story I most often tell begins with a meeting called by Dr. Kathy Skau, department head of Teacher Education and Supervision at the University of Calgary. She called a small group of faculty together to discuss possibilities for an experimental program in teacher education. Teacher education is often a topic at the autumn department retreat, but rarely do department members come together after the retreat to make changes in the program. This is partly because teacher education is a faculty-wide responsibility but also because when they return from the retreat faculty members are immediately caught up in the demands of teaching. The formation of a group to discuss a possible alternative program was something new. The group eventually consisted of Garry deLeeuw, Garth Benson, Suzanne Kurtz, Pat Hogan, and Jean Clandinin. Marilyn Stratton, an instructor in the required educational administration course, also joined the group albeit somewhat later. Bill Hunter worked with the students in a computer course although he stayed at the periphery of the inquiry.

During the fall of 1988 and winter of 1989, the group met to discuss program issues in teacher education and what would constitute an alternative to the present program. We discussed the kinds of experiences we would want student teachers to have, what kinds of parts we would want to play in relation to students, and how we would work with schools and teachers. In our proposal for a small amount of University Special Projects funding we wrote:

> We seek to promote a different relationship between theory and practice. Rather than beginning with the theory and methods of instruction, the proposed alternative program begins its sequence of instruction in practice and, as student teachers begin to develop understanding of practice, various theoretical readings are introduced. Here the starting point of teacher education is in practice because it is from this perspective that individuals construct their own personal knowledge of teaching. This practical starting point gives students a grounded way to make sense of the theories, models and research they encounter in university classes. Furthermore, the proposed program acknowledges students begin teacher education with personal knowledge acquired from their prior experience. Both the experiential knowledge and the practical starting point provide a context in which students can plan, experiment, reflect and read in order to develop their teaching knowledge. Through this process, students construct and reconstruct their own personal practical knowledge.
>
> *(Clandinin & Hogan, 1989, p. 2)*

In the proposal, we attempted to explain the shape of the plot outlines of the imagined new story of teacher education. It was, however, with little understanding of the ways in which each of our stories would be lived out within the new program constraints.

As the small group discussed possibilities, we situated the program in ongoing work in narrative inquiry and personal practical knowledge. Personal practical knowledge is

> a term designed to capture the idea of experience in a way that allows us to talk about teachers as knowledgeable and knowing persons. Personal practical knowledge is in the teacher's past experience, in the teacher's present mind and body, and in the future plans and actions. Personal practical knowledge

> is found in the teacher's practice. It is, for any one teacher, a particular way of reconstructing the past and the intentions of the future to deal with the exigencies of a present situation.
>
> *(Connelly & Clandinin, 1988, p. 25)*

This perspective viewed the knowledge of experienced teachers as legitimate, as something different from theoretical knowledge, although we saw theoretical knowledge as part of teachers' knowledge (Elbaz, 1983; Lampert, 1985). Teacher knowledge was seen as constructed and reconstructed in practice and through reflection upon practice (Britzman, 1990; Clandinin, 1986; Hogan, 1988). Teacher knowledge was described as biographical (Grumet, 1988), embodied in who we are as people, and enacted in our practice.

Our group used this theoretical foundation to help us think about what we might do differently as we structured an alternative program in teacher education. We drew on earlier work where I had imagined that

> by adopting a personal knowledge perspective, reflection gains importance as a critical element in teacher education. By making reflection an integral part of three kinds of teacher education experiences (observation, student teaching and other courses), an intellectual experience is set up. Student teachers have not yet worked out a dynamic relationship between their imagery and other dimensions of their personal knowledge and practices. The significance of personal knowledge in curriculum is that we must go beyond theoretical principles and rules of teaching and beyond practical description of action found in statements of strategies and routines. We would focus on ways of thinking and on plans and programs by which teachers and student teachers may reflect on themselves as knowing, teaching beings. Examining research knowledge, participating in applied research, observing other teachers teaching, trying out ideas developed elsewhere can all be valuable if they are part of a process of professional interaction, action and reflection.
>
> *(Clandinin, 1986, p. 175)*

However, in the program, we wanted to emphasize teacher education as a collaborative inquiry in which collaboration was essential between student teachers, university teachers, and cooperating teachers. We wanted to look at teaching not as the transmission of knowledge but as collaborative inquiry involving students and teachers at all levels. This would involve shared work in a practical setting among student teachers, cooperating teachers, university teachers, and children. We saw this collaborative process as similar to collaborative research in which there is a joint living out of all participants' narratives so that participants are continuing to tell their own stories but the stories are now being lived out in a collaborative setting (Connelly & Clandinin, 1990). The inquiry, however, was not to begin with prespecified problems to which theory or sets of rules were applied, but was to begin with the phenomena of a teacher's classroom practice and a student teacher's intention to develop his or her practical knowledge.

The collaborative inquiry would occur in the practice of teaching through the process of reflection-in-and-on-practice (Schön, 1983, 1987). This would allow our program to recognize that people say and do different things in different circumstances and, conversely, that different circumstances bring forward different aspects of their experience to bear on the situation. According to this view, a person's personal practical knowledge depends in important measure on the situation (Clandinin & Connelly, 1988). Through this reflective process of constructing and reconstructing personal practical knowledge, the temporal and social/cultural horizons of each participant would, we hoped, be expanded and changed.

We imagined this process would be ongoing throughout the practicum year with constant opportunity for reflection-in-and-on-action. The participants would continually construct and reconstruct personal practical knowledge as they engaged in practice. Their ongoing practice would be the framework for understanding theories and for constructing and reconstructing practical knowledge.

Adding other participants to the story

When the group of university teachers had worked out the ideas sufficiently well for Pat and I to write the proposal, it was time to begin work with teachers who might be interested in participating with us. Our group wanted to be able to include their knowing in the ways we structured the program. While we recognized the constraints of the temporal cycles of the university week and year and the constraints of the number and names of necessary courses, we sensed we had flexibility to try out new variations on the themes set by the proposal, the people working in the program, and the temporal cycles of schools and university.

At this point we had set up a weekly cycle for the student teachers that named their courses and gave a temporal sequence to their weeks. They would be in the schools on Monday, Wednesday morning, and Friday. Tuesday and Thursday mornings would be spent in four methods of instruction courses (mathematics, science, social studies, language arts). The methods courses would be integrated with each other as much as possible. Tuesday afternoon would be spent in an advanced computer applications class, and Thursday afternoon would be spent in a required educational administration class. Wednesday afternoon would be spent in small group seminars in the schools. This schedule met the requirements for coursework and practicum in the elementary route professional program.

The yearly cycle had been set in order to have the student teachers begin work with the teachers as early in the school year as possible (late August or early September). They would stay on the school cycle until the end of April. However, we scheduled some full weeks in the schools with no university classes, and we also allowed a one-week break in each term with no university or school expectations. These nonscheduled times were for work on assignments. We hoped student teachers and cooperating teachers could negotiate flexibility around these cycles. We also agreed that students would keep dialogue journals, but we had only tentative discussions on this topic. Other than this framework, we hoped to negotiate the rest of the shape of the story with student teachers and cooperating teachers.

Our university group sent out invitations to teachers and principals with whom we had worked in other settings. We talked with each of them individually to find out their interest and to tell them briefly about what we envisioned. They gave us names of other teachers who might be interested. Friends of friends were invited. The first meeting of interested school people was April 6, 1989. We shared our ideas and, in small discussion groups, we heard theirs. A steering committee of 14 teachers plus five university teachers was set up. Over the spring months the steering committee met. The program began to take shape in these discussions.

The plot of the story began to unfold quickly in April when we spoke to prospective students. We visited classes to distribute brochures and invited students to an information meeting. There we shared the sketchy ideas for an alternative program in teacher education. We provided as much information as we could about the program and talked about what we hoped would be its collaborative nature. We asked them to consider what we had in mind and, on the basis of their intentions, to choose whether or not to work with us. Decisions were out of our hands at that point as registrations for the 28 spaces in our program were to be filled by the admissions office on a first-come, first-served basis. Many of the students who eventually came to work with us in the program stood in line from early in the morning on registration day to ensure a spot. Clearly they too saw a need for an alternative program in teacher education.

In discussions with the university teachers and cooperating teachers, both in the steering committee and in the large group meetings, many issues in the inquiry began to surface. These issues added to the ones our university group had imagined. The issues emerged from the different institutional stories that shaped and constrained each participant's knowing as well as from each participant's narrative of experience.

In these discussions, points of tension were noted. As we analyzed field notes of these meetings, we found issues about the journals. For example, questions were raised about how to have the journals be "true reflections" rather than reflected journals and places to fulfill course requirements or explain classroom activities. Other questions were raised about how to work with cooperating teachers, a university teacher, and student teachers in small journal group settings. These questions were linked to the notion that we needed to be writing and talking together in order for collaboration to lead to changed practice. We talked frequently about trusting relationships as the key to the program. Issues of evaluation occupied a great deal of the discussion early in the deliberations. Questions were raised about how to view evaluation differently given the collaborative nature of the relationships and the reflective nature of the processes with which we were involved. In the field notes we wrote:

> Given that we and the students are trying to make sense of classrooms and our work as practitioners, and that the students are trying to make sense of theory in light of their own experience in our classrooms, much of the evaluation will be a kind of self-evaluation occurring in a collaborative relationship that gives students a great deal of voice.
>
> *(Notes to file, May 18, 1989)*

Those notes drew our attention again to the importance we were placing on this as a collaborative inquiry.

> It is important to keep in mind that in fundamental respects, evaluation is an ongoing process in which all persons involved need to have equal voice. It is important also to remember that we will not be alone, but that we will have many others with whom these questions can and will be explored.
>
> *(Notes to file, May 18, 1989)*

As the stories in our program emerged, these notes took on importance. We began to be aware of the possible tensions in learning to live a new story of teacher education. Other issues that foreshadowed our awareness of the institutional boundaries of our knowing were issues about working with in-school administrators and negotiating new relationships for student teachers with school administrators. In early meetings we discussed the need for continuity and consistency between the schools and the university. In part, this was a concern about the student teachers' weekly and yearly cycle being different from the school's cycle. We all sensed the possible tension that would result from this, but we could not imagine other possibilities that would fit within the university constraints. A frequently expressed concern was how difficult it would be to learn to live out the new story we were creating in the inquiry rather than falling back into the stories we had experienced in teacher education.

Bringing the participants together

By June's end, the yearly school cycle necessitated the calling together of the 28 students, 28 cooperating teachers, and five university teachers for an evening planning session. This was the first meeting of the whole group. After that meeting, it was left to the university teachers to match students with teachers and to inform everyone of the paired relationships. At the meeting some of the cooperating teachers and student teachers made their own matches and let the university teachers know their choices. The matches left to the university teachers were made on some of the standard criteria about geographical location, time and family constraints, and subject matter specialties. The university teachers informed the student teachers and cooperating teachers of their partners in early July. The stage was set for the program to begin with the late August–early September meetings in the schools.

Narrative themes in the inquiry

Narrative themes, in many ways interrelated, emerged from the inquiry. We discuss five important ones here.

An important narrative theme in the inquiry was a view of teacher education as part of the ongoing writing of student teachers' lives, not a separate preparation for something disconnected from what came before and a readying for what is to come after. Teacher education was seen as part of the ongoing storying and restorying of students' lives. Teacher education experiences were part of ongoing narratives of experience, narratives that were being continually revised and rewritten as individuals found new ways of making sense of their work as teachers and as people, and as they found themselves in new situations.

Another narrative theme in the inquiry was a questioning of the separation of theory and practice, a questioning of the view that we learn theory in order to apply it to practice. In our inquiry we tried to make new sense of how theory and practice might be connected; we tried to engage in a dialogue between our practices and theory, a dialogue mutually informing to both theory and practice, to researcher and practitioner. In this view, theory was not seen as superior to practice but as in a kind of dialectical relationship to practice. The dialogue or conversation between theory and practice resulted in new understandings for both.

A third narrative theme was collaboration. In our inquiry we wanted to learn to listen to each other so that together we might all learn to make new sense of practice and learn to live more moral lives in our teaching (Coles, 1989). We engaged in making sense of teacher education with each other, that is, with our student teachers, with cooperating teachers, and with university teachers. When we worked with others, we were able to see more clearly new possible stories. We did not see our work as teachers as changing or transforming children or each other. That was not our project with student teachers. We did not see ourselves as the ones who held the power to transform others. As we worked with each other, our attention was drawn to other plot lines and other ways of living and telling our own stories. This happened because we engaged with each other with intensity, paying careful attention to how others were telling and living their stories. When we became participants in their stories, their stories changed. When they became participants in our stories, our stories changed. The experience was educative for each of us.

A fourth narrative theme was a search for language to talk about the ways each of us made sense of ourselves as people and as teachers. We wanted to develop a language of teacher education that allowed description of ways of finding a place in order to feel part of a personal and professional community. We wanted a language of teacher education to talk about who we were and about what lives we were writing for ourselves.

A fifth narrative theme was improvisation or what Bateson (1989) calls desperate improvisation. We engaged in an inquiry in which there were many ways of knowing, many ways of making sense, and many institutional stories. Yinger (1987) has written about practice as improvisation in which teachers improvise around a theme. Improvisation became a theme for the ways we learned to live new stories of practice. There were many improvisations as student teachers, cooperating teachers, and university teachers tried to figure out what it meant to learn to live a new story.

Purposes for writing the stories

We have several purposes for undertaking to write our stories in this book. We undertook this inquiry into teacher education in part to serve our own purposes as cooperating teachers and university teachers. We wanted to work with student teachers in new ways, ways that would allow them to see a range of possibilities for themselves as teachers. Cooperating teachers also participated, in part, in order to engage in an educative experience for themselves. They wanted to learn to live new stories of practice with the children in their classrooms. As cooperating teachers and university teachers, we also wanted to learn to live new ways of storying our own practices in teacher education. In part, then, when we write down the stories we have lived in this inquiry, it is to record for ourselves the new stories we have learned to live and tell.

But in writing this book we hope to reach a wider audience of practitioners, including cooperating teachers, student teachers, and university teachers. I have written elsewhere about the purposes of writing narratives for a larger audience.

> Narrative inquiries are shared in ways that help readers question their own stories, raise their own questions about practice and see in the narrative accounts stories of their own stories. The intent is to foster reflection, storying and restorying for readers.
>
> *(Clandinin & Connelly, 1990, p. 20)*

These are our purposes. We want to engage readers in considering what our stories of teacher education allow them to see in their stories and practices of teacher education.

In earlier writing (Clandinin & Connelly, 1990) I used Crites's (1975) words to suggest how people should tell their stories in ways that encourage readers to be reflective about their practices and to invite them to engage in a restorying of their stories. Crites (1975) noted that the completeness of a story consists

> in the immediacy with which narrative is able to render the concrete particularities of experience. Its characteristic language is not conceptual but consists typically in the sort of verbal imagery we employ in referring to things as they appear to our senses or figure in our practical activities. Still more important the narrative form reproduces the temporal tensions of experience, a moving present tensed between and every moment embracing a memory of what has gone before and an activity projected, underway.
>
> *(p. 26)*

As I thought about our purposes in writing this book and in telling our stories for others, Crites reminded me that these stories are not models or solutions to the problems of teacher education but are stories that highlight the tensions each of us experienced as we lived out our personal stories embedded within the cultural and institutional stories of teacher education, schools, and universities. I want to foster reflection on the ways individuals and institutions live and tell stories of teacher education. Perhaps our stories begin to do that.

In subsequent chapters, several participants tell their stories. Through these chapters we highlight the ways many of us came to make sense of our experiences in the program and of teacher education more generally. This book has been put together by a small group of practitioners, university teachers, student teachers, and cooperating teachers, who were interested in writing about their experiences in this inquiry into teacher education. What we have done as editors is to offer a range of possible stories of experience. In Part One of this book three student teachers have authored chapters in order to give their accounts of their experiences of learning to teach. Part Two of the book is collaboratively written by student teachers and cooperating teachers in order to tell stories of their experience of working together in teacher education. In Part Three, chapters are written by cooperating teachers who wanted to tell their own stories of new possibility in their practices and in teacher education. Finally as editors and authors of the book, we have written about new insights into teacher education that we hope highlight some possible ways to restory teacher education.

> What matters is that lives do not serve as models; only stories do that. And it is a hard thing to make up stories to live by. We can only retell and live by the stories we have read or heard.
>
> *(Heilbrun, 1988, p. 37)*

References

Bateson, M. C. (1989). *Composing a life*. New York, NY: Atlantic Monthly Press.

Britzman, D. (1990). *Practice makes practice: A critical study of learning to teach*. New York, NY: SUNY Press.

Clandinin, D. J. (1986). *Classroom practice: Teacher images in action*. London: Falmer Press.

Clandinin, D. J., & Connelly, F. M. (1988). Studying teachers' knowledge of classrooms: Collaborative research, ethics and the negotiation of narrative. *The Journal of Educational Thought, 22*(2A), 269–282.

Clandinin, D. J., & Connelly, F. M. (1990). Narrative and story in practice and research. In D. Schön (Ed.), *The reflective turn: Case studies of reflective practice* (pp. 258–282). New York, NY: Teachers College Press.

Clandinin, D. J., & Hogan, P. (1989). *Special projects proposal*. Internal University Proposal. Calgary, AB: University of Calgary.

Coles, R. (1989). *The call of stories: Teaching and the moral imagination*. Boston, MA: Houghton Mifflin.

Connelly, F. M., & Clandinin, D. J. (1988). *Teachers as curriculum planners: Narratives of experience*. New York, NY: Teachers College Press.

Connelly, F. M., & Clandinin, D. J. (1990). Stories of experience and narrative inquiry. *Educational Researcher, 19*(5), 2–14.

Crites, S. (1975). Angels we have heard. In J. B. Wiggins (Ed.), *Religion as story* (pp. 23–63). Lanham, MD: University Press of America.

Elbaz, F. (1983). *Teacher thinking: A study of practical knowledge*. London: Croom Helm.

Elbow, P. (1986). *Embracing contraries: Explorations in teaching and learning*. Oxford: Oxford University Press.

Grumet, M. (1988). *Bitter milk: Women and teaching*. Amherst, MA: University of Massachusetts Press.

Heilbrun, C. (1988). *Writing a woman's life*. New York, NY: W. W. Norton.

Hogan, P. (1988). *A community of teacher researchers: A story of empowerment and voice*. Unpublished manuscript, University of Calgary.

Lampert, M. (1985). How do teachers manage to teach? Perspectives on problems in practice. *Harvard Educational Review, 55*(2), 179–194.

Noddings, N. (1986). Fidelity in teaching, teacher education and research for teaching. *Harvard Educational Review, 56*(4), 496–510.

Schön, D. (1983). *The reflective practitioner: How professionals think in action*. New York, NY: Basic Books.

Schön, D. (1987). *Educating the reflective practitioner: Toward a new design for teaching and learning in the professions*. San Francisco, CA: Jossey-Bass.

Yinger, R. (1987). *By the seat of your pants: An inquiry into improvisation and teaching*. Paper presented at the annual meeting of the American Educational Research Association, Washington, DC.

5

NARRATIVE AND STORY IN TEACHER EDUCATION

Introduction

> Current research on women often focuses on a single aspect or stage of life. Dissection is an essential part of scientific method and it is particularly tempting to disassemble a life composed of odds and ends, to describe the pieces separately.
>
> *(Bateson, 1989, p. 10)*

In *Composing a Life*, Bateson draws our attention to the importance of looking more holistically at our lives. She emphasizes the temptation of trying to make sense of pieces of our lives without understanding the narrative wholes in which the pieces are embedded. While Bateson is looking at women's lives, her words have particular significance for teacher education. Too often we look at teacher education as separate from the ongoing lives of teachers and student teachers. We pull out the years of teacher education to examine them. In so doing, we separate teacher education experiences from the pasts and futures of our student teachers' lives. We do not create spaces to acknowledge either the ways they have already written their lives prior to teacher education or to the ways they continue to live their stories in the context of teacher education. Bateson's words taken into the teacher education context highlight the importance of making sense of teachers' and student teachers' lives as narratives of experience, a living-out of the stories we tell ourselves in order to make meaning of our experience.

In our work with teachers (Connelly and Clandinin, 1988) we came to understand our own lives as teachers and researchers as well as the lives of teachers, student teachers and children narratively. Our work on narratives of experience draws attention to the broad sweep of our lives, to the ways our pasts are connected to our presents and futures as we live out and tell our stories. Looking at life as narrative or storied allows us to see the unities, continuities and discontinuities, images and rhythms in our lives. We take the view that one of the basic human forms of experience of the world is as story and that the storied quality of experience is both

Reprinted with permission. Acknowledgement; Clandinin, D. J. (1991). Narrative and story in teacher education. In T. Russell & H. Munby (Eds.), *Teachers and teaching: From classroom to reflection* (pp. 124–137). London: Falmer Press.

unconsciously restoried in life and consciously restoried, retold and relived through processes of reflection (Connelly and Clandinin, 1990).

> Narrative, for us, is the study of how humans make meaning of experience by endlessly telling and retelling stories about themselves that both refigure the past and create purpose in the future. Deliberately storying and restorying one's life or a group or cultural story is, therefore, a fundamental method of personal and social growth: it is a fundamental quality of education.
>
> *(Connelly and Clandinin, 1990, p. 24)*

Our use of the terms 'narrative' and 'story' draws on distinctions that other researchers have developed. In social science research the two terms are often collapsed with no great loss of precision. Polkinghorne (1988, p. 13), for example, reviews possible uses of both terms and concludes by treating them as equivalent – a position close to that adopted by Carr (1986). We have an in-between usage. When referring to participant situations (such as classroom field records and interview data) we tend to use 'story' to talk about particular situations and 'narrative' to refer to longer term life events. Everyday speech patterns modify this loose distinction and we would more often say 'deliberately storying and restorying one's life . . .' rather than 'deliberately narrating and renarrating one's life. . .'. We would, however, follow Carr and Polkinghorne here and treat the two expressions as equivalent. When we refer to research, research method and researchers we use the term 'narrative' exclusively. For example, we would say 'narrative researchers, as Mishler (1986) shows, are engaged in the collection of stories when conducting interviews'. Our ideas on narrative method are elaborated in Connelly and Clandinin (1990).

Personal practical knowledge as narratively constructed knowledge

To speak of teachers' knowledge of schools and classrooms as personal practical knowledge (Clandinin, 1986; Connelly and Clandinin, 1988) is to capture the idea of experience in a way that allows us to talk about teachers as knowledgeable and knowing persons. We see personal practical knowledge as in the person's past experience, in the person's present mind and body and in the person's future plans and actions. It is knowledge that reflects the individual's prior knowledge and acknowledges the contextual nature of that teacher's knowledge. It is a kind of knowledge carved out of, and shaped by, situations; knowledge that is constructed and reconstructed as we live out our stories and retell and relive them through processes of reflection.

Our work to this point has explored experienced and novice teachers' personal practical knowledge. We do this experientially and biographically by understanding teachers' knowledge as constructions and reconstructions of their life narratives. We see this storying and restorying of each of our lives as going on in our work as teachers and researchers.

Narrative inquiry as research method builds on this process of growth, that is, on these constructions and reconstructions of personal practical knowledge as we story and restory our lives. Narrative inquiry is the storying and restorying of our narratives of educational experience. The narrative account of an educational event that we wrote as researchers constituted a restorying of that event. We saw those accounts, at least to the extent that they were a restorying of the event, as on a continuum with the processes of reflective restorying that goes on in each of our educational lives. We came to see narrative inquiry as going on, therefore, both in researchers' work as well as in each of our educational lives. It is, therefore, less a matter of the application of a scholarly technique to understanding phenomena than it is a matter of 'entering into' the phenomena and partaking of them. For us, we saw narrative as part of the phenomena of educational experience.

In this chapter, I briefly outline the process of narrative inquiry in order to set a context for viewing teacher education as a kind of narrative inquiry for all of the involved participants, university teachers, cooperating teachers and student teachers. In this work, I offer a view of teacher education as a way of composing our lives as teachers, a way to not disassemble but to bring back a more holistic way of seeing experience and teacher education. Seeing teacher education as narrative inquiry is, for me, a way to connect our pasts as children and students in school to our present experiences as student teachers, cooperating teachers and university teachers with our imagined future experiences.

This chapter offers an account of a particular narrative inquiry into teacher education. In the 1989–1990 academic year, a group of university teachers, cooperating teachers and student teachers worked together in order to explore an alternative approach to teacher education as narrative inquiry. This chapter describes how we conceived of teacher education as narrative inquiry and illustrates these ideas through a telling of one student's story in the program. The story of Julie illustrates the storying and restorying between one university teacher and one student teacher as we worked together in the inquiry. I attempt to highlight the growth and change as we both came to new ways of living our stories. The story also highlights the tensions as individuals live out their stories embedded within social, cultural and institutional narratives.

The process of narrative inquiry

Prior to giving an account of teacher education as narrative inquiry, I briefly outline the process of narrative inquiry as we have engaged with it in our research. (More detailed accounts are presented in Connelly and Clandinin, 1990 and Clandinin and Connelly, 1991). Briefly stated, we have noted that narrative is both phenomenon and method. Narrative names the structured quality of experience to be studied and it names the patterns of inquiry for its study. In narrative inquiry, we say that people lead storied lives and tell stories of those lives and narrative researchers describe such lives, collect and tell stories of them and write narratives of experience.

We see our work as narrative inquirers as staying open to continually assessing the multiple levels (temporally continuous and socially interactive) at which the inquiry proceeds. The complexity of staying open to the multiple levels becomes apparent when we realize that people are both living their stories in an ongoing experiential text and telling their stories in words as they reflect upon life and explain themselves to others. For the researcher, this is the smallest portion of the complexity, since a life is also a matter of growth toward an imagined future and, therefore, involves restorying and attempts at reliving. A person is, at once, then, engaged in living, telling, retelling and reliving stories. We have begun to work with teachers and other practitioners to give accounts of the storying and restorying that goes on in each of our lives. For example, in work with Stephanie, a primary teacher, I construct stories that illustrate how her image of the classroom as home is central to her storying and restorying of her classroom practices (Clandinin, 1986). Similarly, in our work with

Phil, a school administrator, we illustrate the narrative unity of community that is a unifying thread through his storying and restorying (Clandinin and Connelly, 1991).

The possible entanglements of seeing and describing story in the everyday actions of teachers and children is particularly acute in the tellings and retellings for it is here that temporal and social-cultural horizons are set and reset. As narrative researchers we add to the complexity of the process for, as researchers, we become part of the process. Researchers' narratives are lived, told and retold in the research process. Thus the narratives of participants and researchers become, in part, shared narrative constructions and reconstructions through the inquiry.

Narrative method involves participant observation, shared work in a practical setting. The process is a joint living out of two persons' narratives, researcher and practitioner, so that both participants are continuing to tell their own stories but the stories are now being lived out in a collaborative setting. We see the initial process of beginning to work together as an ethical matter, a negotiation of a shared narrative unity.

> We have shown how successful negotiation and the application of principles do not guarantee a fruitful study. The reason, of course, is that collaborative research constitutes a friendship. In everyday life, the idea of friendship implies a sharing, an interpenetration of two or more persons' spheres of experience. Mere contact is acquaintanceship, not friendship. The same may be said for collaborative research which requires a close relationship akin to friendship. Relationships are joined, as MacIntyre (1981) implies, by the narrative unities of our lives.
>
> *(Clandinin and Connelly, 1988, p. 281)*

When we conceive of negotiation of entry in this way, we highlight the way narrative inquiry occurs within collaborative relationships among researchers and practitioners (Connelly and Clandinin, 1990). Here I want to emphasize that in the process of beginning to live the shared story of narrative inquiry, the researcher needs to be aware of constructing a relationship in which both voices are heard.

In narrative work on teachers' personal practical knowledge, data originated in researcher observation, participant observation of practice and observations by other participants, as well as through personally reflective methods such as journal keeping, story telling, letter writing and autobiographical work such as those involved in the writing of personal annals and chronicles. In the research process, the researcher adds his or her own reflective voice. For example, the researcher responded to teachers' stories with questions about why the story was told in the way it was. By answering the researcher's question, the participants were able to penetrate more deeply to other experiences to trace the emotionality attached to their particular way of storying events and this, from the point of view of research, also constituted data.

Movement from experience to researcher and practitioner field notes, transcripts, documents and descriptive storying of the experienced narrative, to a mutual reconstruction of a narrative account, characterizes the process of narrative inquiry. Both researchers and practitioners are participants in the research and, as such, engage in the collaborative process. Both work through a mutual reconstruction of the telling of the story in practice that has been captured in field notes, transcripts and documents. The narrative inquiry process is a process of data collection, mutual narrative interpretation by practitioners and researchers, more data collection and further narrative reconstruction. The narrative inquiry process itself is a narrative one of storying, restorying and restorying again.

In narrative inquiry we offer ways of telling individuals' stories – researcher's *and* participant's – as embedded within particular cultures and histories. Accounts of how the individual is shaped by the larger professional knowledge context and also the ways in which the professional knowledge context has been reshaped in the unique situation in which the individual lives and works are constructed. Therefore, in narrative inquiry we both understand and try to give an account of the ways in which the individual is shaped by the situation and shapes the situation in the living out of the story and in the storying of the experience.

There are many risks, dangers and abuses of narrative (Connelly and Clandinin, 1990), including difficulties that arise such as 'narrative smoothing' (Spence, 1986). However, another risk that becomes particularly apparent as we lived out our narrative inquiry in teacher education was the construction of a story by the university teacher-researcher that could be given as a kind of script to student teachers. In situations where some participants have been traditionally silenced, as student teachers have been, this risk becomes particularly acute.

One purpose of narrative inquiry is to foster reflection and restorying on the part of all participants in the inquiry. The first, and central, contribution lies in the interactive relations between practitioner and researcher that lead to a mutual, collaborative telling and retelling of the stories of the participants – both practitioner and researcher. This leads to a consideration of the way in which participation in a narrative inquiry opens participants to understanding change in their practices (Clandinin, 1989; Connelly and Clandinin, 1988). This change and growth occurs for all participants for no-one emerges unchanged from this process. We had begun to explore the ways in which change in practice occurs for teachers and researchers within the collaborative relationships of narrative inquiry as a process of 'giving back a story' (Connelly and Clandinin, 1985).

Teacher education as narrative inquiry

Our insights into understanding narrative inquiry as an educative process that facilitates change and growth through reflective storying and restorying lead us to conceptualize teacher education as narrative inquiry. Some colleagues, both practising teachers and university teachers, worked together to explore the possibility of making sense of teacher education as narrative inquiry. In our inquiry we wanted to explore ways of constructing teacher education that would allow each of us, student teachers, cooperating teachers and university teachers, to tell our stories and, through the collaborative inquiry, to envisage new ways to tell and live our stories in teaching practice. We saw ourselves as engaged in a process of becoming attuned to hearing our own stories as they were lived out in our practice; to hearing others' stories as they were lived out in their practice; and, in hearing our stories as they were given back by other participants in the program, to see possibility for new stories of classroom practice and teacher education. We also wanted to stay attentive to the ways in which the cultural, historical and institutional narratives shaped the telling and living out of our new stories of teacher education.

Making sense of teacher education in this way allowed us to explore the personal knowledge of student teachers and to work with them in collaborative, supportive working relationships as their personal knowledge was made practical in classroom and school situations. As student teachers constructed and reconstructed their knowing, we, as university teachers and cooperating teachers, also engaged in a reflective restorying. We saw ourselves as engaged in learning to hear and tell our own stories as we worked with students in our classrooms and classes. Our work with them both helped us to see the stories we were living and telling even as their participation with us shaped the new stories we were learning to tell.

Our ideas of teacher education as narrative inquiry were shaped by what we understood it meant to engage both in a collaborative relationship and, within that relationship, to respond to another's story. The idea from our work as researchers seemed to fit with the kinds of teaching-learning relationships we were attempting to establish in our exploration of teacher education as narrative inquiry. We wanted to pay close attention to relationships between student teachers, university teachers and cooperating teachers that were akin to friendships, relationships that would be joined by the narrative unities constructed through our shared work.

Giving back stories: a narrative response

Notions about our collaborative relationships led us to explore the ideas of response. We had written about entering into another's story by becoming a participant in the shared story lived out in practice. We had only begun to explore the question of response. What did it mean to offer a response to another's story? What constituted a response that allowed space for all participants' stories? What kind of response allowed for a mutual reconstruction of all participants' stories? We were informed by the work of Belenky and her colleagues, who wrote about what they called a connected teacher:

> As a teacher, she believed she had to trust each student's experience, although as a person or a critic she might not agree with it. To trust means not just to tolerate a variety of viewpoints, acting as an impartial referee, assuring equal air time to all. It means to try to connect, to enter into each student's perspective.
> *(Belenky et al., 1986, p. 227)*

Belenky draws attention to the importance of trying to respond from the perspective of the other, suggesting an attempt to understand the other's way of knowing. While we recognized the importance as educators of hearing the students' voices, we wanted the relationship between university teacher, student teacher and cooperating teacher to be educative for all participants, that is, to include space for all participants' stories. Bateson allowed us a way to make sense of what we wanted to do. She wrote that:

> Today, more than twenty years later, I see the next step in the concept of response. It is interesting that, in spite of the different emphasis, the word 'response' provides the etymology of 'responsibility', whose central place in women's ethical sensitivities Carol Gilligan has so eloquently investigated.
> *(Bateson, 1989, p. 234)*

Bateson drew our attention to the ethical side of response and what it means to respond. It became important for us to consider how our response, that is, our way of connecting both the story given and the story given back, was a question of moral responsibility. Gilligan's work with young girls helped us think about our responses as moral.

> Yet to open oneself to another person creates great vulnerability, and thus the strength of girls' desire for relationship also engenders the need for protection from fraudulent relationships and psychic wounding.
>
> *(Gilligan, Lyons and Hanmer, 1990, p. 21)*

As we worked together, we came to understand the way shared stories were given and given back in the context of relationships. It was important to understand our responses as moral.

We also realized that the stories given back, the responses, were not only personal in the sense of coming from our own narratives of experiences, but were also embedded in particular social, cultural and institutional narratives. Not only our stories but our responses to others' stories were set within all of the contexts in which our stories were lived and told.

Reading and hearing others' stories became ways to help us hear our own stories and to understand the ways our stories are embedded in social and cultural stories. Bateson illustrated how reading others' stories help us become aware of our own when she wrote:

> Women today read and write biographies to gain perspective on their own lives. Each reading provokes a dialogue of comparison and recognition, a process of memory and articulation that makes one's own experience available as a lens of empathy. We gain even more from comparing notes and trying to understand the choices of our friends.
>
> *(Bateson, 1989, p. 4)*

Bateson's words also helped us see other possible ways of considering response. We came to see that it is from hearing the questions of our friends and teachers, that is, from within our trusted relationships that we learn to see new possibilities in living our stories. Her words drew our attention again to thinking about new possibilities for all participants, not only for students.

Initially we thought of our work as teacher educators, both university teachers and cooperating teachers, as giving back student teachers' stories. However, our work became a three-way dialogue between student teacher, cooperating teacher and university teacher in which stories were given and given back between all participants. These three-way dialogues were similar to the kinds of response we had given and received in discussion and narrative accounts written to and with, participants in our research projects. These given back stories picked up on ongoing narrative threads in a person's life and offered back other possible interpretations of these stories.

In our study of teacher education as narrative inquiry we struggled with the complexity of response for not only did university teachers, cooperating teachers and student teachers give back each other's stories but so did children, other colleagues, other staff members, parents and so on. These connected responses, these given-back stories, allowed us to see new narrative threads and tensions in all of our stories. Each of us began to see our work as teachers working with children in uncertain contexts as always living and telling, reliving and retelling our stories. We felt, as Bateson noted, that we needed 'to reinvent' ourselves 'again and again in response to a changing environment' (Bateson, 1989, p. 17).

As we worked together in the inquiry, we saw that each of our lives was being restoried through having our stories given back by others in our classroom and university contexts. Distinctions of role between student teacher, cooperating teacher and university teacher faded as we learned to hear the response of the other, to make sense of the new insights we had into our own storied lives. There were many tensions as we struggled to do this for we were living out our new stories within institutional narratives where teacher-student relationships are not founded on assumptions of equality and mutuality and where the constraints of time, position, power and evaluation shaped our collaboration. We struggled to establish relationships that would provide all of us with 'experiences of mutuality, equality and reciprocity' (Belenky et al., 1986, p. 38). For student teachers and cooperating teachers who have often seen themselves as less important and less valued than university teachers, it was a difficult ongoing struggle to live new but connected stories within traditional institutional narratives.

Paley's (1990) description of Jason, a little boy in kindergarten, captures something of the feeling we all experienced at some time over the year.

> Jason, finally, has figured out his own way to use his most precious possession and private fantasy to enable him to play with others. He has, in a real sense, come home. Which is to say, school is starting to feel like home. He can breathe deeply and open the doors of his helicopter house to others.
>
> *(Paley, 1990, p. 146)*

Paley, in her description of Jason, gave us a way to express our struggle to learn to work together. We too found ways to open our 'doors' to each other, to share our stories and to hear them given back so we could begin to live them with new possibilities.

Giving back Julie's story

The following fragment of a story illustrates one instance of giving back a story in the context of teacher education as narrative inquiry. We have called it Julie's story. Julie was a student teacher in our program who worked in a Grade 3–4 classroom. One of the assignments in our program was to follow one child's development in mathematics for a short period of time. In her work on this assignment, Julie chose to follow a small group of boys who were working on a task that her cooperating teacher called the house project, a project in which the boys were to figure out how to design and cost out a house given a certain set of constraints. This was an enrichment task in the classroom. Julie advised me she was going to work with this group of boys as they worked on the house project. We talked very little about the project in our seminar although, as students worked on their assignments, many did discuss them with me or other instructors. In the first months of the project, Julie and I attempted to establish what I thought was a collaborative relationship. We engaged in an ongoing journal dialogue and met on a weekly basis in a seminar group. However, evaluation, an important thread in the institutional narrative of teacher education, had not become an apparent tension in what I thought was a relationship of mutuality, equality and reciprocity.

In November, Julie gave me her first paper, one she had written on her work with the boys. The paper was a mixture of transcribed notes from the boys' conversations interspersed with various quotations from learning theory texts and quotations from theoretical resources on mathematics learning. I was surprised for I had expected something much different from Julie. My surprise caused me to reflect on what I had expected. I had expected a paper that talked about the particular boys, the particular task and what she had learned from the experience. I gave back in my response to her paper a story of distance from the children, of lack of connection with the subject matter and a lack of her voice as she hid behind the various theoretical formulations displaying a kind of what Belenky et al. (1986) would call 'received knowing'. Julie was angry with me and with herself but she was able to begin to make sense of the given-back story. I began to be aware of the institutional narratives and the ways evaluation shaped and constrained the collaborative relationship that Julie and I were attempting to construct. Julie had, in the face of a university assignment, completed a paper that drew on quotations from experts and that silenced her own voice, accounts of her own narrative knowing.

We talked and wrote and responded to each other in her journal over the next months. Julie's story of mathematics began to emerge. Several months later, in April, she gave me a second paper that offered another account of her story with the young boys. It was a story that began with Julie's story of mathematics, a story of lack of connection, of fear, of humiliation in which she endured teachers who held up her papers as inadequate and of summer holidays spent practising mathematics 'facts'. It was also a story in which she learned to depend on friends to explain to her what mathematics was all about, to help her make the connections to a subject matter story that seemed distant from her. As she retold her own story of learning mathematics, she saw how she had relived that story in her relations with the boys and mathematics. In rewriting the paper she now began to see her choice of working with the house project in new ways as she wrote about wanting to see what would happen when children were allowed to work with their peers on mathematics projects and when mathematics seemed more relevant to real life.

As Julie retold her story of mathematics as a learner and her story of working with the young boys, she made more sense of the way her old story had been relived in the work with the house project. She had not been able to find a connection to either the boys who were doing the project nor to mathematics as a subject matter. She was reliving her story of lack of connection, of silence.

Julie came to understand her story of learning to be a teacher this year as one in which she needed to learn to live a new story of mathematics in order to teach it. She began to involve herself in educational situations, courses in which she could explore a new story of herself as a learner of mathematics. But she also became interested in exploring her experience of mathematics within the context of the larger story of girls and mathematics and science learning. She began to research the topic in the literature and to talk to her female colleagues about their experiences. She began to explore, with her cooperating teacher, her feelings of the need for her voice to be heard in the classroom and the ways in which the young girls in the classroom needed to have space for their voices to be heard as they tried to make connections to the subject matter of mathematics.

As I reflected on Julie's story then and now as I write this chapter, the ideas of giving back stories took on new meaning for me. In my work as a teacher educator, I understand the importance of staying open to other possible readings of story even as I recognize the difficulty of staying open to possibilities. It is a felt tension in how I construct the horizons of my knowing. The institutional narratives in which I am embedded become apparent as I try to live a new story of teacher education. Collaboration becomes particularly important in order that we might have a wide range of stories given back from many participants. The collaborative relationships help us become attuned to the tensions such as those evoked as the evaluation process became part of the stories that Julie and I were living out.

It was important for me to have my story of surprise at Julie's paper given back to me by other participants in our program. Their response caused me to wonder about young women who enter teacher education as received knowers and the challenge of having them become constructed knowers. But their responses also caused one to ask questions about my own lived story as a received knower. I also sensed the importance of telling stories such as my story with Julie so other readers might raise questions about their practices in teacher education. Other students and teachers might see reflections of their stories in the ways we have chosen to tell Julie's story. For us as we think about teacher education as narrative inquiry, we see again the ways in which narrative inquiry leads to growth and change, to educative possibilities.

Educative possibilities in narrative inquiry

Practitioner-participant and researcher-participant goals in narrative inquiry (Clandinin and Connelly, 1991) are meaningful only within a larger social narrative shared by both. Practitioner and researcher continue to work, and so the restorying is expressed in reshaped relations with children, school, community, teachers and so on. A second goal for the researcher involves the more formal aspects of the story – a story in which the researcher has confidence may be read with meaning by others. We have written that the question of audience is what primarily separates the interests of researcher and practitioner-participant in narrative inquiry. The practitioner-participant, in the end, is storying his or her experience and so must live out the experience. The researcher, while also restorying his or her own experience wants others, an audience of other practitioners and researchers, to read narratively the one narrative presented in the research account. A third researcher goal is to develop theoretical constructs, which offer a language for thinking and talking about experience, practice and teacher knowledge.

As we reflect on teacher education as narrative inquiry we see the goals in educative terms. We want student teachers to learn to live their stories in practical situations and to see new possibilities for living out different stories than those they experienced as students. We also want cooperating teachers to live new stories in their practices with the children that allow for change and growth for them and the children. As cooperating teachers and university teachers we also want to live new ways of storying teacher education in our schools and universities.

There is, however, also a need to write narratives of our work in teacher education for a larger audience. We need to pay particular attention to how to write our accounts of teacher education as narrative inquiry and the ways in which such accounts should be read. Something of the spirit of action of the participants, students, teachers and university teachers needs to find a place in these stories. As in the accounts of research, issues of representation and audience are central concerns.

One purpose of narrative research is to have other readers raise questions about their practices, their ways of knowing. Narrative inquiries are shared in ways that help readers question their own stories, raise their own questions about practices and see in the narrative accounts stories of their own stories. The intent is to foster reflection, storying and restorying for readers. Rose (1983, p. 17) remarks that 'the work as a whole will suggest new truths especially the extent to which all living is a creative act of greater or less authenticity, hindered or helped by the fictions to which we submit ourselves'.

To be a reader of a narrative is to be drawn into a story, to find a place or way of seeing through participating in the story. Crites (1975, p. 26) reminds us that the completeness of a story consists:

> in the immediacy with which narrative is able to render the concrete particularities of experience. Its characteristic language is not conceptual but consists typically in the sort of verbal imagery we employ in referring to things as they appear to our senses or figure in our practical activities. Still more important the narrative form aesthetically reproduces the temporal tensions of experience, a moving present tensed between and every moment embracing a memory of what has gone before and an activity projected, underway.

Here Crites gives a sense of what narrative researchers try to capture in their narrative writing. They attempt to have readers understand enough of the participants' experiences so that they can share something of what the experience might have been for the participants. In order to do this a reader must make a genuine effort to share in the experience of the participants. It is something akin to what Elbow calls the 'believing game', 'an act of self-insertion' (1973, p. 149). At its best it is a dialogue that allows a reader to share some qualities of the participants' experience. Narrative researchers need to consider the ways in which readers are drawn into the narrative and see possibility for alternative possible stories.

These issues seem particularly important as we begin to tell stories of teacher education as narrative inquiry. We do not propose to offer solutions or models for teacher educators or student teachers. Rather, we want to tell the stories in ways that highlight the tensions between personal and institutional narratives, between university and cooperating teachers' stories and student teachers' stories, and through these stories to foster reflection on the ways individuals and institutions construct teacher education.

Acknowledgement

This work was supported in part by a grant from the Social Sciences and Humanities Research Council of Canada.

References

Bateson, M.C. (1989) *Composing a Life*, New York, The Atlantic Monthly Press.

Belenky, M., Clinchy, B., Goldberger, N. and Tarule, J. (1986) *Women's Ways of Knowing*, New York, Basic Books.

Carr, D. (1986) *Time, Narrative and History*, Bloomington, Indiana University Press.

Clandinin, D.J. (1986) *Classroom Practice: Teacher Images in Action*, London, Falmer Press.

Clandinin, D.J. (1989) 'Developing rhythm in teaching: The narrative study of a beginning teacher's personal practical knowledge of classrooms', *Curriculum Inquiry*, **19**, 2, pp. 121–141.

Clandinin, D.J. and Connelly, F.M. (1988) 'Studying teachers' knowledge of classrooms: Collaborative research, ethics and the negotiation of narrative', *Journal of Educational Thought*, **22**, 2A, pp. 269–282.

Clandinin, D.J. and Connelly, F.M. (1991) 'Narrative and story in practice and research', in Schön, D.A. (Ed.) *The Reflective Turn: Case Studies In and On Educational Practice*, New York, Teachers College Press, pp. 258–281.

Connelly, F.M. and Clandinin, D.J. (1985) 'Personal practical knowledge and the modes of knowing: Relevance for teaching and learning', in Eisner, E. (Ed.) *Learning and Teaching the Ways of Knowing*, Eighty-fourth Yearbook of the National Society for the Study of Education, Part 2, Chicago, University of Chicago Press, pp. 174–198.

Connelly, F.M. and Clandinin, D.J. (1988) *Teachers as Curriculum Planners: Narratives of Experience*, New York, Teachers College Press.

Connelly, F.M. and Clandinin, D.J. (1990) 'Stories of experience and narrative inquiry', *Educational Researcher*, **19**, 5, pp. 2–14.

Crites, S. (1975) 'Angels we have heard', in Wiggins, J.B. (Ed.) *Religion as Story*, Lanham, MD, University Press of America, pp. 26–63.

Elbow, P. (1973) *Writing Without Teachers*, London, Oxford University Press.

Gilligan, C., Lyons, N. and Hanmer, T. (Eds) (1990) *Making Connections: The Relational Worlds of Adolescent Girls at Emma Willard School*, Cambridge, MA, Harvard University Press.

MacIntyre, A.C. (1981) *After Virtue: A Study in Moral Theory*, London, Duckworth.

Mishler, E.G. (1986) *Research Interviewing: Context and Narrative*, Cambridge, MA, Harvard University Press.

Paley, V. (1990) *The Boy Who Would Be A Helicopter*, Cambridge, MA, Harvard University Press.

Polkinghorne, D.E. (1988) *Narrative Knowing and the Human Sciences*, New York, State University of New York Press.

Rose, P. (1983) *Parallel Lives*, New York, Vintage Books.

Spence, D.P. (1986) 'Narrative smoothing and clinical wisdom', in Sarbin, T.R. (Ed.) *Narrative Psychology: The Storied Nature of Human Conduct*, New York, Praeger, pp. 211–32.

6

CREATING PEDAGOGICAL SPACES FOR DEVELOPING DOCTOR PROFESSIONAL IDENTITY

D. Jean Clandinin and Marie-Therese Cave

OBJECTIVES

Working with doctors to develop their identities as technically skilled as well as caring, compassionate and ethical practitioners is a challenge in medical education. One way of resolving this derives from a narrative reflective practice approach to working with residents. We examine the use of such an approach.

METHODS

This paper draws on a 2006 study carried out with four family medicine residents into the potential of writing, sharing and inquiring into parallel charts in order to help develop doctor identity. Each resident wrote 10 parallel charts over 10 weeks. All residents met bi-weekly as a group with two researchers to narratively inquire into the stories told in their charts.

RESULTS

One parallel chart and the ensuing group inquiry about the chart are described. In the narrative reflective practice process, one resident tells of working with a patient and, through writing, sharing and inquiry, integrates her practice and how she learned to be a doctor in one cultural setting into another cultural setting; another resident affirms her relational way of practising medicine, and a third resident begins to see the complexity of attending to patients' experiences.

CONCLUSIONS

The process shows the importance of creating pedagogical spaces to allow doctors to tell and retell, through narrative inquiry, their stories of their experiences. This pedagogical approach creates spaces for doctors to individually develop their own stories by which to live as doctors through narrative reflection on their interwoven personal, professional and cultural stories as they are shaped by, and enacted within, their professional contexts.

Reprinted with permission of John Wiley and Sons. Acknowledgement; Clandinin, D. J., & Cave, M. (2008). Creating pedagogical spaces for developing doctor professional identity. *Medical Education, 42*(8), 765–770.

KEYWORDS

family practice/*education; *internship and residency; narration; *professional practice; physician–patient relations; humans; male; female.

Introduction

A pressing challenge in medical education, in both undergraduate and residency programmes, concerns helping doctors develop their identities as technically skilled as well as caring, compassionate and ethical practitioners. This is a persistent problem in medical education, as evidenced by the concerns raised by Coulehan (2005). One way of responding to this challenge is to consider narrative reflective practice approaches.

In an attempt to refine narrative reflective practice approaches that work with medical students, residents and doctors in the early stages of their careers, the present authors (Cave and Clandinin, 2007a,b) developed two small-scale studies to explore the most educative approaches. Both studies adopted a narrative view of experience (Bruner, 1987; Bateson, 1994; Carr, 1986) as well as a narrative research methodology (Clandinin and Connelly, 2000a). The educational purpose of this work is to engage residents in understanding their experiences as doctors as narrative life compositions through learning to narratively reflect on their experiences in order to develop a deeper understanding of their professional identity.

In the study reported here, we adopted the process of using parallel charts (Charon, *Changing the Face of Medicine*). Charon also works from a narrative view of experience in which people both live and tell stories of their lives. She asks medical students to write stories of their experiences with patients in parallel charts where students write down those things that 'are critical to care of your patient that don't belong in the hospital chart, but they have to be written somewhere' (Charon, *Changing the Face of Medicine*).

OVERVIEW

What is already known on this subject

Efficacy of parallel charts has been established with medical students.

What this study adds

Narrative reflective practice using parallel charts including dialogue groups with family medicine residents positively impacts residents' professional identity in terms of making them more caring within their professional practice. Using the study process, which includes writing, reading and collaborative inquiry into the charts, creates an effective narrative medicine learning context.

Suggestions for further research

Comparative studies with residents in other medical disciplines as well as studies with medical students in the clerkship years may be valuable.

This paper focuses on developing a pedagogical strategy for engaging family medicine residents in writing parallel charts and participating in small-group sharing and discussion about their charts.

Methods

The researchers invited residents in one family medicine clinic to an information session where they explained that writing parallel charts based on residents' clinical practice and reflecting on these charts would aid the development of residents' professionalism, empathic understanding and self-awareness, and would help to integrate their sense of self with their professional persona. They invited residents to write a parallel chart on one clinical encounter each week for 10 weeks and to attend bi-weekly sessions to share and discuss their parallel charts with participating residents and the two researchers. Exit interviews on what they had learned about their experiences were also scheduled. The two researchers are skilled educators with expertise in narrative inquiry and with experience in working with residents, undergraduate medical students, teachers and administrators in narrative reflective practice. Due attention was paid to the particular ethical concerns involved in using narrative reflective practice in medicine (Charon and Montello, 2000).

In this paper, we include one parallel chart as written and read by one resident. We show the inquiry process into the chart as it was captured in transcripts. The transcription of the first part of the first session with a group of four volunteer residents (Miriam Peretz, Sarah Khorami, Chris Jones, Josh Smith) follows. Names of residents are pseudonyms. Interspersed with the transcription is the researchers' analysis of the pedagogical process. Initially, Sarah read her parallel chart without interruption. The first response was one of affirmation and validation for her sharing. The researchers and residents prompted Sarah to tell more by asking questions, showing interest, and inviting her to expand on what she had written. After the initial reading and questioning by researchers and residents, the chart was used to stimulate others in the group to use the story as a starting point for wondering about themselves as doctors and for considering what the story triggered for them about their own clinical experiences. Part of the researchers' task was to bring other participants into the conversation. A similar process was followed in the remainder of the first session and in subsequent sessions.

Analysis is of the whole process, from the oral sharing of the written parallel chart through the group dialogue about the participants' responses to the chart. The analysis is based on a close reading of both the parallel chart and the reflective and reflexive dialogue that ensued.

Results: reading and negotiating parallel charts in the relational group space

Box 1 shows Sarah's first parallel chart. Sarah read her parallel chart to the group and the reading was transcribed.

Sarah is an international medical graduate who has practised for several years in another country. From these earlier experiences, she has begun to develop a sense of who she is as a doctor; that is, she has a professional story to live by (Connelly and Clandinin, 1999).

BOX 1 SARAH'S FIRST PARALLEL CHART

So excuse my English because this is my second language so there is a problem. Um during a call in obstetric rotation I was called for a delivery of baby at 11 pm. As routine, when a pregnant woman comes to the ward the resident on call will take the history and physical exam and then, later on, the nurse can call the resident into the delivery when it's the time. This time I had no idea who is the pregnant woman. Not knowing her, I entered the room and saw a young and pretty lady in the delivery bed trying to push out the baby. I introduced myself and asked her if anyone is accompanying her. She said, 'No.' I could not see joy, fear, pain or even sadness in her face. The nurses were encouraging her to push harder. By this time my staff on call arrived. After about 10 minutes of labour, the baby's head was out. I was holding the baby's head, everybody saw the baby's head . . . cranium and . . . could not breathe. An on-call gynaecologist shouted at me to raise the baby's head. I did, to suction the nose and mouth. The baby cried. We pulled the rest of the baby out of the mom's body. It was a boy. The Apgar score was not that good. It took about 2 minutes until the baby's colour was a little pinkish but his cry, but his, but his cry was weak and raspy. I was worried. Everybody was, except the mom. She turned her head and looked at the other side. When she was asked if she wants to hold the baby, she nodded no. The nurse took the baby to the NICU [neonatal intensive care unit].

At that moment I had two different feelings. On one hand, I was proud of myself to deliver a baby. On the other hand, I was sad of seeing a new mom with flat emotion in her face and not wanting to even look at the baby. The gynaecologist asked the mom if there is anyone you could call to come to the room. She said, 'I came by myself.' She said that she doesn't want to keep the baby and wants to put him for adoption. The gynaecologist agreed to call the social worker for that matter. When he left I couldn't help myself asking more questions: 'Who is the father of the boy and does he know you are pregnant?' 'How come no one is with you?' She got pregnant after having a date. They broke up after. And the guy had no idea she was pregnant. She said, 'I think for adoption I should tell him about the baby.' She was living with her parents at that moment. Her mom questioned her a couple of times about her big tummy. She denied the pregnancy. She had no prenatal care at all. That was, that day was the first time seeing a doctor for pregnancy, had no feeling for the baby and wasn't sure if she wants to tell her parents about the baby. I ask her, 'If, if you did not, if you did, didn't want the baby, why didn't do abortion?' She said she had talked to someone in supporting group for unwanted pregnancy and was told if she had an abortion she was facing more psychological consequences. I comforted her and came out of the room.

All the nurses and the staff were talking about her. I was very upset. Being a mom, I couldn't understand how come a person can let her baby go for adoption. I had to talk to someone. I called my husband. Almost tearful, but I was telling him this slowly but it wasn't enough. I told one of the medical students about her. He is from India, with close contact to mine. I told him that I have hard time understanding one, why someone could ah be so irresponsible to let get pregnant in the first time and then go through whole pregnancy and then put their own blood and flesh for adoption. He understand me, understood me. I always think of the worst scenario. What if the adopting family are not good enough for the baby? What if they abuse him, sexually or physically? How he would feel when he grows up? How long he would wonder about his mom and asking himself why his mom didn't keep him. For sure he always would wonder why his mom didn't like him because if she did she would not abandon him and one million more questions went through my mind at that night and the following day.

Two days later I saw the girl walking into another unit. She was changed. She was more energetic. I noticed a couple of people surrounding her. I heard somebody said to her, 'That is the best.' What was the best? A few hours later I saw her again, this time face-to-face. I ask her why she was still there. She said, 'The baby is in the NICU and *we* have problem feeding him.' I looked at her and asked, 'What do you want to do about the baby?' She proudly said, 'I will keep him.' I could not believe what I heard. Not thinking that this isn't professional, I hugged her and told her that was the best thing she could do. Obviously she called her parents. They all supported her and wanted to keep the baby.

A few days later, we, the residents and students, were talking about interesting cases we had. I told them this story and how I felt when I knew the baby was going for adoption and how I preferred to have abortion than adoption myself and why not her. One of the female residents commented, not very friendly: 'You can't judge people. You don't know why she did that. She had her own reasons.' Did she? I thought about what she said. She was right. I never had unwanted pregnancy and I never did abortion. I did not know about her family situation, religious, culture, or economical situation. Not everybody had financial and emotional support. Why did I think that she had no feeling for her baby? Of course she had. She was suppressing it. I learned my lesson. I'm not going to judge a person based on what I observe. You always see the tree, not the roots.

I will pay more attention to the roots.

Initially, the researchers affirmed Sarah's reading, and asked questions about the process of writing, encouraging Sarah to give more details about who she talked with, the age of the patient, and the use of drugs. Their purpose was to validate both her telling of the story and the importance of it. The conversation followed this pattern for seven minutes until the researchers began to speak of the importance of finding 'out someone's life story' and needing to 'know more about them before you can make a judgement'. They drew on their work in narrative inquiry, where individual events are understood within the context of a person's whole life story (Bateson, 1990). Their comments made a space for Miriam to pick up on the term 'judgement', and to gently remind Sarah that 'we do have belief systems, we all come with our own and it's important to recognise when we start sort of thinking about those belief systems'. She noted that:

> every day is a judgement call. We see someone, we look at them and . . . we make a judgement call based on their clinical presentation . . . and it is really hard not to judge . . . Especially if it's not your belief system . . . I would have probably approached that entirely differently.

Knowing that Miriam's identity as both a person and a doctor had been shaped on a different cultural landscape than Sarah's, one of the researchers asked Miriam to expand on her different approach, hoping Miriam would offer something of her story in order to highlight her belief system. Miriam put her focus on the future for the baby:

> I'd almost be . . . just as happy or just as satisfied if the mom did give up the child. Because I know it's going to be hard for the child, it's going to be hard for the mom to give it up, but at the same time the mom doesn't want the child . . . She obviously had no prenatal care . . . just because she makes that decision to keep the baby now doesn't make her mom of the year, or make her become super mom all of a sudden . . . And there's a lot of families out there who are very good and could have a child and would really care for it and love it so I would, maybe, would have approached that differently.

Miriam noted that when a patient is making a moral life decision, it is difficult for a doctor to present the options impartially:

> I find that a lot of the way those conversations play out is very much based on our judgements and our belief system . . . but how [do] you let someone arrive at a life choice when you're sort of a snapshot in their life and you don't really know where they come from?

One of the researchers picked up on Miriam's idea that doctors are only a 'snapshot' in the midst of a patient's life. Temporality seemed key, as Miriam suggested that she, as a doctor, entered a patient's life, in the midst of her own life and the patient's life. In the moment of entering, the doctor tries to gather narrative threads that link backwards in time in both the patient's and the doctor's lives and stretch forwards in possibility. Miriam pointed out to Sarah that it was through her questions to the patient that she discovered 'how she'd been hiding it . . . it's very, very difficult'. Sarah agreed, noting there is much we do not know about each patient's life situation and how alternatives come to be chosen. Miriam connected a story of her doctor husband to Sarah's comments about her approach being shaped in a different culture and connected the conversation back to doctor identity.

One of the researchers connected the story back to Sarah's parallel chart as she wondered whether Sarah acted 'by chance or was that deliberate and did you have to go and take care of her after the delivery?' Sarah responded: 'I tried to put myself in her way to talk to her and see why is she still here.'

Having picked up on Sarah's comment that she did not see the patient for '2 days' after delivery, one of the authors tried to get Sarah to speak of the narrative coherence of the unfolding events (Carr, 1986) by asking: 'What do you think happened in between?' Sarah reported that: 'She called her parents and they came and they support her.' Sarah then gave her version of the story: 'They wanted her to keep the baby. That all she needed was some support.'

Picking up on the temporality of events, one of the researchers noted that doctors often 'only just get such a little moment; and what happens in that moment makes such a difference'. At this point, one of the researchers asked Chris what he 'would have done', hoping Chris would think about who he might have been had he been in the situation. Chris responded:

> I try not to make that decision. I might have thought that just because of how the situation presented itself but I don't think that's my role in that situation so I probably wouldn't have asked all those questions and would have gotten very little social history from her; she has no prenatal care, no father and what else we really need to know is [who is providing] the obstetrician service . . . I probably would have invested somebody else as best I could, certainly called social work.

Sarah, recognising Chris's approach as being different from hers, asked: 'How do we know what she needs if you don't talk to her?' Chris responded: 'Okay, I would have asked what are your plans for the baby, and then I would have known and then probably let somebody else sort it out, to be honest.' Sarah persisted with: 'Like who?' Chris responded: 'The social worker.' Sarah continued to question Chris as she reclaimed her story. Under Sarah's questioning, Chris began to see that the situation may be more complex than his first response suggested.

Before the conversation shifted to the next parallel chart sharing, Miriam returned to the importance of knowing as much as we can about each patient and his or her support systems. Sarah returned to affirming the importance of her skills:

> I can communicate with people well, like they talk to me, they trust and they say things that they may not tell someone else. That's why I talked to her . . . I could talk to her, I was a mom myself and I think it helped her a little bit.

The unpacking of the transcript highlights a process through which Sarah tells her story and tries to integrate her practice in this setting with how she practised in another cultural setting. Miriam speaks of the importance of acknowledging living in relationship with her patients and the short moments in which life-changing decisions are made with them. Chris speaks of the technical role of doctors.

Conclusions: the narrative reflective process in shaping professional identities

The narrative reflective process from the writing of the parallel chart, through the reading of the chart in the group, to the response and dialogue about the chart is an evolving, improvisatory process that allows doctor learners to compose their own meanings which shape their identities, their stories to live by. Connelly and Clandinin (1999) conceptualise stories to live by as the threads that link knowledge, context and identity and allow them to be understood narratively.

The process of narrative reflective practice allows each doctor to tell his or her story, which then becomes the starting point for the group's shared narrative inquiry. The group, with the guidance and support of the two researchers, narratively inquires into the story by asking questions that point towards temporality (what happened before, what happens now and what will or might happen), the personal (what was happening to the person), the social (what events were unfolding) and place (Clandinin and Connelly, 2000a). Engaging in this way also directs attention towards the multiplicity of vantage points that can be adopted within the story (Charon, 2000). However, perhaps more importantly, other group members try to make meaning of the story for themselves through narratively imagining themselves into the reader's story. We borrow the idea of narrative imagination from Sarbin (2004). Participants search for meaning for themselves in the story they have heard. One of the key differences from the well-known approach developed by Balint (1964) is the focus on engaging the narrative inquiry process (Clandinin and Connelly, 2000a) to inquire into multiple ways to interpret the story. The Balint (1964) approach, rather than an inquiry process, uses a psychotherapeutic process to engage in reflection. Often there is a focus on a problematic issue (Balint, 1964). Similarities between the processes include working towards honing the doctor as an instrument of healing, and attending to the story and making it a transformative process for the doctor. Salinsky (2007) noted significant differences in group purposes and leaders' intentions for the group. The writing of the chart in the narrative inquiry process represents another layer of reflection.

As the pedagogical space is composed, each writer or teller reads the story into the storied landscape of the group, and each participant sees the story differently. The storied landscape is a metaphor borrowed from Clandinin and Connelly's (2000b) description of the professional knowledge landscape as a place filled with many kinds of stories which create a context that is both intellectual and moral. As the dialogue continues, the multiple meanings of the initial parallel chart are negotiated, and turned over and over as new possibilities for understanding become apparent. The goal is not to come to a shared meaning, but to allow each resident to come to his or her own meanings and thus to develop his or her own professional identity.

In the example described here, Sarah is engaged in crystallising who she will be as a doctor in Canada; she deepens her understanding of who she is as a doctor, identifies the important skills involved in asking questions and learns that relating to the patient results in the patient becoming more energetic and reconnecting with her family. She reaffirms that there is a place for her life experience in her practice.

As Sarah tells and retells her story in the writing and sharing of the parallel chart and in the dialogue around the parallel chart, she is searching for a kind of narrative coherence in her stories to live by, in effect, for her professional identity. In the writing, reading and inquiry into Sarah's parallel chart, we see that she is 'telling and retelling, to ourselves and to others, the story of what we are about and what we are' (Carr, 1986).

Carr notes that the unity of self is 'not a pregiven condition but an achievement' (Carr, 1986) and, as such, creating spaces which encourage the telling and retelling of the stories of who we are, our stories to live by, is vitally important in the development of doctor identity. This pedagogical approach creates spaces for doctors to continue to develop their own stories to live by as doctors, in that it allows doctors individually to narratively reflect on their own interwoven personal, professional and cultural stories as they are shaped by, and enacted within, their professional contexts. The stories of others are an integral part of this process, a process which goes beyond identifying role models. A doctor's role or doctor behaviour can be learned from others and, like a mask, can be worn or taken off, but the shaping of doctor identity is highly personal. Each doctor brings a unique life story to his or her practice, and the meanings he or she derives from the stories he or she tells from those experiences shapes the lens through which he or she views each new clinical experience. As doctors tell and retell stories of their experiences with other doctors, they metaphorically lay their stories alongside those of others. As Bateson (2000) writes, '. . . wisdom, then, is born of the overlapping of lives, the resonance between stories'. Resonant rememberings created by the spaces between stories are what provide us with 'multiple lives to test and shape our own' (Bateson, 1990). Clerkship and residency years are times when each learner doctor is most intensely involved in the shaping of his or her own doctor identity. In writing, reading and inquiring into the parallel chart, a doctor learner reflects on becoming a good doctor, on the learning from an encounter with a patient and on his or her experiences with others involved in caring for the patient, as well as from the discussion with fellow doctors within a parallel chart group. It is often this discussion which elicits increased self-awareness and the pearls of professionalism.

Contributors: both authors contributed equally to data collection, analysis and interpretation and to the preparation of the manuscript.

Acknowledgement

This study was funded by the University of Alberta Hospital Foundation.

References

Balint M. *The Doctor, His Patient and the Illness*. London: Pitman, Medical 1964;1–355.

Bateson MC. *Composing a Life*. Harmondsworth: Penguin Books 1990;1–241.

Bateson MC. *Full Circles, Overlapping Lives: Culture and Generation in Transition* New York: Random House 2000;1–262.

Bateson MC. *Peripheral Visions: Learning along the Way*. New York: HarperCollins Publishers 1994;1–243.

Bruner JS. Life as narrative. *Social Research*, 1987;**54**:1–17.

Carr D. *Time, Narrative and History*. Bloomington, IN: Indiana University Press 1986;1–189.

Cave M, Clandinin DJ. Learning to live with being a physician. *Reflective Practice* 2007a;**8**(1):75–91.

Cave M, Clandinin DJ. Revisiting the journal club. *Medical Teacher* 2007b;**29**(4):365–370.

Charon R. *Changing the Face of Medicine*. www.nlm.nih.gov/changingthefaceofmedicine/video/58_1_trans.html [Accessed 13 October 2006].

Charon R. *Narrative Medicine: Honoring the Stories of Illness*. Oxford: Oxford University Press 2006;1–266.

Charon R, Montello M. *Stories Matter: The Role of Narrative in Medical Ethics*. New York: Routledge 2002;1–242.

Clandinin DJ, Connelly FM. *Narrative Inquiry: Experience and Story in Qualitative Research*. San Francisco: Jossey-Bass 2000a;1–211.

Clandinin DJ, Connelly FM. *Teachers' Professional Knowledge Landscapes.* New York: Teachers College Press 2000b;1–179.

Connelly FM, Clandinin DJ. *Shaping a Professional Identity: Stories of Educational Practice.* New York: Teachers College Press 1999;1–184.

Coulehan J. Today's professionalism: Engaging the mind but not the heart. *Academic Medicine*, 2005;**80**(10):892–898.

Salinsky J. Editorial: the leaders, the group members and the pursuit of change. The *Journal* of the *Balint Society*, 2007;**37**. www.balint.co.uk/journal/. [Accessed 18 October 2007.]

Sarbin TR. The role of imagination in narrative construction. In: Daiute C, Lightfoot C, eds. *Narrative Analysis: Studying the Development of Individuals in Society.* Thousand Oaks, CA: Sage Publications 2004;5–20.

7

SHIFTING FROM STORIES TO LIVE BY TO STORIES TO LEAVE BY

Early career teacher attrition

Lee Schaefer, Charles Aiden Downey, and D. Jean Clandinin

Introduction

We began this research by asking questions about the high number of teachers who leave teaching in their first five years of teaching. The literature on early career teacher attrition (Borman & Dowling, 2008; Guarino, Santibanez, & Daly, 2006; Macdonald, 1999; Smith & Ingersoll, 2004) left us with wonders around the experiences of teachers who leave. The storied experiences of those who leave appear absent, for the most part, in the literature. In order to hear the stories of the experiences of early career teacher leavers we engaged in a narrative inquiry with four teachers who left teaching in their first five years. We are researchers, who are also teachers who have left classrooms. The stories of these early career leavers resonated strongly with us. As we engaged in the study, we awakened to how the early career teacher leavers' stories shifted and changed with each conversation, as the research conversations allowed them to make sense of their experiences with leaving.

A story fragment

We begin with a story fragment from a narrative account (Clandinin & Connelly, 2000) with Natalie, one of the early career leavers that Jean worked alongside. As shown in Natalie's story fragment below, the conversations were imbued with emotion, with regret, and with tension, as her stories to live by shifted to stories to leave by (Clandinin, Downey, & Huber, 2009).

I (Jean) sit at the small table in my office across from a striking young woman. I call her Natalie. We are talking about her experience of leaving K-12 teaching after only four years. She wipes tears from her eyes and I know this is a difficult conversation for her. She tells of coming to Canada as a small child with her parents, of speaking a language other than English, of being identified early as someone who needed help, and of working with an academic tutor through her elementary and junior high school years in order to do well in school. She tells of going into the sciences when

Reprinted with permission is from Caddo Gap Press. Acknowledgement; Schaefer, L., Downey, C. A., & Clandinin, D. J. (2014, Winter). Shifting from stories to live by to stories to leave by: Early career teacher attrition. *Teacher Education Quarterly, Winter, 41*(1), 9–27.

she entered university. She also tells of living within a family story in which she needs to have a career. In order to live up to, or to live out, that family story (Carr, 1986), she tells of her decision to take a dual degree, one where she could earn both a B.Sc. and a B.Ed. As her stories unfold over several conversations, I come to know more and more of Natalie's experiences, her stories of her experiences of coming to teaching, and of teaching. At first she tells stories with lightness. Natalie tells a story of herself as a good teacher who knew her subject matter, was asked to participate in school and government curriculum committees, and was able to help her students learn the subject matter she loved. Natalie was given a tenured position early, a sign of the high regard of her school district. As she said,

> So one of the reasons I still kept going to work and was relatively happy was cause I loved being in the classroom. I loved the interactions there. Different things would happen every day . . . so different dynamic things happen and I like that. That's why I loved the classrooms.
>
> *(Natalie, personal communication, February 13, 2012)*

Natalie also tells of working closely with a small group of colleagues over many hours and weeks to devise an innovative approach to curriculum and how much she enjoyed this work with colleagues.

Then, as we came to know more of each other through further conversations, there are more tears as she tells of her experiences of leaving K–12 teaching. These are hard to tell stories, stories she has not told before in the smoothed over, cover story of how she left teaching to come to graduate studies. She tells of how she and her colleagues were not recognized for their innovative work but that someone else was given the credit. She describes how she was unable to even arrange an appointment to tell the recently appointed principal of the high school where she was teaching that she was resigning.

> I tried to get in to see her all week and I couldn't so finally I saw her in the hallway and I just said, "Oh by the way, I'm leaving next year". So it wasn't official, can book a time with you to come and break some news to you? She said, "Oh I'm really glad that this is where you want to be, so you're going to be achieving your dreams."
>
> *(Natalie, personal communication, February 13, 2012)*

The story that the principal told of her, a story composed around a plotline that she was following a path to achieve her dreams, was not Natalie's story. It was one told of her, and to her, by the principal. This became Natalie's smoothed over story, a story that made it safe to leave teaching for graduate studies, a story with a plotline that she was achieving her dreams. As her stories to live by shifted to stories to leave by, she told this safe cover story. It was this plotline that shaped the first story Natalie told me. It was as we came into relationship over several conversations that deeper, silenced, riskier, and more complex stories of experience began to become apparent.

Before we leave this fragment, we want to let you know that Natalie still tells a story in which she wants to teach. Doing graduate work provides her an opportunity to continue to live a story of herself as a learner and as someone who can change the world. Only now she tells a story that she can change the world through her research and by working alongside people in policy settings. And being an academic will, she imagines, allow her to continue to teach.

As we reflect now on the stories that Natalie was living and telling, we see how difficult it was for Natalie as she tried to carve out spaces so she could be who she imagined she could be as a teacher. Perhaps the only way Natalie could find spaces to be, and become, the teacher she had imagined she would be, that is, the only way she could compose a narratively coherent story to live out, a story that made sense, was by leaving.

Framing the literature on early career teacher attrition

While there is some disagreement about the actual percentage of teachers who leave teaching in their first five years (from 5% to 50%), "one very stable finding is that attrition is high for young teachers" (Guarino et al., 2006, p. 10). There are several large-scale studies, mostly in the US, that document the numbers and reasons why teachers leave teaching within five years (Alliance for Excellent Education, 2005; Borman & Dowling, 2008; Guarino et al., 2006; Ingersoll, 2001). These studies provide a means to see the phenomenon of teacher attrition, studies which allow us to see the phenomenon small in Greene's (1995) terms. However, we do not see "big", that is, we do not see the experiences of individuals who leave within these trends. Few studies focus on the experiences of individuals who left teaching (Buchanan, 2009; Rinke, 2007). This is, perhaps, why Rinke (2007) regards early career teacher attrition as a "silent crisis" (p. 3). Our inspiration for the study reported here was to bring awareness to this silence through inquiry into the lives of early career teachers as they came to teaching, taught, and left K-12 teaching within their first five years.

Natalie's story fragments raise resonances with our own stories of leaving teaching. We, Lee, Aiden and Jean, the co-authors, resonated with her stories of coming to teaching to change students' lives. We also imagined being and becoming teachers who changed students' lives. This resonance continues as Natalie tells stories of tension within the system, of not being able to live out her imagined stories of teaching (Schaefer & Clandinin, 2011). We three also left teaching when we were unable to live out our imagined stories. As we returned to Clandinin et al.'s (2009) work around the shifting landscapes and shifting identities of teachers we began to wonder about the stories that the participants we worked alongside were telling us. We recognized two silences: one silence is the lack of attention to the storied experiences of teachers who leave teaching; other silences live within the stories that early career teachers tell of leaving. It is to both silences that we turn our attention in this article.

"Teachers on landscapes learn how to act and think in appropriate ways, ways that are sanctioned by others positioned in the conduit" (Clandinin & Connelly 1995, p. 158). It seems that just as individuals learn how to act in appropriate ways, they also learn how to leave in appropriate ways. Clandinin et al. (2009) wrote of the cover stories that teachers who leave often tell. These stories of leaving often include agreeable plotlines of departure, socially acceptable ways to leave teaching in the classroom. This notion of cover stories, stemming from Crites (1979), allows us to conceptualize the stories that teachers tell of leaving as safe cover stories; stories that conceal the more difficult stories of leaving that, as we came to see alongside our participants, are permeated with tension. The leavers we worked alongside have shown us that creating spaces for inquiry into leaving awakens 'the roar which lies on the other side of silence' (Eliot, 1874, as cited in Clandinin et al., 2009). As we worked closely with the four participants we began to hear these more complex, less comfortable stories. Natalie began to tell stories with plotlines of not being recognized for work she had done, of taking "one for the team" when she was silenced, and of becoming increasingly alone when collaboration was no longer supported.

Crites' (1979) conception of cover stories is much more nuanced than simply lying to cover up the truth. For Crites "two different renderings of experience can co-exist in a single consciousness" (p. 126), not so much "side-by-side" but rather in layers. One story is what Crites names the "real" story, an "unacceptable" or "unflattering" one we can feel but not face. The difficulty of facing the real story spawns a cover story, a "secondary growth, constantly called into play to counter and suppress the real story" (p. 126). Taken together, the two stories create a "double-storied type of self-deception" (p. 126) with the "the real story, though never avowed . . . the one that is actually believed and acted upon" (p. 126) and the cover story making things easier by providing an "acceptable" alibi. For us, the notion of cover stories offers an opportunity to inquire into the socially acceptable stories that teachers might tell in order to be able to leave safely as well as the more difficult stories that may remain suppressed, covered over by cover stories. We wonder if early career teachers learn to tell cover stories about their leaving, and how these stories might cover over much harder stories, what we see as the 'roar on the other side of the silence.' We saw that as Natalie's new administrator offered her a safe cover story, that is, Natalie was leaving to pursue graduate studies. Natalie did not need to tell her administrator or anyone else the more complex and hard to tell stories. She kept those silent and the "roar" was silenced.

Coming to terms: a conceptual frame

We adopted Clandinin and Connelly's (1995) narrative conceptual framework (Connelly & Clandinin, 1988, 1999) around teacher knowledge. Teacher knowledge, conceptualized as personal practical knowledge, is knowledge "imbued with all the experiences that make up a person's being. Its meaning is derived from, and understood in terms of a person's experiential history, both professional and personal" (Clandinin, 1985, p. 362). Personal practical knowledge, composed in, and lived out in, practice is a narrative concept of knowledge that is grounded in Dewey's (1938) theory of experience, Johnson's (1989) theories of embodied knowledge, Bateson's (1989) and Heilbrun's (1988) theories of life writing. Through further studies (Clandinin & Connelly, 1995) that questioned "how the embodied, narrative, relational knowledge teachers carry autobiographically and by virtue of their formal education shapes, and is shaped by, their professional knowledge context" (p. 3), they developed a metaphoric concept of professional knowledge landscapes, composed of relationships among people, places, and things, and with both moral and intellectual qualities. Clandinin and Connelly (1995) see the professional knowledge landscape as composed of both in- and out-of-classroom places and off the landscape places where teachers live. These off the landscape places are sometimes named personal knowledge landscapes. The stories that shape personal knowledge landscapes are sometimes partially shaped by stories on the professional knowledge landscapes. Attending closely to the "professional knowledge landscape that teachers inhabit creates epistemological dilemmas that we understand narratively in terms of secret, sacred, and cover stories" (Clandinin & Connelly, 1995, p. 4). Stories to live by, a narrative conception of identity, "speaks to the nexus of teachers' personal practical knowledge and the landscapes, [in and out of schools], past and present, on which teachers live and work" (Clandinin et al., 2009, p. 141). Stories to live by are "shaped by such matters as secret teacher stories, sacred stories of schooling, and teachers' cover stories" (Connelly & Clandinin, 1999, p. 4). Professional knowledge landscapes, individuals' stories to live by, are always shifting and changing. In this paper, we draw explicit attention to the interconnectedness of the personal and professional knowledge landscapes upon which individuals compose their lives, and on how teachers' imagined identities, their imagined stories to live by, shaped their experiences in ways that allowed them to stay in, or leave, teaching in schools.

From past work (Schaefer & Clandinin, 2011) with two early career teachers in their first year of teaching, it became apparent that complex identity negotiations took place in and across their personal knowledge and professional knowledge landscapes. These landscapes were so interconnected that, at moments, it was impossible to separate the two. The teachers' imagined stories of teaching, as well as their imagined stories of who they would be as teachers away from the school, created tensions within their stories to live by. Further, from the work with early career teachers (Schaefer, 2013; Schaefer & Clandinin, 2011) we learned that individuals enter teaching embodying stories to live by and, as part of their stories to live by, also carry forward looking stories of their imagined lives as teachers, which are part of their imagined lives as people. We draw attention to the idea that teachers are people in the midst of composing lives, both on and off professional knowledge landscapes. This view shifts the focus away from only the professional knowledge landscape, to include the personal knowledge landscape and the spaces between the professional and personal knowledge landscapes. It is in personal and professional knowledge landscapes, and in the spaces between the two, that teachers attempt to live out their imagined stories of who they are, and are becoming. We imagine the spaces between each teacher's personal and professional knowledge landscape as well as between the real and imagined stories of teaching as borderlands, spaces of disjuncture and dissonance that, while charged with possibility, can also be fertile ground for suppression, for what Crites (1979) calls cover stories that cover over secret stories.

Research design, a methodology, methods: coming alongside participants

Using a methodology of narrative inquiry (Clandinin & Connelly, 2000), we inquired into the experiences of three teachers in Alberta, a Canadian province, and one teacher in Georgia, a U.S. state, who left teaching in K-12 within their first five years. We chose narrative inquiry because

> Narrative inquiry, the study of experience as story, then, is first and foremost a way of thinking about experience. Narrative inquiry as a methodology entails a view of the phenomenon. To use narrative inquiry methodology is to adopt a particular view of experience as phenomenon under study.
>
> *(Connelly & Clandinin, 2006, p. 375)*

Working with narrative concepts of personal practical knowledge, teachers' professional knowledge landscapes, and teachers' stories to live by allows us to inquire into the experiences of those individuals who left the profession in their first five years. Narrative inquiry as a relational methodology allows us to study the stories that beginning teachers tell, over time, and in different situations. As a relational methodology, researchers bracket themselves into the study, that is, researchers' experience in relation with participants' experiences are under study.

Throughout the inquiry process from design to composing final research texts, we were attentive to the three dimensional narrative inquiry space of temporality, sociality and place. Lee had five 1.5 to 2 hour conversations with two participants. Jean had three 1.5 hour conversations with one participant. Aiden had five 1.5 to 3 hour conversations with his participant. Three different methods were used to compose field texts with each participant: each researcher's autobiographical narrative inquiry; transcripts of researcher-participant conversations; and timelines, artifacts, and stories of artifacts. Working from the field texts we composed a narrative account for each participant. Narrative accounts are interpretive constructions of individual experiences attentive to the three-dimensional inquiry space. These accounts were composed around what we identified as narrative threads across each participant's life. The draft narrative accounts were then negotiated with each participant in order to deepen understanding about the participant's experiences, and to continue to co-compose the narrative account.

Ethical matters

Narrative inquiry is a relational form of inquiry and as such needs to be lived with attention to relational ethics from study design through to inviting participants to the study, composing field texts, and moving from field texts to interim and final research texts (Clandinin & Connelly, 2000; Clandinin, 2013). We were attentive to this as we negotiated field texts and interim and final research texts that we co-composed with participants. Confidentiality and anonymity were promised. The names used are pseudonyms and we have negotiated the narrative accounts with the participants.

Fragments of narrative accounts

In the opening to this article, we shared a fragment of a narrative account with Natalie. In what follows we share three fragments of narrative accounts with other participants. Space does not allow us to include four complete narrative accounts. We carefully selected fragments to show something of each participant's imagined story of teaching, their experiences of teaching, particularly the bumps between their stories to live by and the professional and personal knowledge landscapes in which they lived and taught, and the ways they tell of shifting their stories to live by to stories to leave by. Within these shifting stories we play with Crites (1979) notion of cover stories and wonder about the roar that is silenced by safe, socially acceptable, ways of leaving.

Alis

As Alis and I (Lee) began conversations she talked about wanting a more flexible job. Before she left teaching she began a small tutoring business in her after school hours. She liked it because it was flexible. She chose how many and which students she took on, and how much to charge. Alis was in the midst of working on a Masters degree in counseling. She talked about it "opening doors," but also said that at some point she might go back to teaching. At the time of the conversations, she was creating a Shakespeare unit for a high school English class she imagined teaching in the future At first, I wondered if Alis fit the criteria for the study, as I had imagined working with individuals who had left teaching and moved on, left it behind. This did not seem to fit Alis' experience. Further conversations revealed layers of stories, stories in which Alis created socially just classrooms that would, in some ways, change the world; stories that involved tension, emotion, struggle, and regret. Below, Alis speaks to the underpinnings of social justice that infused her imagined stories of teaching.

> I've often thought about where the hell did that come from? I think part of it I owe to my Mom and family meetings. . . . like a certain amount of the family budget was set aside to go to charity. And she would sort of say, OK, like as a family, what are we going to give money to? So I was reading about . . . learning about, you know, water and building wells in Africa, and as a young kid we were hearing that at the dinner table.
>
> *(Alis, personal communication, October 24, 2011)*

In these words, Alis offers a glimpse into her imagined stories of teaching, stories situated within her imagined life stories. Although Alis had wanted to be a teacher for as long as she could remember, her imagined story of teaching was of making the world a better place: "I'm going to change the world"; "I'm going to change the system"; "I'm going to change something" (Alis, personal communication, October 24, 2011). She elaborated, "I had the sense that there were people in the world that were suffering and that were unhappy and that I needed to do something about it" (Alis, personal communication, October 24, 2011).

As Alis voluntarily moved through three different teaching positions to try to find a place where she felt she could work to change people's situations, she felt she was moving farther away from the stories she had imagined.

> I actually would love for the school system to give teachers more time to do a good job and to be the teachers they want to be . . . I feel like if I am not teaching I should at least be trying to improve the school system from the outside . . . I feel like you shouldn't just sit there and participate in this broken system. Because how long can you really stay in the system?
>
> *(Alis, personal communication, October 2, 2011)*

Alis's words show something of what she experienced as the bumping places between her imagined stories of teaching, and her experiences of teaching. Her stories awakened me to her strong stories of social justice that she felt unable to live out. She found the dominant stories on the school landscape she was expected to live by, which she called "playing by the rules," not only hindered her ability to help, but possibly harmed students. "Playing by the rules, it genuinely scares me. What am I allowing to happen that should never happen, if I play by the rules?" (Alis, personal communication, February 2, 2011). Alis was a sought after teacher who was offered, and took, a series of positions. She was always the one who chose to leave positions, not someone who was asked or encouraged to leave.

Alongside Alis's struggle to live out her story of teaching as creating better situations for everyone, she also struggled with how much to give to teaching, as she saw how teaching took her away from attending to life on her personal knowledge landscape.

> I think it is impossible, I genuinely think it is impossible to be a high school teacher and to be decent at your job, and have a healthy home life. I really do think it's impossible. Either you're kind of a mediocre teacher and really on top

> of your family life, or you're a good teacher, or a great teacher, but your family is suffering in some way.
>
> *(Alis, personal communication, February 4, 2012)*

In Alis's words we see the connection, and competition, between the stories that shaped her personal and professional knowledge landscapes. Being a good teacher meant sacrificing being a good person in her family and vice versa.

As we talked over five conversations, the many layers of Alis's stories of leaving teaching became more visible. While the story of leaving teaching to pursue her masters degree or to parent were stories of no regrets, of moving forward, of opening doors, I realized these might be what Crites (1979) called cover stories. As we talked, the layers of not wanting to work if she could not attend to ways to change the world in more socially just ways were stories that sat silently behind the easier to tell and easier to understand stories, stories that do not implicate us as teachers, as teacher educators, as policy makers.

Reid

Reid told his colleagues he left teaching to move to a larger city, and to travel. In smaller Canadian communities moving to a larger city is an acceptable story for younger adults. While this is part of Reid's story, I (Lee) learned there were layers behind what seemed, at least in part, to be a cover story. Learning what brought him to teaching helped us to see there was more to his story of leaving.

> From my earliest memories Uncle Mike was always one of my favorite uncles 'cause whenever you go to his house, you're throwing a ball, you got a football out, you got a baseball out . . . just always had that passion for sport and physical activity. So that was always similar to me, so I was always attached to Uncle Mike and knew he was a teacher.
>
> *(Reid, personal communication, November 2, 2011)*

Reid's Uncle Mike, his favorite uncle, was a physical education and mathematics teacher. At an early age Reid connected to his uncle through movement. He spoke of other family members giving him computer games, or toys, but Uncle Mike, "he always gave things that would contribute to activity. For example, like he would give a Timex watch, a staple for every physical education teacher" (Reid, personal communication, February 2, 2011).

While Uncle Mike played a part in Reid's story to choose teaching, Reid also had positive experiences with his physical education teachers.

> Big things that I can really lean on, I had two awesome phys. ed. teachers in high school. Both these two guys were just awesome role models. I always enjoyed phys. ed. more than just because I got to play hockey, and football, and soccer, and all those games, but more though [because] I could attach myself with these guys.
>
> *(Reid, personal communication, November 2, 2011)*

Reid's attachment to these teachers gave him something solid to *lean on*, a relational form of support for a teenager. Reid considered himself an athlete and grew up with very supportive parents who enabled him to be active. But his experiences with these men stayed with Reid, forming "basically a meld of characters who drove [him] to think about that teacher idea" (Reid, personal communication, November 2, 2011). Although Reid spoke passionately about helping students to be active, his stories of coming to teach physical education were connected with his relationships.

Between coaching and teaching, Reid was extremely busy during his first year.

> I was probably firing off 80 to 85 hours a week at the school but I loved the coaching . . . It was basically every weekend, three times a week practices, so my time commitment had gone up 30 hours a week . . . I was kind of burnt out by the end of volleyball.
>
> *(Reid, personal communication, November 2, 2011)*

And yet he had expected this, even welcomed it. "I was kind of expected to do all this stuff. It was a good shift. It was nothing that blew me away" (Reid, personal communication, November 2, 2011). Although Reid seemed okay with teaching consuming all the hours in his weeks, he was cognizant of how things might be different if his situation were different.

> I didn't really have a family yet. So I wasn't in a committed relationship with anybody who was living with me. So that was better 'cause I didn't feel guilty. I'm not sure if that was ever something that came to you, but I never felt guilty being away from home and being at the school because I really had nothing else to do except for teaching and coaching which made it maybe easier for me.
>
> *(Reid, personal communication, November 2, 2011)*

For Reid the teaching schedule, his busyness, what he called being "burnt out" at the end of volleyball season, were not concerns. He was in a tenured position and was highly regarded. However, Reid knew that he wanted someday to be in a committed relationship, an important part of his imagined life story. He awakened to the difficulty of fulfilling both imagined stories in his teaching assignment. Who he was becoming on the personal knowledge landscape bumped against his imagined story of who he imagined becoming as a person

> The big detriment to me, which you know about, was there was no one there. . . . There was nothing that really made me want to stay. I mean relationship is a big part about where you are and there was nothing even close to that there, just because it's a very transient town.
>
> *(Reid, personal communication, November 2, 2011)*

The thread of relationships again weaves back into Reid's stories. While relationships with students on the professional knowledge landscape were fulfilling, even sustaining, the lack of relationships, or even the possibility of relationships, on his personal knowledge landscape shaped Reid's story to leave by. Reid had imagined teaching in a large city. His move to this small town was imagined as a temporary move. To compose his life the way he imagined, he had to leave teaching in the small town. Reid told his story to leave by as one composed around the lack of relationships on his personal knowledge landscape. We wondered, however, about the lack of sustaining relationships with colleagues. Was Reid's story to leave by shaped by the lack of sustaining relationships on both his personal and professional knowledge landscapes? As Reid left teaching to move to a large city, he did not seek out a teaching job. Was the centrality of relationships in his stories to live by a central thread in composing his story to leave by? Was the focus on needing to be in a place where he could find relationships on his personal knowledge landscape a cover story, one that covered over the lack of sustaining relationships with colleagues on the professional knowledge landscape? We wondered if the story of leaving framed by the lack of personal relationships covered over harder to tell stories, stories that were not told or even named.

Tara

Tara and I (Aiden) met on Tuesdays at a small café that she could walk to from the home she worked in as a nanny. I had known Tara for several years, as she had cared for my daughter Maeve one day a week for over a year. She told me the first day I met her that she had been a teacher but had left to have more time to be creative, to write, and to play music. I came to know Tara is an accomplished singer songwriter who has released several albums, which in many ways made her story of leaving teaching to follow her passion acceptable and safe. Gradually Tara told me another story, one about her passion for teaching and having always seen herself as a teacher:

> the more I've spent time with them (children) the more I realize when you are a child how greatly your identity really is shaped in what you'll become. So like it causes me to more greatly see that connection of, I was an older sibling, I was taking care of my younger sibling, and teaching them.
>
> *(Tara, personal communication, January 17, 2012)*

Tara arrived at my house in an old pickup truck with her guitar, ready to sing with my daughter Maeve, who sat beside Tara and strummed her little guitar, bobbing her head so that her blonde hair fell across her face, just like Tara's. Maeve's favourite song was Tara's 'We are Loved' song:

> We are loved, special, and important,
> We also have learning, changing, and growing to do,
> You get to it and I will too
> And don't forget I hope the best for you
> And you, and you, and you and you.

In our fourth conversation I learned Tara wrote the song the summer before her first year of teaching as her "class motto," that captured "the essence of what I want these kids to take away with them, to know" (Tara, personal communication January 17, 2012). As her home life growing up "was not that good" (Tara, personal communication January 17, 2012), Tara wanted her classroom to be a space of affirmation and belonging for students, an uncomplicated space of acceptance.

Tara's recollections of her first year of teaching were filled with stories of being overwhelmed and exhausted. Alongside these were stories of being supported by her principal, Dr. Martel, as well as several colleagues, all older women. One moment early in that first year stood out for Tara, and she told me the story more than once.

> The first compliment Dr. Martel ever gave me – which I will never forget – it was probably the 2nd day of school and I was like walking with my kids down the hallway or something and she just smiled real big at me and said, "The

> children look happy." I think for her to make that comment spoke right to my heart. Yeah that's it – I want a happy bunch of kids. I want to teach them and I want them to learn but I really want them to be happy little people.
>
> *(Tara, personal communication, January 24, 2012)*

Despite feeling "for about 4 years . . . I basically felt like some of the best, warmest, intelligent, vivacious ladies supported me as a young teacher" (Tara, personal communication January 31, 2012), Tara struggled to meet all-consuming demands of teaching, her students, and the relentlessness of the school year.

> I explain to people that like there's 180 days in the school year and when day one starts and they all come barrelling down the hallway and bust through your door and they're basically like "We're yours. You've got to deal with us every day." You know? There's something about that that like, for the next 180 days it feels like just one big long day . . . one big long day that you're waiting to end.
>
> *(Tara, personal communication, January 31, 2012)*

Tara told of giving so much to her students and teaching that it totally subsumed her to the point where she could not even recall her own emotional state during those years: "I was so in the zone that it's hard for me to even think back and gauge emotionally, was I happy? It's blasting you" (Tara, personal communication, January 24, 2012).

During the spring of Tara's third year of teaching her brother died very suddenly. Tara prefaced telling me this with "on a personal note" (Tara, personal communication, January 31, 2012), a preposition clause that shows how she demarcated the professional and the personal. This tragedy, along with the end of a long-term relationship, caused Tara to begin to wonder about "my own being, my own life, just my own life apart from being Ms. Rose" (Tara, personal communication, February 6, 2012). In the final weeks of her third year of teaching, Tara recalls wondering about her life beyond teaching, about "just what was coming next and more of becoming a person rather than just continuing with this career" (Tara, personal communication, February 6, 2012). Feeling completely drained from her third year, Tara spontaneously decided to spend the summer in New Zealand and Australia, which turned out to be "a breath of fresh air that I kind of needed and then wow, look, you know all of a sudden all this teaching inspiration starts bubbling up" (Tara, personal communication, January 31, 2012). But along with the inspiration for teaching she

> started thinking about . . . taking a break. So my thoughts started to go there – along with brainstorming for the next school year – kind of these parallel thought patterns. Like when might I step away from this season and this school? That might be coming up. But I'm also brainstorming and excited about what I'm going do this next year. So kind of both of those thought waves were taking place.
>
> *(Tara, personal communication, February 6, 2012)*

Tara returned for a 4th year, inspired and invigorated to meet her grade 1 students, with whom, because of the "looping," she would teach through Grade 2. She spoke fondly of that year, and still remembers each student. The administration recognized her as a strong teacher, selecting her for advanced training in a program called the

Literacy Collaborative. However, she was already considering that when these students left her classroom, she might also leave.

Tara's principal, Dr. Martel, planned her retirement for the end of Tara's fourth year. Before Dr. Martel left, she spoke with Tara to tell her what might be in store for her under a new administration, and that she might have to leave the school to continue to be the same kind of teacher. Dr. Martel's concern was grounded in her knowledge that the district was mandating more scripted forms of teaching.

> She (Dr. Martel) gave this little metaphor. She said that I was kind of like a butterfly . . . that I might need to fly away, that there might be a better setting for me. I think she was like "private school or some different type of education that's happening." I think she kind of saw how the education system was heading and did kind of share that with me. Again I think a little bit as a warning of "I've let you do what you've done and it's been wonderful and beautiful. I'm leaving now. I kind of want to tell you that I don't know what this next year's going be like for you with the new administrator coming in, but I just want to put it in your ears, put it in your heart, that at some point in your life there might be a better setting for you to have these freedoms and do what you do well."
>
> *(Tara, personal communication, January 31, 2012)*

Dr. Martel was right about things changing under the new administration. Tara's first real interaction with the new principal let her know things would be different.

> (She) came in to observe me, and all she could be baffled by and make notes on are, "Why did the kids in your classroom take their shoes off? That's a fire hazard." And I got nit-picked for things like that.
>
> *(Tara, personal communication, January 24, 2012)*

Tara felt harassed by the new administration during her final year for teaching in ways Dr. Martel had encouraged. She wishes now that she would have told them at the beginning of the year that she was leaving so they would have left her alone and let her leave on a good note. In March Tara informed the principal in a one-line e-mail that she would not be returning. The principal never asked why.

The hardest story for Tara to tell was of the year-end luncheon to celebrate the three teachers who were leaving: Tara and two teachers who were retiring. Tara told of standing in front of her colleagues, trying to thank them and say goodbye, but feeling like she communicated far more, "the people who were listening to me give that goodbye speech, I think it was kind of revealed that my inner world was in a bit of angst, let's just put it that way" (Tara, personal communication, February 14, 2012). While Tara told her friends and colleagues the same story she initially told me about leaving teaching, that is, to have more time to be creative, this was only part of a larger and more difficult story that started to peek through at that luncheon, that still evokes a "sense of shame or embarrassment" (Tara, personal communication, February 14, 2012) for Tara.

In the conversations Tara and I (Aiden) talked sometimes as former teachers, other times as people. We wonder if it is hard for teachers to talk with each other about lives beyond teaching, about the bumping between their lives on their personal and professional knowledge landscapes. How might the separation of lives lived and told on personal knowledge landscapes from lives lived and told on professional knowledge landscapes lead to two different stories being lived and told, one about a teacher and the other about a person? How might this split or separation between Tara, the person, and Ms. Rose, the teacher, and the resulting tension between the two competing stories (Clandinin & Connelly, 1995), contribute to Tara's looking at life beyond teaching, and for a cover story?

It has been five years since Tara has been in the classroom, but she has remained a teacher. She teaches the children for whom she is a nanny. She is also a musician, and a person. She is still searching for a venue where she can be all three at once, and has come up with the idea of starting a "Folk School" in the mountains that will allow her to be creative, to teach, and to have "more breathing time to be a human" (Tara, personal communication, February 14, 2012). Tara is working on this, but at the same time appreciated our conversations as creating "the space for telling the whole story, so I really appreciate that." (Tara, personal communication, February 7, 2012)

As she sings the last line of her *We Are Loved Song* she points at each child when she sings "And don't forget I hope the best for you, and you . . ." The children point at each other as they sing, too. Tara tells how one little boy ended the song by pointing at himself and singing very loudly, "AND ME!" She now sometimes ends the song with everyone pointing at themselves and saying "And me." As we attended to Tara's smoothed over cover story of leaving teaching to pursue her music making, we wondered if this covered over the conflicts she felt between wanting the best for her students and for herself. Had she told the stories of wanting to attend to her own stories to live by might they have conflicted with stories of good teachers as giving all of themselves to teaching?

The roar: learning from stories of experience

As we read through the participants' narrative accounts and revisited the transcripts of the conversations, we came to understand more of the metaphoric roar that lives on the other side of the silence of the experiences of teachers who leave teaching early. Crites' (1979) words help us wonder about how safe stories around leaving may help, in some ways, to create cover stories to leave by, stories that silence other stories, less acceptable stories. Drawing again on Clandinin and Connelly (1995) it seems that just as our participants learned to tell acceptable stories on the school landscape, they learned to tell acceptable stories as they left the school landscape. When asked why she left, Alis initially responded "to be a mom" or "graduate school." While both are possible ways to tell her stories, they are also cover stories that silence the struggles and bumping places she experienced between composing narratively coherent stories to live by on her personal and professional knowledge landscapes. Her silence about the harder to tell more complex stories could have disrupted the professional knowledge landscape of schools.

We now wonder about Reid's stories to leave by, and what stories might have been silenced by his stories of leaving to travel and to live in a city. His story of leaving a small town to live in a city is a safe story as is his story of travelling. These are expected, acceptable stories. We wonder though if his stories to leave by are also cover stories. Knowing that Reid is not teaching in a city as he could be doing, we wonder if there are layers, other stories, covered over by these stories to leave by. As a teacher who came to teaching because of relationships and who only found sustaining relationships on his professional knowledge landscape with his students, was it too difficult to sustain his stories to live by without being sustained either on his personal knowledge landscape or by colleagues on his professional knowledge landscape? Natalie's stories of not being recognized by her principal for her excellence as a teacher and an innovator became her stories to leave by, ones covered over by the safe story of leaving to return to graduate school.

In the participants' stories of their experiences, they described their teaching lives as "hard." Certainly the long hours, physical, social, and emotional demands made teaching hard, but we began to see that stories shaped around these plotlines, stories that often reverberate in school hallways and early career attrition literature, can also act as a kind of cover story, an easy and acceptable alibi. The less acceptable stories, the ones that reside between teacher and person composing lives on two knowledge landscapes, were harder to tell. The participants told of struggling to find ways to compose and recompose their whole lives, ones that were lived on and across personal and professional knowledge landscapes. Is Tara's story of the boy, who pointed to himself as also worthy of the best, so striking because it is rare to hear teachers make similar statements? Leaving the profession to focus on composing a better life, a more coherent life on two knowledge landscapes, is not an acceptable story, in large part because of what it might imply about the teacher and about the professional knowledge landscape. To share these harder to tell stories has the possibility of disrupting the professional knowledge landscape and disturbing those who live on it. The roar created by attending to these more complex stories may well be deafening.

From a research perspective these ideas of life composing, these narrative understandings of teachers' experiences, cannot be easily measured, cannot be accounted for, and are best dismissed and disregarded. Researchers, teacher educators, and teachers who leave, know this. Teachers who leave also know that most often, if they tell these complex, layered stories, they run the risk of being seen as deficit, as selfish, as not able to "hack it," as "not swimming but sinking." Better to tell the safe stories of less risk.

In the large-scale studies of early career teacher attrition (Borman & Dowling, 2008; Guarino et al., 2006; Macdonald, 1999; Smith & Ingersoll, 2004) it is difficult to see teachers as people composing lives. Yet attending to experiences as temporally unfolding and enfolding, as situated in place and in relationships, we came to understand the stories participants had imagined they would live were shaped by their stories in early landscapes, and by their stories lived both in and out of schools, and as inextricably linked to how they imagined they would compose their lives, including their lives in and out of schools. These ideas, often disregarded or invisible on the professional knowledge landscape, and in research, were strongly evident in the participants' stories to leave by.

We realized that creating spaces for teachers to tell their stories that include their lives as people both on and off school landscapes helped us understand more about the chasms that can open between personal and professional knowledge landscapes, between imagined and lived stories, between who each is as a person and who each is as a teacher, between cover stories and what Crites (1979) refers to as 'real stories.' Paying attention to the muted stories that resided in the disjunctures between teacher and person pushed us to consider what stories were left untold.

The all-encompassing nature of the teaching profession stems back to the one room school house where the teacher lived, slept, and taught; the personal life given up for the good of the vocation. These historical narratives create stories of "good" teachers who sacrifice their lives for their students. They also foster cover stories that are seen as "safe," that cite upward mobility, parenting, and further education as "good" and acceptable stories to leave by. These cover stories seem easier and safer to tell than stories of struggle, of the bumping of imagined stories with stories on the professional knowledge landscape, of guilt, and of regret.

Another way to understand the cover stories that teachers tell as they leave teaching is as veritable permission slips that grant teachers permission to leave. Their stories are safe and recognizable, and therefore permissible not only for them but also for those on the professional knowledge landscape and on the personal knowledge landscape. These stories not only allow teachers to leave schools, they also leave the professional knowledge landscapes unquestioned, and therefore intact, as the stories are about the individual and not about the system. These cover over the harder to tell stories that might, if given voice, challenge the larger cultural and institutional narratives about teachers.

According to Lindeman Nelson (1995), dominant or master narratives work to frame particular groups as deficient. Just as importantly, these narratives also work to silence particular groups, people, and stories. In the case of these teachers, the harder to tell stories give way to more acceptable or permissible cover stories that do not challenge or counter the master narratives about teaching or teachers. Hearing their harder to tell stories, we wonder if they contain the seeds of a counterstory that could, if given a collective voice, call attention to and shift the crossings and relationships between teachers' personal and professional knowledge landscapes. Attending to what lives on the other side of silence, the metaphoric roar that Eliot (1874) refers to, allows us to see that the participants' imagined stories of who they would be, and become, as teachers did not just include teaching. The imagined stories included stories of being, and becoming, in social networks, in families, and in communities. And the imagined stories are stories lived in, and balanced between, personal and professional knowledge landscapes. As we reflected on the imagined stories of participants, we saw that when they were unable to live out their imagined stories in all their complexities over time, place and relationships, they felt powerless to negotiate spaces on their professional knowledge landscapes. Frequently, they left (Clandinin et al., 2012).

Research puzzles, research designs, and research texts develop out of always asking questions concerning the significance, the personal, practical, social, and theoretical justifications, of the research. In our study of the experiences of early career teachers who left teaching we respond to the 'so what?' and 'who cares?' questions by showing that the phenomenon of early career teacher attrition is very complex (Schaefer, 2012). Through inquiring into the stories early career teachers live and tell, that is, their experiences, we are beginning to open up other stories about teacher attrition that may be harder for teachers to tell and harder for policy-makers and teacher educators to hear. We argue that while cover stories may make it easier for teachers to leave teaching and, ironically, for researchers to precisely determine why teachers leave teaching, cover stories may ultimately lead to policies or "fixes" based on teachers' alibis for leaving, instead of their more complex and harder truths.

Acknowledgements

We acknowledge the support of a grant from Alberta Education that funded this study.

We appreciate the careful reading of the two anonymous reviewers whose comments helped us make these ideas clearer.

References

Alliance for Excellent Education. (2005, August). *Teacher attrition: A costly loss to the nation and to the states*. Washington, DC: Author. Retrieved from www.all4ed.org/files/archive/publications/TeacherAttrition.pdf

Bateson, M. C. (1989). *Composing a life*. New York: Grove Press.

Borman, G. D., & Dowling, N. M. (2008). Teacher attrition and retention: A meta-analytic and narrative review of the research. *Review of Educational Research, 78*(3), 367–409.

Buchanan, J. (2009). Where are they now? Ex-teachers tell their life work stories. *Issues in Education Research, 19*(1), 1–10.

Carr, D. (1986). *Time, narrative, and history*. Bloomington, IN: Indiana University Press.

Clandinin, D. J. (1985). Personal practical knowledge: A study of teachers' classroom images. *Curriculum Inquiry, 14*(4), 361–385.

Clandinin, D. J. (2013). *Engaging in narrative inquiry*. San Francisco, CA: Left Coast Press.

Clandinin, D. J., & Connelly, F. M. (1995). *Teachers' professional knowledge landscapes*. New York: Teachers College Press.

Clandinin, D. J., & Connelly, F. M. (2000). *Narrative inquiry: Experience and story in qualitative research*. San Francisco, CA: Jossey-Bass.

Clandinin, D. J., Downey, C. A., & Huber, J. (2009). Attending to changing landscapes: Shaping the interwoven identities of teachers and teacher educators. *Asia-Pacific Journal of Teacher Education, 37*(2), 141–154.

Clandinin, D. J., Schaefer, L., Long, J. S., Steeves, P., McKenzie-Robblee, S., Pinnegar, E., & Downey, C. A. (2012, April). *Early career teacher attrition: Problems, possibilities, potentials*. Unpublished manuscript submitted to Alberta Education.

Connelly, F. M., & Clandinin, D. J. (1988). *Teachers as curriculum planners: Narratives of experience*. New York: Teachers College Press.

Connelly, F. M., & Clandinin, D. J. (1999). *Shaping a professional identity: Stories of educational practice*. London, Ontario, Canada: Althouse Press.

Connelly, F. M., & Clandinin, D. J. (2006). Narrative inquiry. In J. L. Green, G. Camilli, & P. Elmore (Eds.), *Handbook of complementary methods in education research* (3rd ed., pp. 477–487). Mahwah, NJ: Lawrence Erlbaum Associates.

Crites, S. (1979). The aesthetics of self deception. *Soundings: An Interdisciplinary Journal, 62*(2), 107–129.

Dewey, J. (1938). *Experience and education*. New York: Collier Books.

Eliot, G. (1874). *Middlemarch: A study of provincial life*. London, UK: W. Blackwood & Sons.

Greene, M. (1995). *Releasing the imagination: Essays on education, the arts, and social change*. San Francisco, CA: Jossey-Bass.

Guarino, C. M., Santibañez, L., & Daley, G. A. (2006). Teacher recruitment and retention: A review of the recent empirical literature. *Review of Educational Research, 76*(2), 173–208.

Heilbrun, C. G. (1988). *Writing a woman's life*. New York: W. W. Norton.

Ingersoll, R. M. (2001). Teacher turnover and teacher shortages: An organizational analysis. *American Educational Research Journal, 38*(3), 499–534.

Johnson, M. (1989). Embodied knowledge. *Curriculum Inquiry, 19*, 361–377.

Lindeman Nelson, H. (1995) Resistance and insubordination. *Hypatia, 10*(2), 23–40.

Macdonald, D. (1999). Teacher attrition: A review of literature. *Teaching and Teacher Education, 15*(8), 835–848.

Rinke, C. (2007). Understanding teachers' careers: Linking professional life to personal path. *Teachers and Teaching, 3*(1), 1–13.

Schaefer, L. (2012). *A narrative inquiry into the experiences of two beginning P.E. teachers' shifting stories to live by*. Unpublished Doctoral Dissertation, University of Alberta, Edmonton, Canada.

Schaefer, L. (2013). Beginning teacher attrition: A question of identity making and identity shifting. *Teachers and Teaching: Theory and Practice, 19*(3). https://doi.org/10.1080/13540602.2012.754149

Schaefer, L., & Clandinin, D. J. (2011). A narrative inquiry into beginning teachers' experiences. *Learning Landscapes, 4*(2), 275–296.

Smith, T. M., & Ingersoll, R. M. (2004). What are the effects of induction and mentoring on beginning teacher turnover? *American Educational Research Journal, 41*(3), 681–714.

8

NARRATIVE INQUIRY AS REFLECTIVE PRACTICE

Tensions and possibilities

Charles Aiden Downey and D. Jean Clandinin

Introduction

In this chapter we take up the task of exploring the intersections, overlaps and tensions between narrative inquiry and reflective inquiry. We frame our exploration as a journey taken into the unmarked commonplaces and edges of these two methodologies to preserve how we muddled in, and sometimes up, what, at first, appeared to be familiar territory. The metaphor of a journey fits well with our goal to produce a sketch of our travels in, and between, these two methodologies rather than a bird's eye view map. We hope that our journey will open up for the reader what it opened up for us: new ways of thinking about both narrative inquiry and reflective inquiry.

Partly we assumed that this journey would be straightforward as both narrative inquiry and reflective inquiry have roots in Dewey's philosophy of experience. We begin with a brief explanation of how Dewey understood human experience as an unfolding inquiry. From this common ground we will then engage in a showing rather than a telling of narrative inquiry, foregrounding key concepts and terms as we go in order to hold them next to our understandings of those of reflective inquiry. Along the way we keep an eye on where we started by tracing terms and concepts back to Dewey's notion of experience to better understand how each methodology works with it. Finally we turn to consider each methodology in terms of its broader goals – what we have come to call its "end game" – to chart possible intersections, overlaps, and tensions between these two forms of inquiry.

Dewey's philosophy of experience

Reflective inquiry and narrative inquiry both claim Dewey's notion of experience as a foundational concept. While Dewey continued to develop his understanding of experience over his career we will work with his definition in *Democracy in Education:*

Reprinted with permission from Springer Nature: Springer. Acknowledgement; Downey, C. A., & Clandinin, D. J. (2010). Narrative inquiry as reflective practice: Tensions and possibilities. In N. Lyons (Ed.), *Handbook of reflection and reflective inquiry: Mapping a way of knowing for professional reflective practice* (pp. 285–397). Dordrecht, Netherlands: Springer.

> When we experience something we act upon it, we do something with it; then we undergo and suffer the consequences. We do something to the thing and then it does something to us in return: such is the peculiar combination.
>
> *(1916, p. 139)*

For Dewey, doing can lead to undoing in the sense that our actions in a world act on us, with the result being an irrevocable alteration in both "it" and us. Dewey understood "us" and "it" not as distinct entities but rather as parts or aspects of an experiential whole, a point he struggled to make in a language prone to dichotomies. For our purposes we take him to mean that to undergo an experience occurs in the relationship between what we do in the world and what this does to us, the relationship between actions and reactions.

Dewey's two criteria of experience are continuity and interaction. By continuity he means "every experience both takes up something from those which have gone before and modifies in some way the quality of those which come after" (1938, p. 35). While Dewey believed continuity to be part and parcel of all experience, he considered growth to be the overarching goal of any experience, which he understood in terms of the quality and type of experiences any experience leads up and opens into. Critical to Dewey is the emerging vantage point created by the unfolding of experience, with each subsequent situation offering us a novel perspective to look back on the experiences leading up to, and out of, an experience, making "growth" provisional and emergent rather than fixed and found. For Dewey this retrospection is always prospective, a looking backwards in the service of looking, and ultimately moving, forward towards both an immediate and more tangible goal such as getting to work on time and *the* less tangible and more slippery goal of all experience growth.

His second criterion of experience, interaction, involves the interplay between "objective" and "internal" conditions (Dewey, 1938). In *The Child and the Curriculum* Dewey (1902) explains his idea of interaction as a means to argue for a radical rethinking of education as neither child-centered nor curriculum-centered but rather focused on the creation of educative situations. In the same spirit as the explorers whose notes contributed to the making of the map, creating situations meant neither to have students simply follow the finished map nor to wander aimlessly in the wilderness but to find a middle ground on which students learn how to "get the benefit of past effort in controlling future endeavor" (Dewey, 1902, p. 104). Dewey understood well that we each live in, and on, our own experiential middle grounds, always somewhat stuck in the mud of trying to get from here to there, from is to ought, and that this muddling around was something we should work on, as doing so would prepare us for the inevitable muddling that comes with the unknown of the future.

Reflective thinking

While Dewey considered continuity and interaction part of all experience, he believed a particular kind of thinking to be best suited for living in the midst and muddles of experience and as such capable of increasing the overall value of any experience. He termed this reflective thinking and built his entire notion of education around fostering it.

Within Dewey's concept of experience, we understand that for him the goal of reflective thinking is learning to make connections between what we do and what it does to us:

> To "learn from experience" is to make a backward and forward connection between what we do to things and what we enjoy or suffer from things in consequence. Under such conditions, doing becomes trying; an experiment with the world to find out what it is like; the undergoing becomes instruction – discovery of the connection of things.
>
> *(1916, p. 140)*

For Dewey learning from experience is less a connecting of the dots of our doing to what it does to us than a reconsideration of the dots themselves. Most profoundly, this makes education an ongoing "reconstruction" of experience in the service of enhancing its meaning and one's ability to "direct the course of subsequent experiences" (ibid.).

Dewey linked his conception of learning to the inevitable muddiness that comes with muddling along; the turns that shift us from our original course of action, pointing us instead onto unexpected and unmarked routes that we then struggle to learn to navigate. Learning begins only when certainty ends. Following from this view, reflective thinking within Dewey's concept of experience with its criteria of interaction and continuity,

> involves a state of doubt, hesitation, perplexity, mental difficulty in which thinking originates; and an act of searching, hunting, inquiring, to find material that will resolve the doubt, settle and dispose of the perplexity.
>
> *(1910)*

Revisiting Dewey then, we note that while doubt, uncertainty and perplexity are part of situations, the distinction between reflective inquiry and narrative inquiry lives in whether, and how, these can be rung out of situations.

While both narrative inquiry and reflective inquiry are concerned with how humans connect what they do to what their doing does to them, they take different tacks on the ways continuity and interaction impact on what we learn from experience. Perhaps, in our view, reflective inquiry stays closer to Dewey's ideas and pursues "reflective thinking" as the best way to get after the making of connections. Narrative inquiry understands "stories both lived and told" as the connector of the person in the world, framing narrative as both phenomenon under study and method of study (Clandinin & Connelly, 1990). We will return to this distinction later in the chapter but with it in mind we now turn to narrative inquiry.

Narrative inquiry

We begin with what we know best and how we best know it by engaging in a showing rather than a telling of narrative inquiry. We hope to illustrate how narrative inquirers work within a metaphorical three dimensional narrative inquiry space in which they use a set of terms that point them backward and forward (Dewey's continuity), inward and outward (Dewey's interaction) with attentiveness to place or a series of places (Dewey's situation). We see these dimensions as directions or avenues to be explored in a narrative inquiry (Clandinin & Connelly, 2000). We do not see the terms in the same way that others might see them if they were positioned within a more conventional research paradigm, that is, as a set of analytic terms. Thinking narratively means keeping the terms close to their experiential origins, to think of them "not so much as generating a list of understandings achieved by analyzing the stories" (Clandinin & Connelly, 2000, p. 54) but rather thinking with them to understand the lives being lived.

Showing a narrative inquiry: mapping our journey

As we wondered about the intersections, overlaps and tensions between narrative inquiry and reflective inquiry, we were taken particularly with the central concern of reflective inquiry as the interrogation of puzzling or problematic situations involving teaching and learning. Struggling with just what this meant we sought to ground it in own experiences. Jean told a story of a situation that unfolded in a classroom where she was a researcher to illustrate her understanding of a problematic situation. In response Aiden told a story of what he considered a problematic situation from his experience as a student teacher in an inner-city high school that occurred over ten years ago. The story appears below not exactly as he told it but as he wrote it later that same day.

Telling the story

"This is bullshit! Why we gotta know this?" Dewarn's words stopped me in my tracks. He and I were the only ones standing in the class, me inches from the blackboard and him at his lab bench three rows back. All of the students turned to look at him and then fixed their eyes on me. Worse yet this moment was being immortalized, as Janet, the field supervisor for my student teaching, had her eye in a video recorder aimed at me.

Just moments earlier I had been selling atoms, trying to get the students in my ninth grade physical science class interested in what the state said I had to cover, knowing it would all go a lot easier if I could make these little bits of matter to them. About fifteen minutes into my well-planned pitch – one in which I sought, as I had been taught, to create "cognitive dissonance" in the students – Dewarn had slapped his hand on his desk, stood up and torpedoed my lesson plan, which had been designed to spark student questions and avoid this question. What to do, what to do . . . I had been stopped in my tracks. I had created cognitive dissonance to be sure, but now it was my own, as I struggled to think of how to answer the question and not look at the camera, which was closing in on me as Janet made her way up the side of the classroom.

I honestly can't remember what I said next. The "lesson" went on, as it had to, and the film continued to roll. Smiling, Janet handed me the tape at the end of class, but in the ten years since I have never watched it. I am not exactly sure why. But I often look at this tape and have made sure it has moved with me over the years. Dewarn's words have always stuck with me, as I have told endless versions of this story, some to teachers, others to friends, and many to myself. When I think about teaching, learning and curriculum he is there, standing his ground and challenging mine.

Re-telling the story

We worked together to engage in the narrative inquiry into this story. Working within the three-dimensional narrative inquiry space, we first talked our way through what we might do and then decided to write in a relational way about the retelling we were engaged in.

Aiden began in a long ago past as he described the encounter with Dewarn in the midst of enacting a carefully planned lesson with a video camera rolling. He slid even further backward as he described the moments leading up to the encounter and what he had been doing. He then slid even further back to give a hint of what he had been taught to do as a science teacher, that is, to create cognitive dissonance in and for his students. He slid forward again but provided no details on how he completed the lesson. He knew he took the videotape from his supervisor as he has it still, although he has not watched it. He then moved temporally forward saying he has recounted this story many times. He finally arrived at the present where he acknowledged that this moment with Dewarn is always with him when he thinks about teaching, learning and curriculum. The past moment with Dewarn stays with him as Dewarn continually stands his ground and challenges Aiden.

Temporality was interwoven with place for Aiden told Jean the story first as they sat together in the Centre for Research for Teacher Education and Development on a cold winter day. The sky was blue outside but we both knew that the window was holding back the frigid temperatures. Aiden took us to another place, an inner-city high school classroom located far away in time and place. We left the warmth of the Centre place for that place that lives now only in Aiden's memory.

Aiden slid us inward and outward. As we began the story he told of Dewarn standing up and confronting him, slapping his hand against his desk, a move that stopped Aiden and caused him what he called the cognitive dissonance he had hoped to create for his students.

A reflection on our narrative inquiry

At this point in our journey we pause to reflect on the central concepts and terms of narrative inquiry, first tracing them back to Dewey and then considering them in relation to our understandings of those of reflective inquiry.

As we noted above, narrative inquiry takes up Dewey's criteria of experience-interaction and continuity – to create a metaphorical three-dimensional narrative inquiry space:

> our terms are personal and social (interaction); past, present, and future (continuity); combined with the notion of place (situation). This set of terms creates a metaphorical three-dimensional narrative inquiry space, with temporality along one dimension, the personal and social along a second dimension, and place along the third.
>
> *(Clandinin & Connelly, 2000, p. 50)*

These terms point us in directions along the continuum of experience, which we understand as a narrative composition. Through stories humans create coherence though time, between the personal and social and across situations. Stories are not just about experience but experience itself; we live and learn in, and through, the living, telling, retelling, and reliving of our stories (Clandinin & Connelly, 2000).

Narrative inquirers do not live outside of the three-dimensional inquiry space but rather live in it, alongside and in relation with their participants. Narrative inquirers tell stories about the stories they and others live and tell, keeping in mind how their own stories shape how they understand and tell the stories of others. They understand story as the fundamental unit of experience; one that cannot be broken down into smaller pieces without a loss of the wholeness of the life that produced it. In narrative inquiry we try to understand the stories under or on the edges of stories lived and told, as no story stands on its own but rather in relation to many others – including the stories of the narrative inquirer.

Returning to Aiden's told story of Dewarn and our subsequent retelling of it, we see that it has not been reduced to a story about "this or that." We have, rather, traced its movement within the three-dimensional narrative inquiry space to show how Aiden took us to a distant place and time to recount a moment that is anything but distant to him. We pointed to the different places and times Aiden wove into his story as possible avenues for further exploration. In narrative inquiry the story itself stands, shifting the focus of the inquiry to understanding the many stories it stands on, beside or among, in order to render an account of life as it is lived.

A turn toward reflective inquiry

Reflective inquiry also takes up Dewey's notion of experience and reflective thinking to focus on what Dewey himself spent a great deal of time considering: how to best learn from the reactions to our actions. We borrow Lyons (2002) definition of reflective inquiry:

> Reflection is an intentional act engaging a person alone, but especially in collaboration with others – students, teachers, practitioners, other researchers or colleagues – in systematic inquiry, interrogating a situation of teaching or learning, usually one presenting some puzzle, to construct an understanding of some aspect of it. Such an act looks both backwards and to the future. It is in service of understanding and meaning that will shape action. It involves gathering and documenting evidence of the inquiry. It likely involves narrative for it is the story of meaning, and it can raise ethical issues for the people involved. *(p. 99)*

We return to Aiden's story of Dewarn with this definition of reflective inquiry in mind to explore the possible intersections, overlaps and tensions between narrative inquiry and reflective inquiry. We consider each form of inquiry in terms of situation, method, the place of unexpectedness, and perspective.

Situation

Narrative inquiry and reflective inquiry define situation slightly differently. Reflective inquiry usually focuses on a particular situation set within a particular context, such as teaching and learning. In Aiden's story of Dewarn this might be Aiden being challenged by a student about the relevance of learning the atomic model. If we imagine an inquiry soon after this event, it might involve focusing on how Aiden designed his lesson plan and the broader unit. It would certainly ask hard questions about what Aiden might possibly do next in this classroom and what he might do in future classrooms to avoid it. Perhaps it might consider how Aiden framed this situation, focusing on "the problem of a problematic situation" (Schön, 1995, p. 31) to offer Aiden the opportunity to see his thought in the situation.

As we showed in the previous section, narrative inquiry takes Aiden's story as the situation, one filled with multiple and shifting situations. It pays attention to the many places and times visited in the unfolding story and, as such, is focused less on the understanding one can draw from any particular situation than from the many situations that make up a life. Narrative inquiry understands any situation as nested within an almost endless array of other situations and, rather than sort them out, seeks to understand and explore the layers of complexity involved in living a life. We believe reflective inquiry and narrative inquiry take a different view of situation, with reflective inquiry focusing in on a particular situation as a means to further understanding and action and narrative inquiry focusing out from any situation to further understand how it might be woven into a life.

We return to Aiden's story to further distinguish between how narrative inquiry and reflective inquiry define a situation by focusing on the lines of inquiry each might take up in respect to Aiden's story. By focusing on the situation as one event within a larger narrative, reflective inquiry might ask Aiden to consider how he might handle his confrontation with Dewarn differently in the future, probing for alternative ways he might think about it his own teaching, particularly those that incorporate how his students might experience it. In narrative inquiry the framing of Aiden's entire story as the situation opens up questions of what lies at the edges of this framing, or the stories of experience that stand at the edges of this one, that may lead up to, and out of, this story. Possible lines of inquiry might include asking Aiden about his other tellings of this same story, what the tape means to him and why he has, as of yet, not watched it and how this story might shift or shape other ones, such as his story of leaving teaching and becoming an educational researcher,

Method

Reflective inquiry both builds on and aims to foster Dewey's notion of reflective thinking articulated in *How We Think* (1910). In this work Dewey lays out how he thinks we should think in order to best learn from experience. His conception draws heavily on the scientific method, which he believed served as the best model for learning from experience. Yet Dewey was well aware of the problems associated with transporting the scientific method into the uncontrollable uncertainty of everyday life, what Donald Schön (1992, 1995) referred to as the "swamp" of practice. Yet, even as the uncertain messiness of life is acknowledged, reflective inquiry takes a more instrumental path to build on Dewey's notion of the scientific method as an archetype for thinking through the problems encountered in the living of a life.

As we showed in the previous section, narrative inquiry takes a more aesthetic path following Dewey (Jackson, 1998; Granger, 2006). The purpose of method for both reflective inquiry and narrative inquiry is to gain a better understanding of how to proceed. However, in reflective inquiry, the method or path to understanding starts in a puzzling around concrete situations with an intention that this will lead to change in the understanding of a situation. In narrative inquiry the starting point is an attempt to understand an unfolding life in all of its temporal, social, cultural and contextual complexity as a means to better understand concrete situations. In part, then the difference is in the starting point for the inquiry.

From these starting points the two forms of inquiry set off in pursuit of very different, if not antagonistic, ends. In reflective inquiry a story might be sacrificed for the evidence it might contain about a particular situation, while in narrative inquiry the story remains, serving as a starting point for exploring the many other stories that live in and around it and make up a life. The difference here lies in the part stories play in the living out of a life. In reflective inquiry story is a resource for thinking while in narrative inquiry, story is the way we live, tell and inquire into our lives.

Applying this distinction between narrative and reflective inquiry to Aiden's story opens up different lines of inquiry. A more reflective inquiry into Aiden's story might seek more concrete evidence to corroborate his story, such as viewing the videotape or seeing the lesson plan. The line of inquiry would cross the line of the story in the sense of dismantling it with, and for, a more scientific or instrumental form of thinking. It would become a form of evidence to be interrogated like any other. Narrative inquiry would do quite the opposite, honoring the story by inquiring into the stories that live on its edges as a means to better understand the stories that Aiden lives and tells in composing his life. This might mean asking Aiden to tell other stories that have influenced his ideas about teaching, learning and curriculum.

The place of unexpectedness

Dewey's early writings on the role of reflective thinking in experience can be thought of as a field manual for how to deal with unexpectedness, a guide on how to best make our way through the inevitable "surprises" (Schön, 1983) that greet us as we try to get on in the world. For Dewey reflection involved learning to detect, dispatch of and come to expect unexpectedness, as reflective thought best helped us out of and ironically then back into problematic or puzzling situations. As Carol Rodgers (2002) notes:

> The process of reflection, Dewey claims (*1916*/1944), moves the learner from a disturbing state of perplexity (also referred to by him as disequilibrium) to a harmonious state of settledness (equilibrium). Perplexity is created when an individual encounters a situation whose "full character is not yet determined".
>
> *(p. 850)*

Dewey considered living in the world to be living in a "series of situations," many harboring enough unexpectedness to produce perplexity and uncertainty. As noted earlier, Dewey believed education to be the process of putting unexpectedness to work for, and ultimately on, us, harnessing it to foster growth and thereby deepen and direct future experience. Through reflective thought we bring an order to the situation and ourselves, banishing unexpectedness into the future to be met again and again. The "swamp" of practice is momentarily drained, allowing us to stand on the firm ground reflective inquiry yields before the water begins to rise and the ground begins to give way again. As Donald Schon reminds us so well, we can never defeat uncertainty so much as push it in a favorable direction:

> what John Dewey called inquiry: thought intertwined with action – reflection in and on action – which proceeds from doubt to the resolution of doubt, to the generation of new doubt. The inquirer is in, and in transaction with, the problematic situation. He or she must construct the meaning and frame the problem of the situation, thereby setting the stage for problem-solving, which, in combination with changes in the external context, brings a new problematic situation into being. Hence the proper test of a round of inquiry is not only "Have I solved this problem?" but "Do I like the new problems I have created?"
>
> *(Schön,1995, p. 31)*

Inquiry is a sort of Sisyphean task with an important twist: the experiential boulder we push up and to some degree out of doubt rolls down yet another unexpected slope, ending up in another swamp of uncertainty, another problematic situation, waiting to pushed up, out and into another one.

As mentioned earlier reflective inquiry focuses *in* on a particularly problematic situation, aiming to better frame, understand and to some degree solve a particular problem while simultaneously honing our more generic ability to solve problems. The translation of what is learned from solving any particular problem into a more generic "this is how to solve problems" form is crucial here, as learning means our boulders should never roll back down the same hill but rather down new ones that we cannot see until it is too late. Again, as our metaphorical boulder goes careening down into yet another unexpected and unexplored swamp of uncertainty, we are left to consider just what went awry, sifting through our previous efforts to figure out what to leave, what to take and what we must improvise, or make, to move this boulder "onward," which less means forward than in a favorable direction out of this situation, towards growth.

In narrative inquiry unexpectedness takes on a slightly different meaning, as situations are understood less as occurring in a series but rather in parallel, or alongside many other situations. For narrative inquirers, the situation "not yet fully determined" is life as it is lived, replete with situations nested, tangled up in and woven into the complexities of the lives of many others. To inquire narratively is to focus on experience as stories lived and told with an understanding that uncertainty lives in and between the situations or lived and told stories. Concretely this means focusing *out* from any one situation to see peripherally the many situations that compose a life (Bateson, 1994). The process of looking across the many stories that compose a life fosters its own form of unexpectedness, one brought on by seeing not only how we have gone about composing a life, but also how we might now go about composing it differently.

In narrative inquiry unexpectedness also lives in, and through, the unfolding relationship between researchers and participants. Living one's life in the midst of others' lives opens us up to the possibilities of what this experience will call forth and lead into. This unexpectedness is not only expected in narrative inquiry but also one of its goals, as inquiring narratively with others opens up the possibility for growth, by which we mean coming to tell and live what at least seem, in the moment, to be better stories.

While both narrative inquiry and reflective inquiry harness unexpectedness in the service of understanding, they go about this slightly differently. For reflective inquiry the unit of analysis is an unexpected and puzzling situation within a certain context, the systematic interrogation of which can yield understandings that inform both a specific course of action and our more generic ability to inquire. For narrative inquirers any one situation or lived story is understood as a part of many others, as situated within an unfolding life. Unexpectedness lies in the process of inquiry, as it opens up the possibility of seeing, telling and living our stories differently.

Returning to Aiden's story we understand narrative inquiry and reflective inquiry to focus on two different places of unexpectedness. For reflective inquiry the unexpectedness occurs in the story, which is, in part, about an unexpected or problematic moment early in Aiden's teaching career. The story might be viewed as a "case" with which to teach beginning teachers, an example of the bumps and surprises that can occur in a classroom with the intention of helping them learn how to anticipate and solve the surprises that will inevitably occur in their classrooms. In a narrative inquiry, the unexpectedness occurs in the telling, which might mean encouraging new teachers to attend to their own stories of experience that Aiden's story calls forth and opens up for inquiry. Not to foreshadow too much of what is to come, but this is indeed what Jean does by telling a story about a student she has not thought about for many years, a story that returns to her unexpectedly, "catching" her while in the midst of attending to Aiden's story.

Perspective

It is difficult to think of reflection and not think of a mirror, as Dewey, much like Marx's (1964) concept of labour, considered experience an opportunity to contemplate, through our actions and the world's reactions, ourselves in the world. One might consider Dewey's notion of reflective thinking a method for refining this mirror, making it more capable of continuously remaking the connections between means and ends. The better our ability to reflect, the more able we are to make the connections between before and after, self and world, that enable us to deepen and ultimately direct future experience.

We are cautious in our metaphor of thinking as a mirror, as it does not adequately reflect Dewey's idea that we live in both *a* world and *the* world. We always live in our world, living in the midst of a life that won't sit still, one always still unfolding. Experience is just that, the schlepping of our world in the world, a trying or doing that can lead to unexpected outcomes, including a very trying undoing of aspects of our world. Dewey understood this as life itself, an inescapable and often hard fact of experience but yet the harbinger of growth, something to be welcomed and worked with rather than avoided. These Deweyan ideas, up to this point, underpin both narrative inquiry and reflective inquiry. However, playing further with the metaphor of a mirror, we turn to a poetic rendition of a shattered mirror:

> *All Faith is false, all Faith is true:*
> *Truth is the shattered mirror strown*
> *In myriad bits; while each believe*
> *His little bit the whole to own.*
>
> (*The Kasidah of Haji Abdu El-Yezdi, "translated" by Richard Burton, 1880 and as quoted in Appiah, 2006, p. 5*)

We played with the idea of a shattered mirror that, for us, could be an uncertain situation within both narrative inquiry and reflective inquiry in order to show tensions and overlaps between what we see as perspective in both reflective inquiry and narrative inquiry.

In reflective inquiry, there is a process of trying to frame a problem in order to move through the uncertain situation. Knowing that the metaphoric "myriad bits" of the "shattered mirror" can be reassembled in multiple ways, the challenge is to carefully attend to this multiplicity of ways. Reassembled in one way the mirror allows one path forward, reassembled in another offers another way and so on. The process, though, is one of reassembling the bits in order to generate new understandings meant to guide action towards the resolution of the problematic situation, at least for the moment.

In narrative inquiry, there is more attention to the pattern in which the mirror has shattered, seeing the "myriad bits" as a life, as stories lived and told by a person in particular times and places. While there is also uncertainty in this moment, in narrative inquiry we do not intend to reassemble the bits but rather to enter the strewn bits of a person's life in the midst and in relational ways, attending to what is possible in understanding the temporal, social and place dimensions within an ongoing life. Attending to the multiplicity of what becomes visible in the unfolding life, the narrative inquirer attends to the particularities of each "bit" or shard in order to compose multiple possible story retellings or ways to move forward in imaginative and narratively coherent ways.

A tension lives between reflective inquiry and narrative inquiry in how the "strewn" bits of mirror are understood and in the ways multiple alternative perspectives are understood (as multiple possible problem framings or as multiple possible re-tellings and re-livings) as both lead toward action. To us reflective inquiry keeps one eye on the problematic situation while training the other on possible solutions, giving its perspective a certain direction, one oriented towards action and resolution. In terms of Aiden's story this means finding and framing the problematic situation and then charting a careful and considered course towards a possible solution.

By contrast, narrative inquiry focuses one eye on stories lived and told and the other on the stories and lives that live at their edges, creating an orientation that can feel more dizzying than directional, more a muddling around in the myriad of stories that compose a life than making any situation in it clearer with the goal of moving it along. In Aiden's story this would chart a course towards the inclusion of other stories rather than the solution of the perceived problem in this particular story, to better understand where this story, bit or shard, stands in relation to the many others that compose his life. We see this metaphorical muddling as generative, and, as we will now show, narrative inquiry often involves a muddling up of a situation or story with the telling of another one.

Unfolding of the narrative inquiry

In Jean's listening to Aiden's story as a narrative inquirer, she listened first to his story, moving imaginatively to what it must have been like for him as a beginning teacher, to what he was experiencing in the moment. She also listened carefully to how he told the story, attending carefully to the plotline he composed, to how he positioned himself in time, in place, to his feelings, his moral sensibilities, the aesthetic sense in the lived moment. But as many authors have noted, when we listen to stories as narrative inquirers, stories are called forth from the stories of the listeners. This process of calling or catching threads from the teller's story is, as Hoffman (1994) notes, a process of resonant remembering. Hoffman describes resonant remembering as "the kind of palpable precise, personal memory in which the emotional meanings of events is recognized, for subjective thought, and for the probing of survivors' own internal journeys" (p. 2). We take Hoffman's idea of resonant remembering, of remembering what happened within each person, and wonder about how we catch resonant threads as we listen to another's story that call up our own internal journeys. As memory "responds more than it records" (De Certeau, 1984, p. 88), resonant remembering can, we see, be triggered by others' stories.

As Jean worked with the retelling of Aiden's story, she was caught by a story from her own experience, not a story which resonated from her student teaching but an encounter from her first year as a full time teacher in the late 1960's. The experience of moving imaginatively with Aiden calls forth a story in Jean, one she has not thought about for years. It is there, always, as its remembering involves a form of forgetting, one in which a memory is not lost forever but rather lived out *in* who she is. As she and Aiden inquired into his story, she began to tell, and later wrote, the following story.

> Thorpe, a slightly overweight nine-year-old boy, was in my Grade Four classroom, a classroom situated in a "portable" classroom, one of several hauled into the parking lot of this overcrowded suburban school. Alongside the portable where I came to know Thorpe were two other portables with classes taught by two other beginning teachers. Thorpe had already made a significant impact on the story of the classroom by that late September afternoon when I sat alone at my desk, working on plans for the next day's class. The door opened and a big burly man came in and took a seat at the back. He said gruffly, "Oh, they gave him to you, a beginning teacher and a woman. How are you doing?" I, startled at his presence, said, "Pardon me, can I help you?" He responded gruffly, "Thorpe. I'm the assistant principal at the neighbouring school and I taught him last year. Are you having trouble with him? Do you want to know what I did?" I remembered the surprise I felt at the intrusion but responded, "Okay. What did you do?" I recalled the hesitance I felt for I had not told anyone but my husband that I was having trouble with a student. He said, "I tied a rope around his neck and whenever he wasn't paying attention, I tugged it. You might try that. I also kept chalk at my desk and when I wanted his attention, I lobbed a piece at him. That won't work for you because you probably can't throw very well." I said, "well I don't think I will try that but thanks for telling me". The visitor stood abruptly and said, "Well, call me if you want some help." I never called but the moment continues to live with me.

That moment was the moment Jean recalled as she and Aiden worked to retell Aiden's story. It had been several years since she consciously remembered Thorpe but the moment of meeting the vice principal came flooding back as she read of Aiden's encounter with Dewarn. The moment with the vice principal was a moment that made Jean think about teaching, learning and curriculum making, about what mattered to her. Thorpe is always there, first as Jean worked that year to make a relationship with Thorpe, a relationship where they could learn together and where he might learn to see himself as a member of a classroom community, not as someone who did not belong in a classroom, something he had learned from the vice principal.

During the long fall term, Jean recounted that she worked to compose a relationship with Thorpe, calling on the other two new teachers to take Thorpe to their rooms when she could no longer see Thorpe as other than an aggravation and felt her frustration rising. She created spaces where they could talk, she chose books she thought he might like, she gave him responsibilities and slowly, slowly, slowly, he began to live and tell another story of himself as a child in school. And Jean continued to imagine how to live and tell a story of her as a teacher who attended to children's lives.

Re-telling the story

Working within the three-dimensional narrative inquiry space, we saw that Jean began to tell her story working with, and in, Aiden's story, an experience that called forth her story of a student she had not thought of for years. Jean slid back in time to her first year of teaching in a portable classroom outside of an overcrowded school to a particular moment about a month into the school year. Sitting at her desk after school she was visited by the vice-principal from Thorpe's previous school, who had come to offer her advice on how to deal with him. Jean learned that Thorpe, the student she is struggling with, had a rope put around his neck and chalk thrown at him by this man, who not so subtly questioned whether Jean, a beginning female teacher, could control Thorpe.

Jean then slid forward to the present to lay her story of Thorpe alongside Aiden's story of Dewarn, as that moment with the vice principal had, in the moment of living, made her consider what mattered to her as a teacher. As Jean laid her story alongside Aiden's, she then returned to her first year of teaching to tell of her efforts to develop a relationship with Thorpe in which Thorpe could come to see himself as a member of the classroom community. Jean developed strategies to prevent herself from seeing Thorpe as the vice principal did, strategies which included sending him to another beginning teacher's portable when she could no longer see Thorpe as a child. Jean worked hard with Thorpe, and his small progress in terms of coming to see himself as a member of the school community fed Jean's imaginings of herself as a teacher who attended to children's lives. Thorpe's slow transformation showed Jean the difference she made in a student, which in turn fueled her imagination as to how to better attend to students' lives.

Jean's temporal and spatial movement back and forth from the present to a long ago past weaves her story of Thorpe into Aiden's story of Dewarn. Jean's temporal coming and going from the present situation transforms it into something else, something less bounded and quite quickly multiplying in time, social and the place. Her telling continues the unhinging of place and time, opening up the possibility for a new story to be told about an old one. Jean's telling of her story in response to Aiden's story binds them together much like a book. The possible threads attaching them remain to be discovered, making the point of Jean's telling of this story a retrospective endeavor.

Laying these stories side by side allows for further narrative inquiry into their resonances. As these stories were told during Jean and Aiden's conversations about the relationship between narrative inquiry and reflective inquiry, they already resonated in and through their place in an ongoing dialogue, as Aiden's story of Dewarn emerged from Jean's story from an ongoing research project and, in turn, prompted Jean's story of Thorpe. Jean's notion that while working with Aiden's story of Dewarn she was "caught" by the story of Thorpe is powerful and quite apt to the way these stories emerged, as we less fished them from our memories than they caught us in a moment that reminded us of other moments, ones which had not faded with time and appear to us as vivid as if they happened yesterday.

The end game

Schön's (1992) concept of generative muddiness is, perhaps, a way to think about the end game, Dewey's end in view for both narrative inquiry and reflective inquiry. Both forms of inquiry are pointed into the future, toward future action, and both carry within a sense of movement or action. For both narrative inquiry and reflective inquiry there is a living out in further action. Thus, temporality and action are central to both forms.

However, as we sift through the uncertainty, Schön's (1992) muddy messiness, some distinctions become clearer. In narrative inquiry there is no certainty in what future stories will be lived and told, even in the near future. There is no plan that can be implemented in action. People, places, other events, emotions, moral judgments and aesthetic responses continually shift and change the array of possible plotlines open to each person. As narrative inquirers we can map out possible plotlines, hint at that array of possibilities but all we can say is that this is how, inquirers and participants, are living and telling the stories for now. We follow one possible trajectory and move forward into other possible uncertainties. Our research texts point to an array of possibilities.

In reflective inquiry there is also uncertainty but, perhaps, reflective inquiry, with the movement from problem framing through to problem resolution and action, has, at least momentarily, a clearer sense of certainty. There, too, however, as action is taken, new situations open themselves to new tensions, new problems and the inquiry process opens again. We understand the goal of reflective inquiry as standing, if only temporarily, on the firmer ground yielded by thinking about a perplexing situation in a disciplined manner. By contrast, we see narrative inquiry as a muddle through the much more spongy terrain of experience, one which pulls us in, gets us muddy and shows our tracks. In reflective inquiry, there is the possibility, at least for a time, of standing on the solid ground of certainty whereas in narrative inquiry, we find that we continue to compose our inquiries and lives within spongy uncertain ground. We stay, we might say, within the peaty spaces of possibility.

We now turn back to Dewey to better understand the commonplaces and tensions in the end games of narrative inquiry and reflective inquiry. Specifically we draw attention to Dewey's (1916) emphasis on the future-oriented and tentative nature of thinking: "to consider the *bearing* of the occurrence upon what may be, but is not yet, is to think" (p. 147).

Dewey's italicization of the word bearing signals to us his desire for readers to pay close attention to what he might mean by this word. For us, his use of the word bearing opens up the possibility of understanding thinking as simultaneously both an instrumental and artistic endeavour. On the one hand, bearing signals an act of taking stock of our current position or situation, our "here" in relation to a hoped for "there," and charting a new course or direction towards it. On the other hand, bearing points to the fruit borne in the process, which one might consider an artfully composed life, one that coheres in and around the possibilities that open up in a constant state of becoming. If we imagine these two takes on the word bearing as two hands on a clock, we might see the more directional and instrumental take as being the minute hand, one in constant movement in and through the situations that make up our lives. The more artistic take on bearing might more resemble the hour hand, one that is moved by and composed of many minutes. While the little hand moves through situations, the big hand moves situations into a life, weaving them into stories of who we are and still might become. For us this is what we take Dewey to mean by bearing, the double movement of pushing uncertainty and incompleteness in a favorable direction while artfully moving toward the composing of a narratively coherent life.

Thus for Dewey, the necessary incompleteness (Greene, 1995) of life makes thinking a prospective endeavor, one that looks back into the past to look forward in the future:

> For we live not in a settled and finished world, but in one which is going on, and where our main task is prospective, and where retrospect – and all knowledge as distinct from thought is retrospect – is of value in the solidity, security, and fertility it affords our dealings with the future.
>
> *(Dewey, 1916, p. 151)*

For Dewey, the meaning of any event always remains a little beyond us, in the possible futures "it portends." This includes the past, which itself remains undetermined and to a certain extent unmoored, as it too awaits the meanings afforded it by the emerging vantage points of ongoing experience. Much like the two protagonists in Samuel Beckett's play *Waiting for Godot*, our past is always somewhat provisional, always waiting for the closure that will never come, yet in the meantime getting on as best it can.

Yet, much like Godot, the future is not a complete stranger to us, as getting on in the world entails imagining worlds that have not yet been but yet might be, worlds our concerted actions aim to bring into being. The past and future are, as Lissa Malkki (2000) argues, "only different chapters of the same narrative story, informing and justifying one another" (p. 328). What brings them together into a temporal whole is our ability to narratively imagine our lives from many different temporal vantage points. While Dewey does not think of experience narratively, he does emphasize that human time is fluid, as we travel prospectively into possible futures and retrospectively back into possible pasts. The reconstruction of experience involves the reconsideration of not only what happened but also a concurrent reconsideration of what might yet happen, all set within situations that are still happening.

As we have yet to find a way off of the ever-shifting and peaty grounds of human experience we, as narrative inquirers, look for a different sort of terra firma, one much more provisional, prospective and tentative. We play with Jerome Bruner's (2002) notion of narrative as subjuntivizing experience as a way to think about the end game of narrative inquiry:

> Through narrative, we construct, reconstruct, and in some ways reinvent yesterday and tomorrow. Memory and imagination fuse in the process. Even when we create the possible worlds of fiction, we do not desert the familiar but subjuntivize it into what might have been and what might be. The human mind, however cultivated its memory or refined its recording systems, can never fully and faithfully recapture the past, but neither can it escape it. Memory and imagination supply and consume each other's wares.
>
> *(p. 93)*

We would add that for us this is true not only of fiction but also of human experience, as stories lived and told, which is always in the midst of an unfolding life. Narrative inquirers less try to drain the "swamp" of experience though a systematic analysis of particular aspects of situations than try to make its muddiness, if anything, even more generative in the sense of opening up possibilities for it to be otherwise, for different stories to be lived and told.

Conclusion as invitation

We hope the story of our journey through the intersections, overlaps and tensions between narrative inquiry and reflective inquiry will be, in some way, as generative for readers as the journey has been for us. We leave it here, for now, knowing that we have neither fully traversed nor definitively mapped the common and uncommon grounds of these two forms of inquiry. Indeed, we may have, with our stories and metaphors, made the grounds more muddled than demarcated. Our inability to draw sharp distinctions or boundaries is less an unintended shortcoming than an intentional stopping short, as, for us, going further would begin to feel like draining the metaphoric swamp of our experience of what it holds best – possibility.

As we reflect on our journey, we now see the terrain we trudged, and particularly places we bogged down, not as *the* but rather *one* way of traversing the intersections, overlaps and tensions between narrative inquiry and reflective inquiry. We understand the product of this wandering as less a map than a story, one meant to invite others in to these wonders.

Epilogue

Our stories in their retellings and reliving continue, as we continue to narratively inquire into them. As we inquired into Jean's story she began to see threads emerging from, and woven into, her ongoing passion for understanding how curriculum can be re-imagined as a curriculum of lives, a way of conceptualizing curriculum-making with children's and teachers' lives at the heart. But narrative inquiry offers both forward and backward looking stories, backward looking stories that allow Jean to see these interwoven narrative trends but also forward thinking stories that take up these re-imagined shifting stories as ways of living in the world. Without knowing with certainty which of these multiple possible stories might be called forth by new situations, Aiden sees students' responses as calls for him to live differently in relation to each student, attending more closely to what matters in the space between him and a student.

References

Appiah, A. (2006). *Cosmopolitanism: Ethics in a world of strangers* (1st ed.). New York: W.W. Norton.

Bateson, M. C. (1994). *Peripheral visions: Learning along the way* (1st ed.). New York: HarperCollins.

Bruner, J. S. (2002). *Making stories: Law, literature, life* (1st ed.). New York: Farrar, Straus and Giroux.

Clandinin, D. J., & Connelly, F. M. (1990). Stories of experience and narrative inquiry. *Educational Researcher, 19*(5), 2–14.

Clandinin, D. J., & Connelly, F. M. (2000). *Narrative inquiry: Experience and story in qualitative research*. San Francisco, CA: Jossey-Bass.

De Certeau, M. (1984). *The practice of everyday life*. Berkeley, CA: University of California Press

Dewey, J. (1902). *The child and the curriculum*. Chicago, IL: University of Chicago Press.

Dewey, J. (1910). *How we think*. New York: Heath and Company.

Dewey, J. (1916). *Democracy and education: An introduction to the philosophy of education*. New York: The Macmillan Company.

Dewey, J. (1938). *Experience and education*. New York: Collier Books, Macmillan.

Granger, D. A. (2006). *John Dewey, Robert Pirsig, and the art of living: Revisioning aesthetic education* (1st ed.). New York: Palgrave Macmillan.

Greene, M. (1995). *Releasing the imagination: Essays on education, the arts, and social change*. San Francisco, CA: Jossey-Bass Publishers.

Hoffman, E. (1994, January 23). Let memory speak. *The New York Times Book Review*, pp. 1–4.

Jackson, P. W. (1998). *John Dewey and the lessons of art*. New York: Yale University Press.

Lyons, N. (2002). The personal self in a public story: The portfolio presentation narrative. In N. Lyons & V. K. LaBoskey (Eds.), *Narrative inquiry in practice: Advancing the knowledge of teaching* (pp. 87–100). New York: Teachers College Press.

Malkki, L. H. (2000). Figures of the future. In D. Holland & J. Lave (Eds.), *History in person: Enduring struggles, contentious practice, intimate identities* (pp. 325–348). Santa Fe, NM: School of American Research Press.

Marx, K. (1964). *Economic and philosophic manuscripts of 1844* (1st American ed.). New York: International Publishers.

Rodgers, C. (2002). Defining reflection: Another look at John Dewey and reflective thinking. *Teachers College Record, 104*(4), 842–866.

Schön, D. A. (1983). *The reflective practitioner: How professionals think in action*. New York: Basic Books.

Schön, D. A. (1992). A theory of inquiry: Dewey's legacy to education. *Curriculum Inquiry, 22*(2), 119–139.

Schön, D. A. (1995). The new scholarship requires a new epistemology. *Change, 27*(6), 27–34.

SECTION III

Journeying with narrative ideas of curriculum making

Coming alongside teachers, children and families

9

NARRATIVE UNDERSTANDINGS OF LIVES IN SCHOOL

In the paper I share with you tonight I sketch a kind of narrative overview of the research program I have been involved with over the past 20 years or so. In so doing I compose a narrative thread that connects what has come before with current work I am engaged in with a group of graduate students, teachers, children, parents and administrators in one school. I begin with my work in a school in Toronto, Bay Street School, in 1981 and end with another school in Edmonton, Ravine Elementary, in 2004. I pick up on moments and tensions that connect these diverse projects with what I am trying to understand about lives in school. My purpose is to show the need for more multilayered, multivocalic research in curriculum studies made possible within a narrative view of curriculum. However, as a kind of prologue, I give a very personal account of how I saw the landscape, the research context in curriculum studies, in which I began.

When I began my doctoral work in the late 1970's at the Ontario Institute for Studies in Education, University of Toronto, it was at an exciting time. Michael Connelly and Freema Elbaz had just begun their work on teacher knowledge. Their ideas of teacher knowledge bubbled out of what was then a fairly new field, that is, the field of teacher thinking. I was a brand new doctoral student, but as a former teacher and school counselor, I found the discourse of teacher thinking refreshing.

As a fledgling curriculum theorist, I was concerned about how much research being done focused on implementation of curricular reforms. While I recognized how one could see teachers as the ones who failed to implement school reforms and new school policies when school change did not happen as planned, I wondered how teachers would give an account of what happened. These abstract teachers I was meeting in the literature were supposed to be the generalized representations of the people I had just left in school. I wondered if teachers' practices did shift, just not in the ways that reformers planned. I wondered what teachers would say about those curricular reforms and how they interacted with their ongoing practices. What if researchers took a different view, I wondered, not one that constructed teachers as deficit "other" in the way the curriculum implementation and development literature was doing?

Clandinin, D. J. (2009). Narrative understandings of lives in school. In A. Pitt (Ed.), *Keynotes in teacher education: CATE invited addresses* (pp. 11–20). Ottawa, Ontario: Canadian Association of Teacher Education.

I knew teachers were knowing people who made choices and decisions that seemed appropriate to their understandings of the children and youth with whom they worked, to the contexts in which they worked and to the subject matter they were teaching. I worried about how teachers were portrayed in the curriculum implementation and reform literature. I began to wonder if I could become a curriculum theorist after all.

I was just as troubled, however, by how teachers were being portrayed in a very different literature, a literature I will call the critical theory research literature. Michael Apple's (1971) research on what he termed the hidden curriculum was all the talk around my graduate study hallways. In much of that work that I loosely grouped together, teachers were also seen as not knowing, as not understanding the complex issues of race, class and gender and as mindlessly reproducing social structures (Anyon, 1981; Popkewitz, 1977). This, too, was deeply troubling to me. While I found the ideas compelling and even a bit seductive, I realized that in none of the discourses did teachers appear as the hard working, thoughtful people with whom I had shared my school life. I told a story of myself as a wide-awake teacher and yet I could recognize some of my practices in some of the critical theory discourse. I knew that literature was helpful to me in reconsidering what I knew about teaching. However, in this literature, I still felt teachers were constructed as deficit "other," as not being quite "good enough." I was having difficulty finding a place where I could continue to name myself as a teacher and to maintain respectful relationships with former teacher colleagues. I wondered if there was a way to understand teachers within curriculum research that was more respectful of the lives teachers were composing within the contexts in which they lived and worked.

The research on teacher thinking (Clark & Yinger, 1977) with its focus on the ways that teachers made decisions and with an underlying assumption that teachers thought before they acted seemed a first opening for me. But these ideas that teachers thought, that we should attend to teacher cognition, did not go quite far enough. The work on teacher knowledge (Connelly & Elbaz, 1980) gave an even more expansive starting point. Now I saw a way to engage in research that began with a view that teachers were knowing people, that they held knowledge born of their experience, reflected upon and expressed in their practices. It was an exciting break from what had been evident in research on teaching and in curriculum research.

As I began to understand what it meant to be a curriculum theorist, I positioned myself in a tradition of curriculum research grounded in John Dewey's (1938) ideas of experience and in Joseph Schwab's (1970) ideas of curriculum. It was Schwab's influence that led Michael Connelly and me to write of four curriculum commonplaces, that is, teacher, learner, subject matter and milieu. In a 1988 description of the curriculum commonplaces, we wrote

> The commonplaces are a set of factors or determinants that occur in statements about the aims, content and methods of the curriculum. Taken as a whole they serve to bound the set of statements identified as being curricular. They comprise the simplest model for looking at curricular problems.
>
> *(Connelly & Clandinin, 1988, p. 84)*

We described some characteristics of the commonplaces in the following way: one, "they are commonplace in the usual sense of the word, i.e., they appear and reappear in curricular statements. We cannot escape them. An adequate curriculum statement must say something about each of them"; two, "many arguments tend to focus on a single commonplace. If so the role played by the others will be, in part, determined by the focal commonplace" (e.g. if organized knowledge is the focus, then the learner may be treated largely as a receptacle', the teacher as a dispenser and the milieu as the housing for the old knowledge and the accumulator of the new); three, "there are a number of different possible foci within a single commonplace (e.g. learner as an inquirer, learner as a social organism, learner as a recording machine) (Connelly & Clandinin, 1988). Establishing this way of looking at curriculum, that is, in terms of the four commonplaces, we acknowledged our starting point as with the curriculum commonplace, teacher. We worked from

> a Deweyan view of the curriculum from a teacher's vantage point (Clandinin, 1986; Connelly & Clandinin, 1988). Dewey's (1938) notion of "situation" and "experience" enabled us to imagine the teacher not so much as a maker of curriculum but as a part of it and to imagine a place for context, culture (Dewey's notion of interaction), and temporality (both past and future contained in Dewey's notion of "continuity").
>
> *(Clandinin & Connelly, 1992, p. 365)*

Further we wrote,

> teachers and students live out a curriculum; teachers do not transmit, implement, or teach a curriculum and objectives; nor are they and their students carried forward in their work and studies by a curriculum of textbooks and content, instructional methodologies, and intentions. An account of teachers' and students' lives over time is the curriculum, although intentionality, objectives, and curriculum materials do play a part in it.
>
> *(Clandinin & Connelly, 1992, p. 365)*

This way of thinking about curricular situations became the way I thought about my work in teacher education, both preservice and in-service. But it also became a way of thinking about the research I was doing for I wanted the research I did to be profoundly curricular research. Thinking about curriculum making in classrooms and schools was an important way for me to connect what I was doing in the university and in my research with my colleagues and other practitioners in schools, colleagues with whom I wanted to maintain relationships and alongside of whom I hoped to make a difference in the ways they and I were able to compose their and my lives in school.

This, then, was the beginning point of learning to live and tell a story of myself as a researcher, of beginning to engage the difficult questions of understanding teachers' lives in classrooms as connected not only to their experiential knowledge, what we have come to call their personal practical knowledge (Connelly & Clandinin, 1988; Clandinin, 1986) but also to their professional knowledge landscapes (Clandinin & Connelly, 1995). As I engaged in research, I continued to see the research I did as curriculum research even as many traditions in curriculum research moved farther and farther from teachers' and children's lives in school or became more and more subject matter specific.

When I began my doctoral research I lived alongside one teacher, Stephanie. In the context of a larger project, we were interested in the reform context in which Stephanie and others in her school were living and working. In the larger study we asked what happened to teachers' knowledge, to their practices, when a new policy was being heavily implemented in their school. My doctoral research focused on Stephanie, a primary school teacher and her knowledge. I studied her knowledge as it was expressed in her practices. In order to understand how her knowledge was held, Michael Connelly and I came to terms such as image (Clandinin, 1986), rhythms (Clandinin & Connelly, 1986b), metaphors (Connelly & Clandinin, 1988), and narrative unities (Connelly & Clandinin, 1986a) as ways to give an account of her knowledge and, perhaps, as a way to talk about teacher knowledge more generally. We defined personal practical knowledge as:

> a term designed to capture the idea of experience in a way that allows us to talk about teachers as knowledgeable and knowing persons. . . . Personal practical knowledge . . . is in the person's past experience, in the person's present mind and body, and in the person's future plans and actions . . . It is seen and found 'in our practices'. It is a particular way of reconstructing the past and the intentions for the future to deal with exigencies of a present situation.
>
> *(Connelly & Clandinin, 1988, p. 25)*

Returning to the curriculum commonplaces, my initial curriculum research focus was on teachers with students as learners, subject matter and milieu forming an interactive backdrop. Of course, teachers such as Stephanie were also seen as learners in this view. Students as learners were seen as co-composers of their lives within milieus that were understood as evolving, shifting, moral, epistemological contexts, shaping and shaped by teachers, children, administrators, parents and larger social, cultural and institutional contexts. We came to define these contexts in which teachers lived using a landscape metaphor as professional knowledge landscapes.

> A landscape metaphor is particularly well suited to our purpose. It allows us to talk about space, place, and time. Furthermore, it has a sense of expansiveness and the possibility of being filled with diverse people, things, and events in different relationships. Understanding professional knowledge as comprising a landscape calls for a notion of professional as composed of a wide variety of people, places and things. Because we see the professional knowledge landscape as composed of relationships among people, places, and things, we see it both as an intellectual and a moral landscape.
>
> *(Clandinin & Connelly, 1995, pp. 4–5)*

Of course, I continued to focus, in further research on beginning teachers' knowledge, on how teachers came to have personal practical knowledge, on how school contexts interpreted in terms of a professional knowledge landscape came to shape teachers' knowledge, on how teachers' identities, their stories to live by (Connelly & Clandinin, 1999), shaped and were shaped by their positions on different professional knowledge landscapes.

Tonight, however, I return to the field texts or data (Clandinin & Connelly, 2000) from my research with Stephanie at Bay Street to help develop an understanding of curriculum puzzles that were apparent in that first study but, for a number of reasons, some of them methodological, I could not yet study. My argument, in brief, is that what I first became aware of in Stephanie's classroom was the bumping up of children's life experiences with the dominant stories of school and with my own storied life experiences as I worked as participant researcher alongside Stephanie. In curricular terms, I was aware, in that first study, of the need to study the moments of intersection between children's experiences and teachers' experiences as curricular moments.

I return with you to that first classroom, Stephanie's primary school classroom at Bay Street School, where I spent more than a year living in relationship with Stephanie and the children. Her classroom was an inner city classroom in multicultural Toronto. Her students were children of many cultures, ethnicities, first languages and religions. The students and their families came from homes classified as in the lower socioeconomic range. Many were from families in transition, families engaged in kinds of nomadic searching for home places as they came from refugee camps, other countries, other places in Toronto and Canada.

I was new to Toronto, new to teaching classes with such a range of cultural backgrounds and such a diversity of religions. I was familiar with children living in poverty, but the children from the refugee camps seeking havens in Canada were a new phenomenon for me. I was not accustomed to the inner city of a huge city like Toronto. It made Edmonton where I had been teaching seem small and uncrowded. My early life was spent on a farm with space and quiet to spread out. I knew acres of farmland, small groves of trees, running creeks and prairie skies. But I had come to know urban life in Edmonton as I studied and later taught there. I was, however, just awakening to an understanding of the Christian emphasis in our schools and how Christian holidays shaped school holidays and some school activities. I was new to discussions of Festivals of Light and what it meant to live alongside children of multiple faiths and religions such as Judaism, Buddhism and Islam.

When I return now to my field notes, I see that I was in a space of wonder. My field notes are filled with wonders about children who had not known the experience of planting and growing seeds in soil because their world was a concrete one. My field notes are filled with notes about the many languages children spoke in the hallways and in the playgrounds. I wondered at their lives composed within the noises of sirens, traffic, and street cars, crowded apartment homes and rows of townhouses and older houses jammed into crowded spaces.

At one point I wondered if I could characterize my experience as being in a kind of liminal space (Heilbrun, 1988; Kennedy, 2001) and in some ways I could. However, while I was new to the children's lives and new to what it meant to be a researcher in someone else's classroom, there was much that I recognized about life in Bay Street School. Stories of school were bred into my bones by this time in my life. I had been a student, teacher, counselor and psychologist in urban and rural Canadian schools. I knew in my bones the dominant story of school. And I knew how to compose a story of success within stories of school. While many of the storylines of the children's lives were unknown to me, the story of school was a felt known with its rhythms, cycles of teaching, assessing and reporting cycles, the physical structure of long corridors and isolated classrooms as separate box-like spaces with closed doors.

On my first day in Stephanie's classroom, April 21, 1981, I met Dimitra, a child of the Greek Orthodox faith, who was coming up to her Easter celebration; Michael had just arrived from Guatemala and was paired up with Dennis, a Spanish speaking child from Ecuador. Stephanie pointed these children out to me as she went about her classroom work, and we negotiated how I could be useful in the context of the ongoing classroom life. The next day, April 22, 1981, I listened in awe as the librarian worked with a class of students, only 4 of whom had been born in Canada. As I began to live alongside the children at Bay Street I found myself wondering who these children were, what their lives were like outside of school and what sense they were making in school.

At first I felt just wonder but soon I began to experience the places of bumping up as Stephanie asked me to teach. She wondered if I could plan and teach a science unit attentive to the changing seasons, something I later learned was an important rhythm in Stephanie's yearly curriculum planning. The choice was easy for me. In early May, 1981, I started an extensive planting unit, something I had experienced in Edmonton classrooms and something embodied in me as a child who had grown up on a farm attentive to the cycles of planting, growing and harvesting. While my notes of May 4 indicated "I was not sure how many seeds the children have actually looked at before" and on May 8 "I noted my impression that the students have not much contact with seeds and growing things," I did not stop in these curricular moments to attend to these as moments of tension. I kept on creating experiences that were comfortable for me and that fit within what I saw as the mandated curriculum of science. My focus was on fulfilling Stephanie's request for my involvement. Rereading my field notes I now know I was in a moment, a place of discontinuity (Carr, 1986) for many of the children.

On May 11, 1981, I wrote in my field notes

> I called the remaining three groups back to work with me. The children were very excited about what we were planting. A number of the students, particularly Sanish, enjoyed playing in the soil. He expressed amazement over finding pieces of root, stones, little pieces of wood in the soil. Denise, a little girl of African-Canadian heritage, dug up her bean seed and was very excited that it had started to grow. Shuk-Shan, a little girl of Chinese heritage, was the student I chose to water the bean plants first. We spent some time together learning how to water them.

And on May 25, 1981, I wrote

> Perhaps the most interesting event happened when I had table two at the back. Denise was having a good deal of difficulty settling down. She wanted more seeds so she could take them home. She didn't want to plant the seeds that I gave her. She dropped her seed and made a fuss about finding it again. She really wanted to take them home to show her mother. [My field notes do not show if I created that opportunity for her.]

The unit continued: the children and I planted bean seeds, measured their growth, recorded our findings in journal record books, wrote experience charts about what we were doing, read books, both fiction and non fiction, about plants, created a miniature garden in the sand box and worked on an integrated subject matter approach until mid-June. While my field notes illustrate the bumping up, the tensions between my stories to live by and theirs, I did not attend to the tensions. Neither did I attend to the children's lives. Their lives were not my research focus. My research focus was on how to understand and give an account of Stephanie's knowledge (Clandinin, 1986). In the research representations, the research texts, I attended to Stephanie's knowledge. Any accounts of the children were given through my account of Stephanie's knowledge. In terms of the curricular commonplaces, my attention was on the teacher commonplace. Learner, subject matter and milieu were understood from the vantage point of Stephanie, as teacher. But the living of the curriculum in the classroom was richly described in the field notes which were filled with children's experiences, integrated subject matter, a teacher, all nested within vibrant school, community and cultural milieus.

The children in Stephanie's Bay Street classroom live not only in the field texts but also in my memory. Those children awakened me not only to the diversity of children's lives but also to the complexity of attending narratively to curriculum in research. The silences I now see in the research texts are what bring me to the current research with which I am engaged with Shaun Murphy, Anne Murray Orr, Marni Pearce, Janice Huber, Vera Caine and Marilyn Huber.

In 1996 Michael and I began to attend more directly to the ways in which teachers' and children's lives intersect, into the ways that children shape teachers' stories to live by, their knowledge and their contexts at the same time as teachers' stories are shaped by children's stories (Connelly & Clandinin, 1999; Huber, Huber, & Clandinin, 2004). I realized as I framed that research that I was turning back on that early research in Stephanie's classroom, on those children of diversity who had so puzzled, amazed, captivated me.

In other research I listened to children's stories, but in that research again it seemed one-sided. I heard the children's stories, but the teachers' stories were silent. This time I wanted to stand alongside, amongst children, teachers and administrators to hear stories in a multivocalic kind of way, a kind of listening to the stories of many participants positioned differently on the landscape as stories being lived and told swirled, bumping, shifting, changing and evolving. Trying to attend to these curricular moments where the stories of children, families, teachers, administrators and stories of school intersect is difficult work. Writing theoretically about narrative understandings of curriculum seemed easy compared to trying to empirically study these curriculum moments. In what follows I detail only four of the methodological challenges we faced as a group of researchers attempting to do this work.

The first challenge is intricately involved with knowing that narrative inquiry is relational inquiry (Clandinin & Connelly, 2000; Connelly & Clandinin, in press; Huber & Clandinin, 2002). By that I mean that as narrative inquirers we enter into landscapes and attempt to negotiate ways of living alongside research participants. In the Bay Street work, I entered into Bay Street and negotiated ways to live alongside Stephanie, the primary school teacher in whose classroom I worked, as well as some other school staff members. My main relationship was with Stephanie, and it was through my involvement with her that I came to live in the classroom. My relationships with the children and families were mediated by my relationship with her. However, in this new work we wanted to negotiate relationships that allowed us to live alongside teachers, administrators, children and families and to hear their stories in their own terms, following their own plotlines. Each researcher tried to position him/herself so we could hear, for example, the stories of a teacher and administrator or a teacher and several children or a teacher, several children and some family members. This involved the negotiation of multiple relationships that evolved over time.

A second challenge involved the need to negotiate thoughtfully ways to enter into the midst of an ongoing story of school and to learn to stand alongside multiple people as they lived their lives. As we begin to work alongside participants we need to understand that individuals are also in the midst of their lives. Participants' lives do not begin when we, as researchers, arrive nor do they end when we leave. As we entered into those spaces, we needed to attend thoughtfully to who we were in those relationships and to how we might shape the lives that were being composed alongside of us. We also needed to attend thoughtfully to how we would move away from those lives at the end of the study. Because we knew that we would be in fairly intensive relationships for at least one year and, as it has worked out, we have been in these relationships for more than two years now, we needed to attend to how we were shaping the lives both by our presence and by our imagined absence from those lives.

A third challenge was learning to live with a skin-tingling kind of awareness to all that was happening. When Maxine Greene (1995) writes of wide awakeness, it was this kind of wide awakeness that needed to live within and among us. As a group of researchers we all knew a story of school and we all had a deeply felt embodied sense of school. We knew it was possible that we would "sleep through," that is, be inattentive to, the tensions that might seep through the ongoing stories to live by as they were lived out in schools. As you will see below we employed diverse methods to compose field texts with participants in order to allow us to hear and see and feel the tensions as children's, families', teachers', administrators' and our storied lives bumped against one another and against institutional, social and cultural stories. In addition to working with a range of field texts, we also worked closely with each other. For the 2002–2004 study in Ravine Elementary we were there as a group, working alongside each other and those in the school. As a research group we came together often to share stories, transcripts, field notes and other field texts and to respond to each other's stories. In that way we stayed awake to possible moments and places of tension.

A fourth methodological challenge was imagining kinds of field texts that would allow us to attend closely to children's, families' and teachers' stories to live by. I will outline three ways we composed field texts in addition to the field notes of classroom, school and home participation, taped conversations with small groups, individual teachers, children and administrators and our own research journals and writing.

Anne Murray Orr (in progress) created an innovative approach of working alongside small groups of children reading children's literature with them. Her intent was to use the children's literature to create spaces for the children to share their stories to live by. Her research, situated in the context of a grade one/two classroom, is still a work in progress as she is in the midst of writing about their work together. Working from her relational knowing of children in the classroom, she carefully selected literature that would draw out their stories. Attending to the children's lives in the classroom, she watched their friendships, their writing, their talk and, based on what she imagined would be a narrative thread in an unfolding life, she chose books to share with children in small groups, books such as *A Gift for Gita* for a girl of Pakistani heritage, *Red Parka Mary* for a girl of Aboriginal heritage and so on, opened up conversations and spaces for the sharing of life stories.

Shaun Murphy (2004), working with a group of grade 5/6 students, developed several ways to come to hear the students' stories as they intersected with their teacher's stories of them. One of them involved the use of students' report cards. In this classroom, as in classrooms all over Canada, report cards are written three or four times a year. As Debbie Schroeder (1996) so eloquently wrote "report cards are a teacher's way of giving back student stories and are powerful in shaping children's stories to live by."

Shaun used the occasion of report cards both as an opportunity for the grade 5/6 students to tell what story they heard/read of them in their report cards but also to create a space for them to retell their teacher's story of them. After the November report cards were sent home to parents and conferences were held, Shaun and Lian, the classroom teacher, returned the children's report cards and asked them to create found poetry from the words in their report cards. Found poetry is an arts-based research process written about by Lynn Butler-Kisber (2002) and Laurel Richardson

(1994). The process of composing found poetry involves working with transcripts and other written texts to pull out key or meaningful words to create an interpretive reading of the text, a reading that is both poetic and deeply meaningful to the person creating the text. It was this process of creating found poetry of their report cards that Shaun and Lian engaged in with the children. In creating this space for the students, Shaun was able to hear the children's stories to live by as they tried to come to a narrative coherence of who they were with the story that their teacher told of them. As with Anne, much more of this work will be found in their dissertations (Murphy, 2004; Murray-Orr, in progress).

The third approach to composing field texts that allowed us to study this moment/place of intersection was created by Vera Caine. In her master's work (Caine, 2002), Vera worked with young women of aboriginal heritage who were HIV/AIDS positive and who lived in an urban centre away from their home communities. Vera gave each young woman a camera and asked her to engage in a visual narrative inquiry (Bach, 1998) with her, composing photographs of their lives and telling their stories over a year or more long study. Vera wanted to continue her work with the use of visual narrative inquiry and to use photographs as a way to compose field texts with children similar to the work of Wendy Ewald (2001).

Vera joined our research group and came to work with a special needs classroom at Ravine Elementary, a classroom with 14 boys. They worked with one teacher, Kristi. The classroom was engaged in the study of a provincially mandated social studies unit on community during the time that Vera was first involved in the classroom. At first, Vera did preliminary camera work with the children. With the support of the research project she provided each child with a camera and black and white film. Their task was to take photographs of community. After the photographs were developed Vera heard each child's stories of the photographs, including details about their purposes for taking them and how they connected to their understandings of community.

Tonight, I focus on one child, a child of aboriginal heritage, a child I call Josh. I had a particular interest in Vera's work with visual narrative inquiry and often stopped down to speak with Kristi, Vera and/or the children in the classroom when I was in the school. As soon as I knew the children's photographs of community were back from the developers, I stopped down to speak with Kristi and to ask to see the children's photographs. I asked to see Josh's. Kristi initially told me she thought Josh had not understood the task. In her words "He must just have taken pictures of the first things he saw." Kristi's sense was that Josh had misunderstood the meaning of the task as he did not understand he was to take photographs of community. For Kristi, as detailed in the mandated curriculum, community is seen in terms of interdependence, in terms of goods and services. Some of the children in the classroom took photographs of schools, churches, supermarkets, gas stations. For Kristi, these children had understood the photography assignment as well as the concept of community. Josh, she thought, had not.

However, as I looked at Josh's photographs, I sensed he *had* understood the task and that in these photographs we could learn much about Josh's story to live by, his story of community and the rubbing points between his story and the teacher's story to live by. One photograph particularly stands out in my memory. It was a photograph of three guitars leaning against a sofa. The photograph was carefully composed and was a striking example of photography. I felt the sense of aesthetic composition and the care that had gone into the photograph design. He had understood what Vera had been teaching about photographs. But I knew there was more at work here.

I knew we were about to learn something of the bumping up places between stories of school and our dominant stories of community with Josh's story to live by in his community.

When Vera and he sat down to talk about the photographs, he spoke of the three guitars as being a community because "one belonged to my dad, one to my uncle and one is mine, and sometimes we play together". There were, of course, other stories of the other photographs, but this one serves as a marker of a moment when we see the interaction of a child, a learner, with his teacher, also a learner, with the subject matter of community as part of a social studies unit all within the nested milieus of classroom, school, cultures and social narratives.

It is moments such as this one that we need to study as curricular moments if we are to understand what it means to compose lives in schools. When children of diversity come to our schools living their life stories, it is such moments that teach us all how to be attentive to what we are doing in these educative or miseducative places we call school. As we are asking in our current study, are schools interrupting children's and teachers' stories to live by? Are their stories to live by interrupted for educative or miseducative reasons? It is in trying to understand educative moments revealed in a photograph of three guitars that perhaps we can begin to understand.

In summary I want to come back to where I began. As I looked back over these more than twenty years as a curriculum researcher I realize that I am just now being able to engage in some of the most pressing curriculum research, research that attends to those moments of interaction among the four curriculum commonplaces as they intersect in the lives of the children, teachers, administrators and families in our Canadian schools. In 1988 we wrote:

> [W]ith the narrative perspective, we understand the child's education in terms of the child's and the teacher's dominant narratives embedded within cultural and historical narratives. The child's education, for instance, is seen in terms of his or her personal narrative and of the meaning this conveys of his or his learning experiences in a particular classroom. The child's education is seen temporally in terms of past, present, and future.
>
> *(Connelly & Clandinin, 1988, p. 111)*

My hope is that this current research offers a way to begin to engage these questions about the lived curriculum in our schools where diverse children and families lives are shaped.

References

Anyon, J. (1981). Social class and school knowledge. *Curriculum Inquiry, 11*(1), 3–41.

Apple, M. (1971). The hidden curriculum and the nature of conflict. *Interchange, 11*(4), 27–40.

Bach, H. (1998). *A visual narrative concerning curriculum, girls, photography, etc.* Edmonton, Alberta: Qualitative Institute Press.

Butler-Kisber, L. (2002). Artful portrayals in qualitative inquiry: The road to found poetry and beyond. *Alberta Journal of Educational Research, 48*(3), 229–239.

Caine, V. (2002). *Storied moments: A visual narrative inquiry of aboriginal women living with HIV.* Unpublished Master's Thesis, University of Alberta, Edmonton, Canada.

Carr, D. (1986). *Time, narrative and history.* Bloomington, IN: Indiana University Press.

Clandinin, D. J. (1986). *Classroom practice: Teacher images in action.* London: Falmer Press.

Clandinin, D. J., & Connelly, F. M. (1986a). The reflective practitioner and practitioners' narrative unities. *Canadian Journal of Education, 11*(2), 184–198.

Clandinin, D. J., & Connelly, F. M. (1986b). Rhythms in teaching: The narrative study of teachers' personal practical knowledge of classrooms. *Teaching and Teacher Education, 2*(4), 377–387.

Clandinin, D. J., & Connelly, F. M. (1992). The teacher as curriculum maker. In P. Jackson (Ed.), *Handbook of Research on Curriculum* (pp. 363–401). American Educational Research Association. New York: Macmillan Press.

Clandinin, D. J., & Connelly, F. M. (1995). *Teachers' professional knowledge landscapes.* New York: Teachers College Press.

Clandinin, D. J., & Connelly, F. M. (2000). *Narrative inquiry: Experience and story in qualitative research.* San Francisco, CA: Jossey-Bass.

Clark, C. M., & Yinger, R. J. (1977). Research on teacher thinking. *Curriculum Inquiry, 7*(4), 279–304.

Connelly, F. M., & Clandinin, D. J. (1986). The reflective practitioner and practitioners' narrative unities. *Canadian Journal of Education, 11*(2), 184–198.

Connelly, F. M., & Clandinin, D. J. (1988). *Teachers as curriculum planners: Narratives of experience.* New York: Teachers College Press.

Connelly, F. M., & Clandinin, D. J. (1999). *Shaping a professional identity: Stories of educational practice.* New York: Teachers College Press.

Connelly, F. M., & Elbaz, F. (1980). Conceptual bases for curriculum thought: A teacher's perspective. In A. W. Foshay (Ed.), *Considered action for curriculum improvement: ASCD Yearbook* (pp. 95–119). Alexandria, VA: ASCD.

Dewey, J. (1938). *Experience and education.* New York: Collier Books.

Ewald, W. (2001). *I wanna take me a picture.* New York: Beacon Press.

Greene, M. (1995). *Releasing the imagination: Essays on education, the arts, and social change.* San Francisco, CA: Jossey-Bass Publishers.

Heilbrun, C. (1988). *Writing a women's life.* New York: Norton.

Huber, J., & Clandinin, D. J. (2002). Ethical dilemmas in relational narrative inquiry with children. *Qualitative Inquiry, 8*(6), 785–803.

Huber, J., Huber, M., & Clandinin, D. J. (2004). Moments of tension: Resistance as expressions of narrative coherence in stories to live by. *Reflective Practice, 5*(2), 181–198.

Kennedy, M. (2001). *Race matters in the life/work of four, white, female teachers.* Unpublished Doctoral Dissertation, University of Alberta, Edmonton, Canada.

Murphy, M. S. (2004). *Understanding children's knowledge: A narrative inquiry into school experiences.* Unpublished Doctoral Dissertation, University of Alberta, Edmonton, Canada.

Murray Orr, A. (in progress). *Stories to live by: Book conversations as spaces for attending to children's lives in school.* Unpublished Doctoral Dissertation, University of Alberta, Edmonton, Canada.

Popkewitz, T. S. (1977). The latent values of the discipline centered curriculum. *Theory and Research in Social Education, 5*(1), 24–40.

Richardson, L. (1994). Writing: A method of inquiry. In N. K. Denzin, & Y. S. Lincoln (Eds.), *Handbook of qualitative research* (pp. 516–529). Thousand Oaks, CA: Sage.

Schroeder, D. (1996). *Reclaiming our teaching lives: The curriculum of middle space.* Unpublished Doctoral Dissertation, University of Alberta, Edmonton, Canada.

Schwab, J. J. (1970). *The practical: A language for curriculum.* Washington, DC: National Education Association, Center for the Study of Instruction [Reprinted in Westbury & Wilkoff, *Science, curriculum, and liberal education: Selected essays.* Chicago: University of Chicago Press, 1978].

10

THE INTERWOVEN STORIES OF TEACHERS, FAMILIES, AND CHILDREN IN CURRICULUM MAKING

Simmee Chung and D. Jean Clandinin

> Human lives are not pieces of string that can be separated out from a knot of others and laid out straight. Families are webs. Impossible to touch one part of it without seeing the rest vibrating. Impossible to understand one part without having the sense of the whole.
>
> *(Diane Setterfield,* The Thirteenth Tale, *p. 59)*

Setterfield's quotation calls us to consider the complex interconnections when lives meet or become interwoven. As teachers and researchers in schools, we see our lives and our families' lives as interwoven with the lives of our students and their families, as well as other teachers and administrators. These intertwined and fluid sets of lives seem to ripple and shift as they bump against social, cultural and institutional narratives. Setterfield's words illuminate a frame for this narrative inquiry of how curriculum can reflect the lives of all those it affects.

We began this narrative inquiry (Clandinin et al., 2006) with research puzzles around children's experiences both in and out of school. As we attended to children's lives we necessarily attended to the stories they lived and told (Clandinin & Connelly, 1992). We wondered about how teachers experienced making curriculum attentive to the diverse lives of children within achievement - focused stories of school.

During our inquiry, we became aware of some of our assumptions about the lives of children and their families. We became attentive to the gaps and silences in children's and families' "lived" and "told" stories of school as they bumped against our teacher stories (Clandinin et al., 2006). Considering ourselves in relation with children and families helped us see how they often experienced school and classroom landscapes as places of tension.

In this chapter we focus our research on one child, newly arrived to Canada, and her mother's lived and told stories. We consider how these stories shaped in-classroom curriculum making as well as how the in-classroom curriculum making

Reprinted with permission from Teachers College, Columbia University. Acknowledgement; Clandinin, D. J., & Chung, S. (2010). The interwoven stories of teachers, families and children in curriculum making. In M. Miller Marsh & T. Turner-Vorbeck (Eds.), *(Mis)understanding families: Learning from real families in our schools* (pp. 179–195). New York, NY: Teachers College Press.

shaped the lives of this child and her mother. The elementary school in which the study was undertaken was in an urban, upper middle-class community composed of children from multicultural backgrounds. In the 2006-07 school year we lived our lives alongside children from a Grade-3 classroom, a year when the children have their first set of provincially mandated standardized tests.

Our research puzzles became a journey of unknowing and knowing (Vinz, 1997) through which we became aware of the need to consider the diverse voices and lives of families, too often absent in schools. Vinz (1997) suggests the practice of "shifting valances of dispositioning" (p. 145) in which educators move between "unknowing, giving up present understandings (positions) of our teaching, to not knowing" to acknowledge ambiguity and uncertainty (p. 139). Vinz's concept of dispositioning became important to us as we were dispositioned from attending to "planned" curriculum, attending that blurred our vision of the "living" curriculum (Clandinin & Connelly, 1992; Aoki, 1993). We wondered how children's and families' stories were given space in curriculum making in schools.

In our view, we are a "living" curriculum, not a curriculum laid out by mandates and plans, but rather one composed of lived and told experiences. This view of curriculum, as composed of children's and teachers' lives, allows us to notice complexities that are not otherwise visible as they meet in the nested milieu of classrooms, schools, and communities around particular subject matters.

If children and teachers are cocomposing curricula of lives in schools and classrooms, in what ways does the story of each child's family become part of this cocomposition? By listening more closely to each child's and each family's lived and told stories, might we better understand the tensions children and families experience in curriculum making? Our work is situated with Clandinin and Connelly's (1995) understanding of school landscapes that include both in-classroom and out-of-classroom places. We imagine landscapes, not as static sites in which people's "stories to live by" (Connelly & Clandinin, 1999)—their identities—are fixed, but rather as temporal places that shape and are reshaped by those who live within them.

Vibrations on the Family Web: A Narrative Inquiry Methodology

Entomologists tell us that a spider feels every vibration on its web (Mason, 1999). Revisiting Setterfield's metaphor, we imagine a child and their family as a web, and we realize that when we touch one part of a child's life, we set off vibrations in the rest of the family. By the same token, when the family touches its child, the child's life vibrates into classroom curriculum making. In this view, we see the place of families in curriculum making in new ways.

Too often when we think of curriculum making, we think about only the visible lives of the children and the teacher. Setterfield's notion of family webs help us think about what is invisible. Could it be that even though we do not usually know about families' stories, they create vibrations in our classroom curriculum making? We wonder if, like a spider, a child feels every spiraling vibration from her family web, then conversely, do the vibrations that bounce off a child shake the family web to its core? By being attentive to our unfolding, narrative inquiry research puzzles, we became aware of the importance of seeking out and listening more closely to not only children's and teachers' stories, but to families' stories as well.

Clandinin and Connelly (2000) describe narrative inquiry in terms of a three-dimensional inquiry space with dimensions of sociality, temporality, and place.

By inward, they mean toward the internal conditions, such as feelings, hopes, aesthetic reactions, and moral dispositions. By outward, they mean toward the existential conditions, the environment. By backward and forward, they refer to temporality past, present, and future. Narrative inquiry consists of being in the field, writing field texts (data), and composing research texts. A variety of field texts were constructed and collected for this study: oral histories, memory-box items, photographs, student- and teacher-generated documents, transcripts of individual conversations with children, parents, and teachers, and field notes.

By considering family stories, we focus in on how one mother's lived and told stories shape her relationship with her child both in and out of the classroom and out of school altogether. Setterfield (2006) wrote, "I shall start at the beginning. Though of course the beginning is never where you think it is . . . Our lives at the start are not really our own, but only the continuation of someone else's story . . ." (pp. 58–59). Setterfield draws attention to how we are always in the midst of living and telling the stories of our lives and that our lives are always composed in relation to family and cultural stories. As we worked together in the move from field texts to research texts, we composed fragments of a child's story and her family stories as they vibrated against each other without clear beginnings or ends, but rather, as story fragments "lived and told". We selected six story fragments from our field texts to show how we have come to understand the ways that vibrations, as stories bump together, can touch the child's life, her family's life, the teacher's life, and other children's lives in the classroom.

Story Fragment 1: So Korean

As Simmee Chung engaged in conversation with Elizabeth's mother in the fall, 2006, Mrs. Han, who had begun to feel comfortable with telling stories to Simmee, told stories of Elizabeth as well as stories of her own uncertainties. Mrs. Han fiddled with her hands as she nervously told our translator, (Dr. Ji-Sook Yeom):

> I don't know if you want to listen to this story or not . . . Elizabeth had a bit of a problem with a friend in her classroom. This child gave Elizabeth a hard time on how she dresses, talks and how she behaves, all kinds of things.

The friend, also Korean, was born in Canada whereas Elizabeth immigrated to Canada. Mrs. Han described how Elizabeth went home crying that day as the other child told her that she "talked funny" and should not act "so Korean" but more like everyone else. Through telling the story, which had strained their family, Mrs. Han began to fill in gaps in Simmee's ways of knowing this family. Simmee realized Elizabeth was now dressing more like the other children. Rather than wearing her unique clothing from Korea, Elizabeth now wore clothing purchased locally. Intrigued by Elizabeth's new style choices, Simmee asked her why she wore her jeans with one pant leg rolled up. Elizabeth shrugged as she stated she did not know why, only that she had seen others wearing their pants like that. Simmee now understood why Elizabeth had given her a "cover" story—that is, a story that she composed and told to help her fit into dominant stories of school (Clandinin & Connelly, 1995).

Mrs. Han's voice was barely audible as she described how she confronted the other child's mother, who responded, "This is Canada, but same in Korea." The other child's mother explained that, similar to Korea, teachers and families see the children differently according to how much money the family has. She said people judge others by "how they dress", and said that she agreed with her daughter's advice to Elizabeth, as they, too, being Korean in a predominately affluent White community, were also learning to fit in. Her daughter was helping Elizabeth fit in. Still shaken, Mrs. Han wondered if her Korean friend was right. She asked Chung if this was true in Canada. For Elizabeth and her mother, Elizabeth's living curriculum was at the forefront.

What could have been overlooked or seen as small vibrations between her and her friend marked an important moment of tension for Elizabeth as she questioned who she was, and perhaps who she could be, while she negotiated her living curriculum alongside her peers. These vibrations gained momentum as they touched those she loved. Attending to the vibrations in these family stories, we began to see the threads that connect the two mother's stories. Elizabeth is told how to dress and behave in school by another child. She then tells her mother who speaks to the other child's mother. These family stories, in turn, vibrate forward to the children, and their stories of who they are. The children's stories vibrate onward, and shake the classroom's living curriculum.

If we look at children and families as part of their own family webs and as possibly threaded together with other children's families' webs, we imagine how strong these collective vibrations might be within families and between families. As we trace through the threads of stories, traveling forward and backward among a child's stories, her mother's stories, and the family stories of another mother and child, these vibrations become visible.

Story Fragment 2: A Bouquet of Flowers

It was the week of Thanksgiving when Elizabeth secretly handed Simmee a gift with a card attached. The card, with no words on the cover, was illustrated with a beautiful bouquet of flowers. Elizabeth shyly told Chung it was from her mother.

> Dear Teacher,
>
> I appreciate that you always look after my daughter, Elizabeth, with love. Since the first day of school she has enjoyed everything with pleasure. Because she has come to Canada not even a year ago. She would have some problems with English and with Canadian Culture. Please understand that and Elizabeth and I will do our best to help her to get along with it well. I always hope to see you at school someday, but due to my lack of English, my cares weigh heavily on my chest. I feel sorry that although I'd like to see you at school, my lack of English makes me worried. I wonder if Elizabeth doesn't bother you during classes.

When Simmee finished reading the card, Elizabeth explained how her mother had asked a Korean neighbor to translate and write this letter in English. Simmee began to understand how important it was for Mrs. Han to connect with her, the teacher, to share her fears and hopes for her daughter. Simmee found herself shifting backwards and forwards between the stories she had initially "told" of Elizabeth and her mother. Simmee was surprised to hear that Mrs. Han felt tension about who she and her daughter were on the school landscape. For Simmee this contradicted her story of seeing Mrs. Han on the first day of school. Before dropping Elizabeth off in the classroom, she smiled at Simmee and they bowed politely to one another.

Now Mrs. Han's words on the card interrupted Simmee's first stories of Elizabeth as she began to wonder more deeply about the other stories Elizabeth and her mother lived by.

Simmee felt compelled to respond to Mrs. Han, a mother who cared so deeply about her child. She realized Mrs. Han wanted to be visible in composing the classroom curriculum.

> Dearest Mrs. Han,
>
> I am so touched by your words and acts of kindness. You are too generous and do not need to give me anything as the best gift is having Elizabeth in my class. Elizabeth is doing so well in grade three, you do not need to worry about her. Elizabeth is an excellent student. She is loving, helpful, hardworking, and kind. I could not ask for a more thoughtful student as Elizabeth always puts a smile on my face. I wish I could speak Korean because you are so lovely. Thank you again for your gift. Have a wonderful Thanksgiving and Chusok day. Elizabeth told us all about this special holiday.
>
> Always,
> Simmee

Story Fragment 3: Living a Presence of Being Korean

When Simmee first met Elizabeth, her thoughts were ones in which she admired Elizabeth's strength. Simmee recalled the first day of school when Elizabeth bounded into class holding her mother's hand. Elizabeth excitedly waved goodbye to her mother. Simmee was struck by how grown up Elizabeth was in a tailor-made coat covering a plaid dress. Simmee remembered commenting on her outfit and Elizabeth confidently responded that her outfit was from Korea, where she was from. As Simmee got to know her, she marveled at how she took the initiative to bring in various collections of Korean dictionaries and information books which complemented classroom resources. In the first month of school, Elizabeth even participated in a schoolwide writing task about traditions and wrote two pages about a special Korean moon festival called Chusok celebrated every October. She volunteered to read it aloud to her classmates.

Elizabeth explained to the class that she and her mother wrote it together. Her mother described the tradition and Elizabeth translated it in to English. Elizabeth told Simmee they wanted other people to learn about their Korean traditions. Simmee continued to be fascinated by what she saw as Elizabeth's courage. Once, on a field trip, Elizabeth offered Simmee a homemade Korean sushi roll that she brought as lunch. As they ate together, Simmee noticed other children staring at Elizabeth's lunch. Elizabeth munched happily on her seaweed snack and didn't seem to notice the stares. Simmee wondered how Elizabeth and she were so different for, when Simmee was a little girl, she hid her culture and heritage. She did not dare eat authentic "smelly" Chinese food at school, nor did she choose to share her heritage with her classmates.

During one art lesson as the children studied Van Gogh, Elizabeth brought in a Korean version of a book about Van Gogh and excitedly translated the book to English so her classmates could understand. A classmate asked if Elizabeth could read it aloud in Korean and she did. Some classmates were in awe as she read. Simmee thought she and Elizabeth lived out very different stories as children who immigrated to Canada. Elizabeth seemed to be a confident, carefree child with little tension and few worries in her life.

During one snowy recess Simmee began to see herself in Elizabeth's lived stories. Elizabeth asked if she could read an information book about space, the topic of study in language arts, outside. Simmee thought it a strange request to bring a book outside when it was so cold; most children opted to make snow angels. Elizabeth explained she wanted to get an A in language arts so she was learning as much as she could about space. Simmee agreed to Elizabeth's request and later, when Simmee was outside walking with the children, she noticed Elizabeth sitting by herself, clutching the book in her bare hands. Concerned, Simmee asked another student to bring Elizabeth some gloves. As she looked at Elizabeth with her nose pressed against the book, she began to retrace her own memories of herself as a little girl. She wondered if there could be multiple and more complex plotlines in Elizabeth's life. Simmee recalled how she, too, had wanted to belong, to fit in, to not to stand out. As a child, she had found solace by immersing herself in books, imagining herself in other worlds, imagining what could be otherwise. Simmee began to see how Elizabeth and she were not so different after all.

Story Fragment 4: Tensions on the Family Web

As we listened to children's stories, teachers' stories, and family stories, we began to understand the importance of attending to tensions that may impact a child's and their family's lives.

Around Christmas time, the children composed letters to Santa Claus. Simmee found herself traveling back to a familiar childhood landscape as she read Elizabeth's letter. Elizabeth wrote:

> I don't know what I want. But the first thing that I want is for my family to come to Canada because everybody in my class has their family in Canada.

Simmee reflected on the landscape on which Elizabeth lived, a landscape similar to her own. Simmee and her family, too, once had to leave a homeplace. She could feel Elizabeth's words in her letter. She began to listen more closely in the classroom as Elizabeth revealed many stories about aging grandparents, cousins, and close friends who still lived in Korea. Elizabeth longed for her extended family to be living in Canada. Simmee understood how Elizabeth felt for she, too, had once longed for her extended family to be close by. Elizabeth wrote the following letter to Chung at Christmas,

> Thank you Ms. Chung for teaching me and loving me. I want to be like you because you are smart. Have a Happy Christmas! Ask Santa if he has a good present for you. P.S. Be healthy. Your Friend, Elizabeth

Simmee was surprised as she read that Elizabeth wanted to be like her for she wished she had been as brave as Elizabeth when she was a little girl. Revisiting Setterfield's words, "Impossible to understand one part without having the sense of the whole" (2006, p. 59), we are reminded that we cannot fully understand a child without listening to the interconnected vibrations of her life in the context of her family. Simmee found herself thinking about their stories lived and told as immigrant children, as well as the stories of her own mother; her mother had also felt the vibrations as they bumped against stories of school and school stories. When Simmee was four, her family immigrated to Canada from England in the hope for greater opportunity. During her childhood, her family transitioned to three small rural communities, each time opening and closing a Chinese restaurant. In every town, Simmee remembers being the only Chinese family. She remembers moments of tension in her childhood as she struggled to fit in and make sense of who she was. She recalls her mother's anxieties and worries for her. Now, recollecting her childhood stories and her mother's stories, Simmee wondered if the tensions in her family web were similar to the ones Elizabeth and her mother were feeling.

Story Fragment 5: Naming the Tensions on the Family Web

Simmee gathered the children in the classroom sharing corner. Acknowledging the diversity within her classroom, Simmee read the children her latest favourite book, *The Name Jar* (Choi, 2003). On the cover is a picture of a Korean girl staring into a jar filled with names written on pieces of paper. The story began with the little girl, Unhei, reluctantly saying goodbye to her grandparents at the airport in Korea as she leaves for North America. Wiping away Unhei's tears, her grandmother gives her a tiny pouch, which held a wooden block carved with a Korean character. "Your name is inside," her grandmother tells her. As Simmee read the book, Elizabeth inched closer, at one point even reaching out to touch a page. Afterwards, Simmee and the children engaged in a discussion about whether or not the main character should have kept her Korean name—a name others found difficult to pronounce—or have taken a common English name.

Many stories about belonging were told by the children that day. Elizabeth revealed her name was not Elizabeth at all, it was Ji-Sook. Shortly after reading the book, Elizabeth wrote a note to Simmee, "Well I didn't pick my English name so I just want to be called my Korean name (Ji-Sook). Ji-Sook proudly shared that, on her mom's side of the family, all children's names end in Sook and their last name goes in the front. As Elizabeth explained this, Simmee recalled wondering when she first saw Elizabeth's report card with the name Ji-Sook. When we learned of the significance of Elizabeth's Korean name, we began to use her English name and Korean name interchangeably in the classroom. Simmee had not questioned why Ji-Sook went by an English name as her own parents had also changed their names in order to belong in Canada. Accepting the silence at that time, Simmee had not thought to ask why, for she made assumptions as she forwarded her own stories of belonging.

The day after reading the book, Simmee had another research conversation with Mrs. Han. She asked Mrs. Han if she had heard about Elizabeth wanting to use her Korean name. Mrs. Han told Simmee that when Elizabeth came home the day before she said, "Oh mom, I just don't like my name, Elizabeth." In response, Mrs. Han firmly told her daughter that everybody wants that name; she was named after English royalty. As Elizabeth debated with her mother, Mrs. Han stated, "So that's a good name and you'll be a good person. I think about it a lot when I give you that name". Elizabeth settled by agreeing with her mother.

After listening to Mrs. Han's account of the conversation, Simmee asked how she would feel if Elizabeth still wanted to use her Korean name. Mrs. Han said she wanted her daughter to be "common" and "the same as other children". Simmee and Mrs. Han shared more stories as they wondered about what "belonging" could mean. Mrs. Han began to realize how brave and strong her daughter was to want to use her Korean name. She wondered if it connected Ji-Sook to their culture. Simmee shared her experiences of inclusion as a child immigrating to Canada and how she once felt that belonging meant being like everyone else. Simmee and Mrs. Han came to a shared appreciation of Ji-Sook's strength as she struggled to hold on to her Korean name, a name that gave a story of who she was. Simmee told Mrs. Han that Ji-Sook was a special little girl who stood out. Standing out, being different, is good. As Simmee said this, Mrs. Han smiled and nodded.

Simmee later spoke to Ji-Sook while they were playfully making outfits for Ji-Sook's teddy bears. Not knowing the earlier conversation Simmee had had with her mother, Ji-Sook shared that she felt very sad when she arrived home after thinking about *The Name Jar.* The book reminded Ji-Sook of leaving Korea and her family. She felt particularly sad about the airport scene at the beginning of the book. Simmee asked Ji-Sook if she wanted everyone to call her by her Korean name,

> Ji-Sook: I don't care what I'll be called. Uh just, it doesn't really care for me.
> Chung: So a name isn't really important to you? So how come yesterday you told me that you wanted them to call you Ji-Sook?

As Simmee reflected, she understood the tensions Ji-Sook was experiencing around using her Korean name. Although Ji-Sook previously shared with her classmates the tensions around her name, Simmee wondered if Ji-Sook would feel comfortable sharing the tensions that occurred between her and her mother around the name.

We wonder if it is possible or necessary to pinpoint where vibrations first begin, for the vibrations in a web reverberate strongly to every thread, in every direction. As curriculum makers attentive to children's and families' lives, we know, regardless of where vibrations begin, we need to attend to them all. By attending closely to negotiating a curriculum of lives in the classroom, there are safe spaces for the children to engage in inquiry into their stories to live by. However, the vibrations that began through reading the book and engaging in the discussion left lasting imprints on Ji-Sook's life, vibrating onwards, touching the story of who Ji-Sook is and may become. As Ji-Sook wondered about who she was becoming in choosing to use her Korean name, she bumped against a story her mother wanted for her.

SIMMEE: Do you think that your mom wants you to use an English name?
JI-SOOK: Yeah.
SIMMEE: What do you want?
JI-SOOK: I can't just . . . my mom. We don't like to be or disagree.
SIMMEE: You said some of the other kids were calling you your Korean name today? Did you like that?
JI-SOOK: Yeah. Kind of they're learning from me and I'll try to learn their names in Chinese or like lots of stuff. So I'm trying to memorize all of them so I can like work on other languages.

Ji-Sook's words stayed with us, "I can't just . . . my mom. We don't like to be or disagree." Although the vibrations were first noticed in the classroom as Ji-Sook identified with the book, these vibrations traveled to touch Ji-Sook's story of who she was and who she wanted to become. Reverberating from her family web of stories to the classroom curriculum making, the vibrations of stories lived and told, inevitably lingered, touching webs of lives.

As spaces were opened in the conversation between Simmee and Ji-Sook, Ji-Sook once again began to share stories where she imagined herself and others to be otherwise. Although her story of "being otherwise" bumped against her mother's story of who Ji-Sook was, Ji-Sook revealed she loved her Korean name and wanted to use it more. While she feared that some people would have difficulty pronouncing Ji-Sook, her Korean name was important to her and she was determined to use it.

Over the year, we saw Ji-Sook waver between using her English and Korean names. She signed her name Ji-Sook or Elizabeth, depending on how familiar a friend was to her. Ji-Sook was mainly used for those who were closer to her and Elizabeth for those who still called her Elizabeth. Ji-Sook continued to struggle with what name to use. One day she ripped up a beautiful butterfly title page on which she had written, "by Elizabeth." She redid the entire assignment, writing instead "by Ji-Sook". Ji-Sook frequently chose to reread *The Name Jar* during independent reading time. Each time we saw Ji-Sook with *The Name Jar* in hand, we wondered about the impact it had on her and her mother's lives.

At the end of the year, Simmee gave Ji-Sook her own copy of *The Name Jar* as a gift, inscribed:

> Dearest Ji-Sook (Elizabeth),
>
> Ji-Sook, thank you for teaching me about following your dreams and how to be strong. You make me smile every day with your warm heart. I have learned so much about your special Korean culture and I think you are a brave little girl. I think you will change the world with your kindness-you already do. You remind me of this special girl in this book. When you write the book about your life one day, I want to be one of the first people to read it. You and your mother have special stories to tell. Keep dreaming and imagining . . . Thank you for making everyone feel like they, too, belong.
>
> Love always,
> Ms. Chung

Story Fragment 6: Gaps and Silences In and Between Webs

> "While I wash dishes, I cry . . ."
>
> –*Mrs. Han, 2007*

Mrs. Han's voice quavered as she described her part time job at a fast food restaurant. In Korea she was a vice-principal of a kindergarten. In Canada, she worked as a dishwasher and sandwich maker. We sensed sadness in Mrs. Han's voice as she shared her and her husband's hopes for their daughter. They came to Canada so Ji-Sook would learn more English. Mrs. Han's eyes lit up as she described how she hoped, one day, to return to Korea where Ji-Sook would attend university and then, eventually, a university in the United States. She wondered about their decision to come to Canada. She wondered if Korean families do too much for their children. She wondered if she was putting too much stress and pressure on Ji-Sook to succeed.

As Simmee listened, she realized how little she really knew about this family. Mrs. Han continued to fill in the gaps as she described firmly telling Ji-Sook, "Although you work very, very hard there is discrimination because we are strangers in this society." She shared that Ji-Sook cried when she said this and responded, "I can do very well. I will do my best!". Ji-Sook shared her dream of attending Harvard University. Mrs. Han, surprised at her daughter's knowledge, asked how she knew of

Harvard. Ji-Sook replied, "That is the best University in the world. You trust me, I will work very hard to get into Harvard University".

In our inquiry into the tightly interwoven stories in this family web, we saw how each thread vibrated and, inevitably, touched other threads. Simmee found herself returning to the image of Ji-Sook reading a science book outside on a cold winter day. Attending to all of the story fragments, we began to better understand how the family's web of stories was, in part, threaded around dreams of Ji-Sook's academic achievement.

We felt the vibrations, the tensions, as Simmee apologized for not being able to talk much to Mrs. Han during the grade three parent information session. This session, given by teachers, was intended to alleviate parents' and children's anxieties around provincial achievement tests. Mrs. Han shared how she did not want to go to the session because of her lack of English. However, Ji-Sook begged and pleaded, saying "Mom if you don't come, I won't be able to graduate my grade three". Mrs. Han gave in. Ji-Sook was worried that she would "lose information or miss something that other children might know". Although Mrs. Han would not understand what was being said at the session, she agreed to attend as she wanted to help her daughter find success in a foreign school landscape.

Mrs. Han shared that, at first, she did not think these government tests were important but her Korean friend told her that usually only the "elite" are well-educated people and are known to do better at these "tests". Resonating in Mrs. Han's mind were her friend's words, "This is the same kind of society as Korea. In Korea we have a lot of gap between the poor families and the rich families. The higher scores are from the 'elite' [rich], they are known as the well educated people". Mrs. Han's fears were cemented as the other Korean mother told her that the results of these "tests" in grade three determined children's placement in junior high. As Mrs. Han shared this story of tension, Simmee shared her stories of growing up with limited financial resources. Moving through a series of small towns, the last place she remembered living with her parents was above their restaurant in a place they would eventually see as a home. Simmee's story brought forth tension for her as an educator for she hoped that teachers, like families, would not be judged by their financial status. As Simmee and Mrs. Han continued to share their stories, their journey of knowing and unknowing connected their lives.

As we understand family stories as intergenerational and interwoven, we realized it was important to inquire into Mrs. Han's stories of her experiences of school as a child. More silences were revealed. When Simmee asked Mrs. Han about her experiences in elementary school and her relationship with her mother, Mrs. Han began to cry as she traveled back to her childhood experiences.

Mrs. Han spoke of her stories which ultimately shaped her daughter's curriculum of life.

> I grew up in a small country. There was not much competition in academic areas, so if somebody is doing really better than other children, that person is really stands, stands outs. When I look at my mother's younger face, my mother is like me. The relationship between my mother and me is like the relationship between me and Ji-Sook. I want my daughter to stand out and my mother was like that to me.

Mrs. Han tearfully explained that she wished her mother had pushed her more academically because she felt she missed out on opportunities, having only gone to a two-year college rather than a four-year University. "I tell Ji-Sook to work hard and then later you choose what you want to be and that's your choice . . . I don't want her to blame me later".

As Mrs. Han opened up to tell her childhood stories, she became mindful of how her storied landscape was affecting her daughter's life:

> One day Ji-Sook came home and then she sighed, 'oh tomorrow is reading test'. I told her to not worry and just be comfortable and you can do your best. Then that night, Ji-Sook threw up everything.

Although Mrs. Han had come to new ways of knowing during our time with her, a knowing where she tried to put less stress on Ji-Sook, Ji-Sook still put pressure on herself to succeed. Family stories appear to be so deeply and tightly woven that, even when we try to loosen the strands, each story in the web continues to reverberate through each child's curriculum of life. We wondered about how the stories of assessment shaped and reverberated through each family's web. We wondered about possibilities in our stories as we shared our hopes. In our conversation with Mrs. Han on the last day of school, she reaffirmed the need for spaces in our lives to re-imagine new possibilities for ourselves and for our children.

SIMMEE: What are your hopes for your daughter?
MRS. HAN: Respect. If people don't listen to you, you cannot have . . . but if you have reputation or respect then other people will listen to you.
SIMMEE: Is that how you can make a difference?
MRS. HAN: Yes.
SIMMEE: My last question. What are your hopes for yourself?
MRS. HAN: I didn't think about that. Here in this country, in this situation, I do not have any room or any energy to think about that hope.

A Sense of the Whole: Creating Spaces for Families in Curriculum Making

Relational knowing is a primary aspect of narrative inquiry (Clandinin & Connelly, 2000). In our inquiry, we became aware of the importance of listening to family stories as they influenced their child's interactions with the mandated curriculum as well as their unfolding life curriculum. We realized that we needed to be intentional about creating spaces where the interwoven personal stories of children existing within their family stories could be told and retold through shared narrative inquiries. In the classroom, we worked together with the children and their families to create what became known as a project in citizenship education. In this 7-month long narrative inquiry project, children composed annals, took photographs of places and people where, and with whom, they belonged. They also took photographs of objects that symbolized "belonging" in their lives and made collages of who they were and who they were becoming. Working in small-group and whole-class response groups, the children and we became aware of the ways family stories were present in classroom curriculum making.

Through attending more closely to one child's story, her mother's story, and other family stories, we learned more about making spaces to cocompose a curriculum of lives. For example, we wondered about the stories of achievement testing that are shaping stories of school. As we heard in Ji-Sook and her mother's stories, vibrations from these stories can travel backwards to parents' earlier experiences of assessment. In turn, these earlier experiences may vibrate forward to a child's life. We wondered how often parents are caught in their own spaces of tension and thus live out their stories through, and with, their children. We wondered about how we could more intentionally create spaces for such stories to be told so that we could understand how assessment could be shifted from assessment of learning to assessment for learning and assessment as learning (Adamson, 2008). These latter ways of thinking about assessment fit more seamlessly within our view of curriculum making.

We remain hopeful that school landscapes can be otherwise as we attend to family stories and begin to make spaces for cocomposing a curriculum of lives alongside children, families and teachers. As Mrs. Han and Simmee continued to imagine otherwise with one another, Simmee responded, "Yes, I think that hope is all we have." To create change in our ways of knowing, we need to attend to all vibrations, especially those that are invisible upon first glance. By listening to the voices of families, we can acknowledge and appreciate the diversity in our classroom webs and in our webs of lives.

By attending to family vibrations lived and told, we can begin to interrupt and rewrite dominant stories of school (Clandinin et al., 2006). Through listening closely to vibrations within these intergenerational webs of lives, we can cocompose a curriculum in schools where all involved feel like they belong. Simmee's conversation with Ji-Sook on the last day of school reminds us of the importance of creating spaces in schools where families can tell, and retell, compose their stories in the most important curriculum of all, a curriculum of lives.

SIMMEE: What are you looking up?

JI-SOOK: Belonging. (She reads the definition in the dictionary). I don't get it. It's too hard the words for me. Just that it takes a long time to think what really belonging means. Like you can't use the dictionary that you could see what belonging means. Can you just figure out what belonging means. Feels like I'm a crazy dictionary.

SIMMEE: Do you think we might just have to figure out what belonging means ourselves?

JI-SOOK: Yeah. (She sighs, slowly closing the dictionary).

Discussion questions

1) In what ways do stories such as those told in this chapter create disruptions in how each of us use our knowledge in our teaching practice?
2) What challenges do you imagine educators will face as they adhere to the planned/mandated curriculum but also try to integrate stories from their students' lives into the curriculum?
3) How can teachers work with parents and children to create spaces that make lives (children's, families', and teacher's lives) more visible in classrooms?

References

Adamson, D. G. (2008). *Shifting the professional landscape: Professional development and assessment for learning*. Unpublished Doctoral Dissertation, University of Alberta, Edmonton.

Aoki, T. (1993). Legitimating lived curriculum: Towards a curricular landscape of multiplicity. *Journal of Curriculum and Supervision*, *8*(3), 255–268.

Choi, Y. (2003). *The name jar.* New York: Dell Dragonfly Books.

Clandinin, D. J., & Connelly, F. M. (1992). Teacher as curriculum maker. In P. Jackson (Ed.), *Handbook of research on curriculum* (pp. 363–401). Toronto: Macmillan.

Clandinin, D. J., & Connelly, F. M. (1995). *Teachers' professional knowledge landscapes.* New York: Teachers College Press.

Clandinin, D. J., & Connelly, F. M. (2000). *Narrative inquiry: Experience and story in qualitative research.* San Francisco, CA: Josey-Bass.

Clandinin, D. J., Huber, J., Huber, M., Murphy, S., Murray Orr, A., Pearce, M., & Steeves, P. (2006). *Composing diverse identities: Narrative inquiries into the interwoven lives of children and teachers.* New York: Routledge.

Connelly, F. M., & Clandinin, D. J. (1999). *Shaping a professional identity: Stories of educational practice.* New York: Teachers College Press.

Mason, A. (1999). *The world of spider.* Canada: San Francisco: Sierra Club Books.

Setterfield, D. (2006). *The thirteenth tale.* Toronto, Canada: Bond Street Books.

Vinz, R. (1997). Capturing a moving form: Becoming as teachers. *English Education*, *29*(2), 137–146.

11

A NARRATIVE INQUIRY INTO FAMILIAL AND SCHOOL CURRICULUM MAKING

Attending to multiple worlds of Aboriginal youth and families

Sean Lessard, Vera Caine and D.J. Clandinin

Introduction

'He phones me or I text him and we meet at school but he also does that for me when I sleep in or don't feel like going to school,'[1] Lane explains as we sit together over a cold drink at the mall.

Lane and Donovan are two youth of Aboriginal heritage with whom we engaged in a narrative inquiry. These words, spoken to Sean early in the study, occurred in one moment when the youth talked about the evolution of their friendship formed within a school and described how the relationship shifted and sustained them in school. Lane and Donovan shared stories of how they first met in the midst of a dodge ball game early in their Grade 7 year. They laughed when they recalled stories of their experiences and, in writing this paper, Sean shared stories of how Lane and Donovan told of negotiating the beginning of their friendship as they dodged balls in the game, amidst the noise and confusion of 30 twelve-year-old youth and many hard-flung balls. The relationship between Lane and Donovan evolved as they made spaces within school where they connected and sustained each other through conversations, activities, and, eventually, text messages. They shared it was not the same when one of them was not at school. As Donovan told Sean: 'If it wasn't for Lane I would have a hard time going to school.' Both Lane and Donovan texted each other, sustaining the relationship through the coaxing and reminders to come to school, to meet each other there, or to wake up because it was a school day. It was not the subject matters or the teachers that sustained their relationships with school, it was their evolving relationship that sustained them and resonated within both of them. As Lane told Sean, 'Donovan looks out for me he always helps me.'

Reprinted with permission. Acknowledgement; Lessard, S., Caine, V., & Clandinin, D. J. (2014). A narrative inquiry into familial and school curriculum making: Attending to multiple worlds of aboriginal youth and families. *Journal of Youth Studies, 18*(2), 197–214.

Aim of study

Our aim is to show the educational and school experiences of two urban Aboriginal youth, who were part of a larger study conceptualized around familial curriculum making (Huber, Murphy, and Clandinin 2011). While curriculum making usually focuses on the experiences of children and youth in schools as students' and teachers' lives meet in the context of subject matter and within nested milieus (Connelly and Clandinin 1988), familial curriculum making is situated and composed in experiences outside of school, within family, and community places. What is called familial curriculum making is educative as it shapes and reshapes the lives of youth and their families. What we share in this paper is an account into the familial curriculum making of Lane and Donovan, two youth of Aboriginal heritage who participated in the research. By sharing the experiences of Lane and Donovan conceptualized around a concept of familial curriculum making, our intention is to make their experiences more visible, more animated, perhaps filled with more possibility and wonder, and to resist the ways in which their lives could be defined or reduced to numbers and deficits.

Coming to the research

The reverberations of previous studies alongside youth who left school early (Clandinin, Steeves, and Caine 2013), and children and families in schools (Huber, Murphy, and Clandinin 2011), shifted our attention to the intersections between home, community, and school. From our study alongside youth who left school early (Clandinin, Steeves, and Caine 2013), we realized that the early school-leaving rate was particularly high for youth of Aboriginal heritage, as well as for some immigrant and refugee youth. We also knew that the move from junior high school to senior high school was a difficult time for many youth and, for some, the transition was just too difficult. They left school.

For Lane and Donovan, the transition included a shift to a new school that was larger in school population and entailed increased subject matter specific demands. In the Canadian context where we work, there are two major school transitions, one between elementary school and junior high school and one between junior high school and senior high school. These transitions are times marked by rhetoric of increased academic expectations and increased student responsibility for learning. Lane told Sean, 'It was difficult . . . I didn't know what this new school was like and it is hard starting junior high. It was difficult.'

Working within the theoretical framework of multiple curriculum-making worlds (Huber, Murphy, and Clandinin 2011) we saw possibilities to shift our attention to the complexity of a curriculum of lives (Clandinin, Lessard, and Caine 2013) both in and out of school, at a time marked by transitions. As we turned to understanding multiple curriculum-making worlds, we wondered, in particular, about the youth and their families of Aboriginal heritage we had been privileged to meet in earlier studies. We locate our study in the area of youth studies, as we are most interested in the relationship between, and intersection of, multiple worlds that youth inhabit. Our intention is to explore the spaces that move beyond prescriptive boundaries that are narrowly focused and/or that suggest a certain pathway or direction for lives. Our work with Lane and Donovan is not meant to be a model for future schools or a lesson for how programs should operate in practice. Our intention through narrative inquiry is to honor the multiplicity of Lane and Donovan's lives lived out within both the school and familial curriculum-making worlds. Like Smyth, Robinson, and McInery (2014), we wonder about the role education plays in the lives of young people, particularly for youth who often live on the margins of school (Pless 2014; Camilleri-Cassar 2014).

Aboriginal youth and their families

Together with culture, education is recognized as an instrumental social determinant to the health of Aboriginal peoples[2] (NAHO 2007). More than half of the Canadian Aboriginal population is under the age of 25, which places an urgent need to collaboratively inquire into the lives of Aboriginal youth. Children and youth of Aboriginal heritage represent 15% of the total population in public schools in the large metropolitan area where our study unfolded, which, at present, is the second largest Aboriginal student population in a Canadian urban center (EPS 2009). The cumulative effects of colonization, residential schools, and the Indian Act changed traditional ways of life significantly and this adds to the complexity of Aboriginal youth's experiences in provincially funded schools. These cumulative effects changed traditional ways of life for many Aboriginal peoples as well as made visible the distinction between schooling and education in the lives of Aboriginal people. The institutional spaces of schools have significantly shaped the experiences of Aboriginal youth and their families. While the relationships between Aboriginal peoples and schools continue to evolve, the relationships between Aboriginal peoples and schools have been irrevocably marked as tension-filled and as lacking meaningful reciprocity between schools and the lives of Aboriginal peoples. These ruptures were shaped from the beginning days of residential schools. Prior to institutional schooling in residential schools, education was within the community and family. When the rupture between schooling and education occurred, and schooling became a dominant force in the lives of Aboriginal peoples, the familial voices and presence of Aboriginal peoples and their distinct history were no longer attended to. It is within this current context that we attend to the lives of Lane and Donovan as their families, like other families of Aboriginal heritage, continue to negotiate the world of school. Intergenerational reverberations from the stories of residential schools shape many Aboriginal people's stories of school (Young 2005).

'Public education provides a rich site for contestation and struggle especially for those whose backgrounds and aspirations are positioned outside those of mainstream society' (Riecken et al. 2006, 266). Simultaneously, Riecken et al. (2006) showed that the 'strength of Aboriginal people is derived from their sense of identity, of knowing who they are and where they come from. A sense of pride provides a resistance to assimilation' (280). Yet, we also understand it is not helpful to create dichotomous groups of those whose identities are nested within traditional authentic ways of being and those who are seen as socially assimilated; we see greater diversity and understand that culture is continuously evolving; traditional ways are dynamic (Brass 2009; Hollands 2004). In many ways Aboriginal youth 'live in a complex world of multiple loyalties – a world that challenges, sustains, and sometimes destroys them but seldom removes their Indianness' (LaFromboise, Trimble, and Mohatt 1990, 637).

Others have recognized that the experiences of Aboriginal youth are embedded within place, family, and community (Friedel 1999; Kirmayer, Tait, and Simpson 2009; Restoule 2008). Yet, little research considers the intergenerational impact of family stories on youth's past experiences, their present and forward looking stories, as well as the longitudinal impact of school engagement on Aboriginal youth's experiences (Royal Commission on Aboriginal Peoples 1996), as well as youth's voices themselves (Friedel 2010). Contemporary Aboriginal youth reinforce and extend their traditional cultural practices and youthful identities (Hollands 2004); they also resist them (Friedel 2010). Like Wilson and Peters (2005), who explored how migration between reserve and urban communities challenges First Nations peoples identity, we wonder how urban experiences shape their relationships to their and their families' cultures, education, and schooling experiences.

We continue to think about identity and the multiplicity within this definition (Connelly and Clandinin 1999) as we attend to the experiences of youth we have come to know in an urban setting. The experiences within urban landscapes affect them as they move back and forth between their home communities and the urban settings, holding on to their home communities as they are being shaped by the necessary in-between-ness of the two worlds they are negotiating. In this work we did not make assumptions or categorize youth as we continued to see their experiences as contextual and shaped by distinct memories of home places with language, protocols, and intergenerational teachings that shaped who they are and who they are becoming in an urban setting. As Lane told Sean, 'I go back and forth between the reserve and the city, with my brother, dad, mom, and auntie is where I live, it depends on what is going on.' Donovan said:

> I have many brothers and sisters, they live in different places, there are so many to list but they are all my brothers and sisters. Where I am living right now is with my dad and in this place I have two brothers and two sisters and share a bedroom with my brother. That is why I go to a lot of schools. It depends on what is happening in my life where I live.

Similar to Friedel (2010) we, too, are aware that the schooling experiences of Aboriginal students and their families are deeply shaped by pervasive issues of marginalization, exclusion, surveillance, and oppression. Turning from understanding the multiplicity of worlds Aboriginal youth and their families experience, to the social and personal contexts of their lives, shifted our attention to a new research puzzle; a puzzle that guided our current narrative inquiry. The multiplicity within the lives of Aboriginal youth and their families are timely sites for narrative inquiry as they are in the midst of a difficult and challenging time period within schools. The challenge lies in the undercurrents of sorting and categorizing within models of schools that are based on set numbers and scores that shape narrow definitions of achiever and underachiever. Many Aboriginal youth and their families currently carry the latter definition, that of underachiever. Seeing Aboriginal youth as only underachievers is a heavy categorization that does not make visible the wholeness, the multiplicity, the deeply nested set of experiences of the youth we came to know. As Lane said, 'It takes me 2 buses to get here' and 'I wake up on my own, and sometimes I am hungry . . . coming to school is hard.' Lane's words make visible his experiences of the structural inequities around housing, transportation, and food that shape his life on a daily basis.

Narrative inquiry as research methodology

> Arguments for the development and use of narrative inquiry come out of a view of human experience in which humans, individually and socially, lead storied lives.

> People shape their daily lives by stories of who they and others are and as they interpret their past in terms of these stories. . . . Narrative inquiry, the study of experience as story, then, is first and foremost a way of thinking about experience. Narrative inquiry as a methodology entails a view of the phenomena. To use narrative inquiry methodology is to adopt a particular view of experience as phenomena under study.
>
> *(Connelly and Clandinin 2006, 477)*

This definition of narrative inquiry links narrative inquiry as a research methodology with narrative conceptions of experience. As described by Clandinin and Rosiek (2007, 42), narrative inquiry begins with 'respect for ordinary lived experience' as it explores both individuals' experience as well as 'the social, cultural, and institutional narratives within which individuals' experiences were constituted, shaped, expressed, and enacted.'

The research design of narrative inquiry enables the formation of intensive relationships with each youth and their family to hear how their educational (home/school/community) stories unfolded over, and in, their lives. As narrative inquirers we both listen to the stories participants tell about their experiences, as well as we live alongside participants as we inquire into their experiences, as we compose field texts and interim research texts and as we find ways to share the final research texts (Clandinin 2013). Spaces of narrative inquiry are attentive to what it means to live as researchers in ethical relationships, to live in collaborative ways.

The stories we tell of ourselves in relation to the Aboriginal youth and their families are also relevant in narrative inquiry. Working within narrative inquiry, a relational research methodology, our experiences shape who we each are and are becoming and how we attend to the stories of the youth and families we work alongside. Sean was a teacher and an Aboriginal consultant within the school system. School matters deeply to Sean and he frequently attends closely to school completion rates for youth of Aboriginal heritage as he learns from families and youth. Jean worked for many years as a teacher, counselor, and researcher in schools. She also attends to children's experiences of schooling through her experiences as a mother and grandmother, experiences that shape her understanding of the intersections between home and school. Vera entered this study as her son began Grade 1, a time when Vera's familial curriculum-making world bumped against school curriculum-making worlds. These experiences shaped, and continue to shape, Sean, Jean, and Vera's experiences alongside participants.

Shaping a research puzzle

In 2010 when we began the narrative inquiry, our research puzzles were around the schooling and educational experiences of youth and families of Aboriginal heritage. In order to undertake the puzzle, we needed to find ways to come to know youth, as well as to have youth take us to their families in order to learn more of who they were in the educative experiences of their families. Our intention was to work from understandings of their familial curriculum-making worlds (Huber, Murphy, and Clandinin 2011). Our research study was informed by earlier research around the experiences of early school leavers. Working with the early school leavers, we came to understand some of the youth's experiences, particularly about the complexity of their lives as their experiences in school and their experiences outside school intersected. Definitions of family and early school leaving became more visible as youth told stories of experiences that shaped them, experiences lived outside of the time and places of school. Our work with these youth shaped our puzzles about youth's experiences outside of school, particularly their experiences lived in relation with their families.

Nested within the research puzzle was a deep sense that in order to attend to the tensions and lives in multiple curriculum-making worlds, we needed to find ways to hear the stories of youth and families in order to attend to the intersections of the youth's curriculum-making worlds.

Living out the narrative inquiry: finding our ways to a field of inquiry

As we imagined our way into the narrative inquiry, we negotiated with a school district and with a school, to create a space in a school, outside of mandated school hours but within the physical place of school. We negotiated, with the permission of the school principal, to meet in a mostly unused classroom at an after school time, a time when other school clubs were held. We initially imagined that if we created a space with art making as the central focus we would be able to make initial contact with youth and we would also be able to build the youth's art-making skills so that they could represent their experiences in a range of esthetic ways. Our design meant that we were not in school classrooms, nor did our time with the youth need to be accountable to mandated provincial curriculum.

We gained permission from the University Ethics Board and local school district to work in a junior high school with a fairly high population of urban Aboriginal youth (40% of youth self-identified as First Nations, Inuit, or Métis). In Canada, based on legal descriptions, Aboriginal people are categorized as First Nations, Inuit, or Metis. As narrative inquirers, we were mindful that these categories existed, but also learned from the youth and their families, that they self-identified by their home communities or by their linguistic backgrounds, as these were more significant to them.

Lane and Donovan told Sean of how they came to name themselves in relation to places and their families. Lane shared stories of his reserve, Sunchild First Nation, calling it 'one of his homes.' It was a place where he grew up and lived, on and off, throughout his life. It was a place where his family had lived. He spoke of the times when he returned, he stayed at his auntie's. Donovan shared that he wanted Lane to learn drum making with him, noting, 'It is important in his community and to many within his family.' As Donovan shared these stories, he spoke of the unique protocols and teachings within his community that are different from the ones lived in Lane's community.

They noted these unique protocols within communities by saying 'in my community' or 'in my family, we do it this way but I think Lane's family celebrates differently.' There was an understanding between them of the commonalities in their Cree heritage but also the differences that resided in their experiences in their different home and community stories. Donovan said in a conversation with Sean that, 'I say I am Cree or First Nations and sometimes Aboriginal but it depends on where I am and who I am talking to. My name is different in each place.' These spaces between the home places and the school places are noted as Donovan spoke of traveling between places. 'The hardest part of the rez to city schools is the getting up in the mornings . . . the toughest part of the rez life for me is leaving behind my family in the city.' As he said, 'The city wasn't bad for me because I liked art and music and gym and we don't have all those things at the reserve school.'

In our original conceptualization of the study we conveyed an almost utilitarian sense of the space we were creating in the school, that is, it would be a space where we could meet junior high students and form relationships with them. It took time to shift our understanding of this space, a shift that was facilitated by the youth. We learned to bring substantial food, rather than light snacks, to the club, as well as we negotiated activities and ways to be in the space. Over time, with the youth who joined us, we came to call this space the art club. Establishing the club was a complex undertaking that required both imagination and careful persistent attention. In negotiations with the youth over time we filled the one and a half weekly hours of club time with activities such as painting, drawing, beading, mask making, drum and rattle making, photography, or collage making.

We engaged in the club space between September 2011 and June 2013; with some of the seventeen youth and their families we continued to engage in conversations and inquiry into their told and lived experiences until the spring 2014. Diverse field texts (data) were composed, including conversations, field notes, artifacts, memory box items, documents (such as school files that were shared with us by parents), and artwork created in the club space. These diverse forms of field texts invited participants into the research in ways that enabled them to actively document their unfolding lives so that the complex connections between their experiences in particular times and places were more deeply understood. Field texts were interpreted alongside participants from within the three-dimensional narrative inquiry space (Clandinin and Connelly 2000), with attention to temporality, the personal and social contexts, and place.

While we initially met youth in this space, we also moved into new places where youth were comfortable, such as malls, restaurants, public venues, and alongside their families in their homes. As the youth allowed us to walk alongside, they taught us gently within their home places, taking care of us in places to which they invited us. During our time together, it was important to attend to the told and lived stories, as well as to the silences and gaps within and between their experiences (Clandinin and Caine 2008). It was within the art club space that we came to know Lane and Donovan, two youth who began to come to the club early in their Grade 7 year.

Sean describes the stories he heard from other research team members about Lane and Donovan before he was able to come to the art club to meet them. He noted that he was told 'you have to meet Lane . . . he is such a leader . . . he has such a wonderful sense of humour.' After the first day when Sean was able to come to the art club he wrote the following field note:

> This was the first day that we had a video camera in the club. Lane brought the camera over to me and started asking questions, urging me to step on stage through the video he was creating with his friends, including Donovan. He continued to ask me questions with the video rolling and then it happened. He said, 'I am telling you that you are now Chief in this movie and your name will be Chief Chitsalot!' We looked at each other and the boys watched for my response. We all burst into laughter.

As Sean continued to spend time with the two boys, both in and out of the club space, he learned more about the humor evident in the exchange in the club and the ways that humor shaped the lives of the two boys. As Sean learned from his conversations with Lane and Donovan, it was Donovan that brought Lane to the club. Donovan came because his sister and her friend came to the club in our first meeting in September.

A theoretical frame of multiple worlds

As we turned to inquire into the storied fragments of Lane and Donovan's experience in the opening section, we worked to understand their experience in terms of Lugones' (1987) concept of world. For Lugones, a world may be a construction of a tiny portion of a particular society, inhabited by just a few people. Some worlds are bigger than others:

> In a 'world' some of the inhabitants may not understand or hold the particular construction of them that constructs them in that 'world.' So there may be 'worlds' that construct me in ways that I do not even understand. Or it may be that I understand the construction, but do not hold it of myself. I may not accept it as an account of myself, a construction of myself. And yet, I may be *animating* such a construction.
>
> *(Lugones 1987, 10, italics in original)*

Lugones described world traveling as living in different worlds where we construct ourselves, and are constructed by others, differently. For Lugones, as a woman of color, an 'outsider to the mainstream' (3), world traveling, that is, living in or traveling to, different worlds was a necessity. Lugones wrote 'those of us who are 'world'-travelers have the distinct experience of being different in different 'worlds' and of having the capacity to remember other 'worlds' and ourselves in them' (11).

As we turn back to the experiences of Donovan and Lane thinking with an understanding of worlds and world traveling, we awaken to their co-construction of a world between them through their sustaining relationship, a world co-constructed and negotiated through conversations over time. Their conversations in text messages and in moments of meeting were part of their world making. This world they co-composed between them was of particular importance in the school curriculum-making world. It seemed their co-composed world allowed them the possibility of coming to the school world. Their work in co-composing was an active and intentional process for each of them.

Working with Lugones' concepts of worlds and 'world'-traveling, Huber, Murphy, and Clandinin (2011) conceptualized two worlds of curriculum making, that is, a familial curriculum-making world as distinct from a school curriculum-making world. The notions of curriculum that allowed their conceptualization were ones of curriculum as a life-making process and of curriculum as a course of life (Clandinin and Connelly 1992; Connelly and Clandinin 1988).

Through the text messages and conversations Lane and Donovan shared, it became increasingly evident that it was their relationship, their co-composed world that sustained each of them in their school curriculum-making world, not teachers or subject matters they studied. In co-composing their world over time, they shared knowledge from other worlds, knowledge that rarely included stories of their experiences within their school curriculum-making worlds. Stories of who they were and were becoming in their other curriculum-making worlds, that included stories of other constructions of who they were, were told. The stories of what it meant to each of them to be a young person who was Cree living in a large urban center was a continuing conversation. Within their evolving relationship and the co-construction of a world within a school place, they found resonance in each other's stories and of what they knew from other places. The intricate details of people within places, and memories of extended families shaped the early moments of their sharing within the world that they were composing in a school world.

Working with the concepts of worlds and world traveling and the concept of curriculum making as a life-making process, Huber, Murphy, and Clandinin (2011) showed how children engage in 'world' traveling over days, weeks, months, and years as they move back and forth between home and school and, in this movement, experience multiple moments when they bumped against the dominant stories of school. Living in both worlds, shaped by different stories, meant they needed to live within different constructions of who they were in each world. Lugones described this 'shift from being one person to being a different person' as 'travel' (11). As Huber, Murphy, and Clandinin (2011) wrote:

> Similar to Lugones' sense of herself as needing to 'travel' to different worlds, worlds in which she constructs herself and worlds in which she is 'stereotypically' or 'arrogantly'perceived or constructed by others, we see that not only are children's worlds of familial and school curriculum making shaped by differing physical places but also by differing ways of being and interacting and, therefore, of knowing and knowledge.
>
> *(108)*

Huber, Murphy, and Clandinin (2011) showed the importance of understanding children and youth's experiences both in and out of school as a process of world traveling from a world or worlds of familial curriculum making to a world of school curriculum making each day; worlds in which children and youth both constructed themselves differently, and were constructed differently. We wondered, as we inquired into Lane and Donovan's morning texts to encourage them to move from their familial worlds of curriculum making to their school worlds of curriculum making, if their texts were a way of easing their way into the school curriculum-making world. Did it help them remember they had a co-composed world of friendship, a world in which their constructions of each other helped them feel more at home in the school curriculum-making world? Using these ideas of Huber, Murphy, and Clandinin (2011) helped us begin to see Lane and Donovan's embodied tensions as they lived in, and between, different worlds of curriculum making.

Coming alongside Lane and Donovan

In the club we became more awake to the multiple worlds that the youth were composing. In the comfort of the club Donovan and Lane and other youth slowly let us into their worlds showing us in multiple ways who they were and who they were becoming. Lane spoke to Sean of the complex familial cultural and community relationships. 'We honour people who have passed at our wakes and in our ceremonies. You can't fall asleep when honouring, that was what I was taught.' Lane's words of honor come from a place of education. He learned in his familial curriculum making:

> that culture matters. I get away from culture in the city. It is why I like going home to visit . . . I guess I miss it a bit if I think about it more. I mostly learned in Sunchild at my reserve. I used to spend time with my grandparents.

> We took language classes at school, people spoke our language in their homes and culture events are where you get together with everyone.

As Lane talked about his experiences in his familial curriculum-making world, he again makes evident that his familial curriculum making shaped how he lives alongside Donovan. 'I met Donovan and that makes it easier here. Loyalty is important to me. I have good friends and I have between 6–8 brothers and sisters in my family.'

It was in these moments of coming alongside youth like Donovan and Lane that other worlds became visible and we began the hard work of inquiry conversations that helped us understand the layers within the lives of the youth and their families. For several weeks Donovan was only able to attend the club for a few minutes, as he needed to look after his younger cousin at home. He did not want to miss time in the art club, nor did his friends in the club want to miss his presence. The following field note describes the way they continued to keep the relationships alive:

> One of the youth arranged to SKYPE Donovan in during art club time; she placed a computer in the middle of the room and throughout the afternoon people stopped and talked with him, shouted across the room to inform him of what was happening, or simply brought their work or ideas to him on the screen. At the same time, all of us met part of Donovan's family and we became part of looking after his little cousin.

As the field note shows, in this moment Donovan allowed us to physically travel to his familial world of curriculum making via technology, something that made us aware that he was beginning to feel at ease in Lugones' sense in the co-composed world that we were creating in the art club.

Donovan and Lane made visible what they knew from other worlds most often through their actions and in the moments of relationships. Through attending closely to the relationships between them, among them and other youth in the club, and within the evolving relationships between them and the researchers, we became more awake to the world traveling that was being lived out. The knowledge that they carried forward, and knew within themselves, was knowledge they had learned from within the places where they had traveled. The places included the people in their lives who taught them within contexts of family and community relationships. Within the club space we recall times when Elder Isabelle Kootenay, one of the Elders who worked closely with us, visited and shared teachings she had learned from her parents and grandparents and from within the context of her community. The following field note shows her presence in the art club:

> Elder Isabelle entered the club space and was met with a flurry of the youth's activities in the form of laughter, energy, movement and creative processes. Food, paint, beads, papers, projects and video cameras encompassed the space as the youth busily moved around in ways that signified the comfort and ease within this co-composed world among the youth and the researchers. The youth's activities and how they interacted within the club were not clearly defined by time, specific rules, outcomes or a certain level of participation. Elder Isabelle Kootenay was greeted with kindness and welcomed in with a handshake and a hug. The youth and researchers worked to reshape the physical space as the youth began moving the tables and chairs to form a circle together as she prepared to share her teachings.

We watched Elder Isabelle Kootenay over multiple days as she carefully created and composed, alongside the youth, the circular process of the medicine wheel, sharing teachings about the seasons, plants, and animals and how these teachings connect to the youth and their lives in the present. Elder Isabelle Kootenay, alongside the youth, co-created a space to help us think with the teachings as we sat in a circle during these times of sharing. Within the space of the circle Donovan and Lane knew within themselves at this time and in these moments that this process was meant to be different. The club was now a space for teaching and listening, observing and respecting in ways that they knew from other worlds, from other places, from other times. The following field note speaks to this:

> The quiet presence of Elder Isabelle Kootenay shifted the space with her invitation to participate in a different way. The club space, which in one moment was filled with the energy of junior high students, moved in a different direction at this time and with a different rhythm alongside Elder Isabelle Kootenay.

We wondered what triggered these shifts within the club space and within the youth. Did this club space trigger memories of other places for them? Did they recognize these relational protocols alongside an Elder? Did the invitation to participate in a different way call forward familial and cultural knowledge recognizable from other places and relationships?

Donovan and Lane helped us become more attentive to the gradual shifting space within the club as they knew within themselves the responsibilities of taking care of an Elder through relationship. Small, but meaningful, shifts occurred in the quietness and slowing down process alongside Elder Isabelle Kootenay. Donovan and Lane moved in relation and responded in ways familiar to them from other places. As we observed, we knew that they had been in similar situations and knew what was expected at this time.

We are reminded of conversations shared with both Donovan and Lane on multiple landscapes. It is only through time and evolving relationships that we became more awake to the stories that were nested deeply within both Donovan and Lane. We realized that these stories are often not visible in the world of school curriculum making. Donovan helped us to think more carefully about this as we came to understand some of the important people within Donovan's home place and within his community. Donovan shared stories of remembered experiences that were not visible or known within the school curriculum-making world. The experiences that he shared were made visible as we walked alongside him both in and outside the arts club. He spoke to Sean saying:

> I used to always visit my Kookum Muriel. She has passed yes . . . she was a good woman, she was kind to everyone, she was an Elder to everyone. She passed away in 2010. I still think of her. I went and visited my brother after when my Kookum died. I tried being so strong . . . but when I got to my brother's I just felt it . . . and then I started to cry. She was my dad's mother. Muriel was her name. She would teach me Cree and all the animals and numbers in Cree but now I forget. But the best memory of her is that she would just spend time with me.

Donovan's love for his community and his vivid recollections of this home place became more visible over time. At first his stories were short and gentle recollections of family situated within his community. Eventually we came to know of people and other places from across time. Through these stories of community and longing for his home place that we came to know of Donovan's Kookum Muriel. Kookum Muriel, the grandmother within his stories, is the person whose memory he carries forward from other places. Her teachings, embodied in Donovan, became more visible as they echoed and stretched across multiple places and spaces. Kookum Muriel and the stories Donovan shares of her are visible in the ways that Donovan moves in relation, in the ways he recognizes teachings from other places.

Donovan shared his memories of his home place and how this home place calls to him in different moments within the present. He shared of his long walks as a young boy down the gravel roads of his community, skipping and throwing rocks into the adjacent pond during these solitary moments of youth. He shared his memories of these walks by himself. He moved and carried himself down the gravel road and toward his destination place, traveling many miles. Donovan had a singular focus on these solitary walks within his community, his home place, for at the end of the gravel road was where his grandmother lived. Kookum Muriel was his home place, a place where he found comfort and meaning. In a conversation with Sean he said:

> across the lake is where she lived she had a big house and she made a farm so I would play with the animals-the chickens and the horses. I would go there, by myself just walking down the road to her house by myself.

Donovan described his grandmother, his Kookum, as a traditional woman and an Elder within the community who taught him about language, protocol and culture. He described her as a gentle person who ran and played with him and taught him how to take care of the animals on her farm. At his Kookum's house is where he felt 'the best.' This was his home 'because she would just spend time with me.' It is through Donovan's memories shared of his relationship with Kookum Muriel that we begin to imagine these teachings, protocols, and relational commitments embedded deeply within him and connected to a home place within a community. Through his stories of experiences we learn what matters to Donovan and what calls to him in the present. It is with good feelings that he shares his memories of Kookum Muriel, but there is also sadness as he finds it difficult to recognize a home place, now that she is no longer alive. He clings to the memories of her, knowing in his body the teachings that shaped him. The pain of loss is evident as Donovan shares that the place, her home, does not feel the same as it did when she was physically present. He said, 'When I drum . . . when I close my eyes and I feel happy and wonder if Kookum Muriel is looking out for me. I have had a lot of loss in my life.' He finds it hard to return to the place now that she is not there. It was, we imagine, his embodied knowing and his memories of Kookum Muriel that were called forth in the art club when Elder Isabelle joined us.

We also recall Lane's response to Elder Isabelle's teachings in the arts club. We recall certain experiences alongside Elder Isabelle Kootenay and how she carefully prepared for teachings to share with the youth and researchers, as the following field note shows:

> Today as Isabelle prepared sage and other medicines for a cleansing ceremony, she quietly asked Lane to be her helper in this teaching process, asking him to be the one to pass the smudge bowl around the circle. It was evident he had

> an intimate knowledge of this experience, of protocol, and of the intricate details of being a helper when asked. It was more visible to us that he had walked alongside an Elder in this way before. He moved with confidence and a deep sense of understanding of the importance of what was being asked of him. In this cleansing ceremony, amongst youth and researchers, he took his responsibilities seriously alongside an Elder. He lit the match and prepared the medicines, carefully fanning them, gently, slowly, and purposefully. He moved with ease, as he brought his knowledge from one world to this art club world that we were co-composing.

We, researchers and youth, observed Lane in a different and new way. We saw his ease in this art club world in this moment. We wondered if the youth also saw him in new ways, the ease with which he animated who he was in one world, his familial cultural curriculum-making world, in this other world. Lane moved around the circle to each one of us, offering the smudge and creating a welcoming space within the circle as we prepared for teachings.

We carried this knowing of Lane into the conversational relationships that evolved over time between Lane and Sean. Through these conversations outside the art club, we began to understand more of the multiple worlds that Lane lived within. Sometimes he told of the important members of his family and how they were teachers to him in different ways. His brothers were often in his stories. He told how, as a young boy, he spent significant amounts of time with his brothers and his family within the community, within a home place far from the urban center where we came to know him. Through time spent alongside his older brothers and other family members, he learned many teachings both cultural, in the form of protocol and ceremony, and contemporary, in the form of music and art. Over time Lane shared what he knew from the places and the people within his life. He shared stories of music making and song making and spending time carefully practicing and learning on his brother's guitar. In a conversation with Sean, he spoke of being comforted 'by playing the guitar, I often play late at night to keep myself company when I can't sleep.' It is through the guitar that he moved to the piano and taught himself to make music in this way as well, learning to bring the various instruments and creative processes within him alive.

As Lane shared stories of traveling between places he often returned to memories of mountains and white waters rushing. For it was within his memories of his ancestral home that he remembered the teachings from his family and what language and protocol and ceremony looked like within this physical place. He recalled the beauty and the majesty of the mountains overlooking the territory and the raw and lasting images of animals that lived within his home place. The stories shared are memories as he longs for a place that was filled with good moments of growing up within a family and a community. It was here in this place amongst the giants in the background and the wildness within the trees and his memory that he learned so much.

Lane only shared these stories over time and through the conversational relationship. The process of becoming awake to what was important in Lane's life became visible first as we watched him alongside Elder Isabelle Kootenay, as he gently and carefully taught us within the club space what he knew deep within himself from other worlds, amongst teachers who had shown him the important details of walking alongside an Elder in relation and the importance of protocol and teachings that are situated within place, over and across time.

So what: moving forward to create possibilities

As we engage in this narrative inquiry with the youth and their families, we hold open questions of the personal, practical and social significance of our work. Questions of significance reflect questions of so what? and who cares? (Clandinin and Connelly 2000). One way of thinking of the so what of this work is to see it as a call to intensify the expectations of teachers in one more way, or to see this work as asking teachers to do more, to be more involved with families, to somehow engage in the familial curriculum making with children and families. We do not see our work in this way and it would be a misreading of our intentions.

We see, rather, that the forward looking story from this research asks those of us who work with children and youth in school curriculum-making worlds to acknowledge, to name, other curriculum-making worlds that families engage in with their children. It is here that we turn to work that is located in youth studies, work that emphasizes the multiple worlds youth live within. In our conversations alongside Donovan and Lane and their families, they spoke of not being asked about their familial curriculum-making worlds in schools. They seemed to know somehow that their experiences in their familial curriculum-making worlds would not be honored in respectful ways in the school curriculum-making worlds. As we moved alongside the youth into their worlds of home and community, we heard stories of their lives as dancers, grandchildren, siblings, and those who attend to, or are cared for by, others. Lane and Donovan told of 'not telling' stories of who they were in their school curriculum-making world, rather, they knew to hold silent the stories they lived in their familial curriculum-making worlds. We came to know not only diverse stories the youth tell of themselves and/or their families, but also of stories they leave behind because there is no safe place to tell them, share them, or celebrate them. How would Lane's love for his brother with developmental delays that shaped so many of his stories in his familial curriculum-making world be reshaped in the school curriculum-making world? Would his love for music and dance shaped in his familial curriculum-making world be changed were he to make it visible in his school curriculum-making world (Lessard 2014)? How would Donovan's experiences of loss in his familial curriculum-making world be understood or taken up in the school curriculum-making world?

Those of us who work in school curriculum-making worlds often do not understand how the experiences of youth in their familial curriculum-making worlds sustain them in schools. If curriculum making can be understood as life making and if an understanding of curriculum making can be broadened to understand curriculum making as occurring in multiple worlds, both in schools and outside of schools, then we can more intentionally engage questions and wonders about the multiple curriculum-making worlds that any one particular child/youth lives within.

This calls all of us, those in and out of schools, to trust that multiple educative worlds exist within each child and within families and communities. Honouring these educative worlds is important as children and youth, like Lane and Donovan, not only live in these worlds, but also these worlds will continue to shape who they are, and are becoming, in their multiplicity. These multiple worlds, as we learned, sustain their lives in the school curriculum-making world. Young (2005) reminded us of intergenerational reverberations, and the importance of attending to them. As we came to know Donovan and Lane, these reverberations across generations became visible. The walk on the edges of the reserves, an experience Donovan returned to physically, as well as in his memory and imagination, to stories of time spent with his Kookum Muriel and other elders in his home community continued to live within him. The home place with his grandmother called to him often, both to physically return but to also return in his imagination. These multiple returnings shape who Donovan is and is becoming, in his multiple curriculum-making worlds. These familial curriculum-making worlds too often bump up against school curriculum making or remain invisible in his school curriculum-making world, shaping his experiences but not being attended to by those who work with him.

While acknowledging the multiplicity of worlds is a first step in coming to understand the richness of children's and youth's multiple worlds, we see that we also need to learn to honor the richness of multiple worlds of curriculum making, neither to erase or write over other worlds nor to privilege one world over another. This, we imagine, is particularly important for children, youth, and families whose lives are usually seen in more stereotypical and deficit ways through what Dewey once called 'the crust of conventionalized and routine consciousness.' Sean, who lived as an Aboriginal consultant with a mandate to increase high school attendance rates, experienced tensions as he learned of the complexities that Lane and Donovan negotiated as they world traveled to their multiple curriculum-making worlds. At times, as Lane struggled to find places to live, he could not attend school. At one point, Lane experienced difficulty when he was asked to leave school and found himself out-of-school and also without a family home in which to live. He named Sean as someone who understood the multiple curriculum-making worlds that he was negotiating as his worlds collided. He spoke from his heart when he said, 'I am tired. I can't see a way out in life anymore.'

Sean wrote in his field notes:

> He told the social worker that removed him from his home that he would only talk to me at this time. I only had a cryptic message on my cell phone 'can we meet' and then silence. I could not find him . . . he was not at home and not at school. People were searching for him throughout the city. He had been missing for weeks, some even say sleeping outside.

Sean awakened to the impossibility of Lane's world traveling between curriculum-making worlds as he asked, 'Are you alright little brother?' (Lessard 2014) as Lane told him these stories. In these moments Sean attended to Lane's familial curriculum-making world first. As Clandinin and Connelly (1995) noted, the most educative experiences in lives are often not ones situated in school curriculum-making worlds.

Greene reminds us of the importance of breaking 'with the taken-for-granted, to see and to say [. . . to strive] toward significant inclusion [. . . and avoid] the brutal marginalizations, the structured silences, the imposed invisibility so present all around.' (Greene 1993, 211) We see that it is important for us and for others who come alongside Lane and Donovan to imaginatively stretch past taken-for-granted assumptions, to see the richness of their experiences in home communities with kookums and moosums, in cultural protocols and knowledge, and in their relationship building with family and community members and each other. In order to break with the taken-for-granted, to see who we are alongside youth and their families, to wonder about our own constructions of Aboriginal youth and their curriculum-making worlds, we realize the intensive processes of self-facing (Anzaldua 1987). We awakened to how important and difficult it is to continuously resist the stereotypical story of being Aboriginal, to resist categorizations and single stories.

In our work with the youth, their families, and with each other, we often wondered about the relationships between the multiple curriculum-making worlds within which each youth and we lived. As we thought about the lives of some youth, we wondered if the curriculum-making worlds lived in some kind of harmony, that is, there was a kind of seamlessness as the youth world traveled. Most often, however, the multiple curriculum-making worlds seemed to live in parallel ways, in a kind of competing, but not conflicting, relationship. Youth moved from one world to the other and could world travel in multiple worlds. We saw that with some of the youth, some of the times. However, too often the worlds the youth inhabited were worlds where they were constructed and constructed themselves in conflicting ways, so much so that it was impossible for the youth to world travel. When their experiences in their school curriculum-making world were so filled with strife, with the impossibility of composing narrative coherence, that is, of making sense of their lives in the two worlds, they did not world travel but avoided traveling to the school curriculum-making world. They left school, at least for a time.

As we lived alongside the youth and traveled to their curriculum-making worlds, we too struggled to navigate the youth's experiences in the familial and school curriculum worlds. As they shared their stories with us, we could not make sense of the complexities they were trying to make sense of. In these moments Donovan and Lane reminded us how important it was to sustain their, and our, familial curriculum-making worlds, to not let the school curriculum-making world dominate their, and our, life making. Alongside the youth, we saw how they, at times, turned away from the school curriculum-making world to sustain themselves. We knew this was what mattered most to them and we validated their life-making processes. Thinking about Donovan and Lane allowed us to think about the educative spaces within our familial curriculum-making worlds.

We also see that it is important to know the difficulty at times that youth had in forcing themselves to travel to the school curriculum-making world. Lane and Donovan co-composed a world between them as they lived within the school curriculum-making world. As they lived within the school curriculum-making world that may have constructed them as two Aboriginal boys in Grade 7, they created for themselves a world in which the layers of their complexity could live. Without their shared world, as friends, as youth, who saw narrative coherence across their experience as youth from diverse worlds, could they continue to travel to their school curriculum-making world? We recognized how in our work as professionals in nursing and education, and as researchers, we, too, co-compose worlds with others who sustain who we are and are becoming. We see the importance that in our lives as researchers, teachers, parents, nurses, friends, and colleagues, we continue to think narratively, to continue to co-create with others spaces for living, telling, retelling, and reliving stories. It is in these moments that we too wonder how the worlds youth inhabit are shaped by institutional, social, political, and institutional narratives; narratives that bring forward the intersections between neoliberal agendas and education (Smyth, Robinson, and McInery 2014) or social inclusion and marginalization in schools (Pless 2014).

We wondered, as we worked alongside each other and the youth, how the absence of meaningful and attentive spaces lead us, sometimes, to turning inward and to silencing the stories that we live and tell in multiple curriculum-making worlds. Disrupting or interrupting these silences is difficult work. Only by being privileged to come alongside, over time, and in multiple curriculum-making worlds have we come to these ways forward. Only by attending closely to the multiple worlds of youth will we, as researchers, as professionals, as people, be able to understand the experiences of youth, in and out of school. This close attention to life making is slow, patient work where we come to understand not only more about the youth but also more about ourselves and the dominant narratives that structure schools and communities.

Acknowledgements

We would like to acknowledge the youth and their families who became part of this work; the elders for helping us; and the members of the larger research team for their commitment.

This work was supported by the Alberta Centre for Child, Family, and Community Research and the Social Science and Humanities Research Council of Canada.

Notes

1 All italicized text are words spoken by participants, which were recorded between September 2011 and June 2013, or field notes written by us.

2 'Aboriginal peoples' refers to the indigenous peoples of North America; the Canadian constitution recognizes them to be First Nations, Métis and Inuit.

References

Anzaldua, G. 1987. *Borderlands/La Frontera: The New Mestiza*. San Francisco, CA: Spinsters/Aunt Lute.

Brass, G. M. 2009. "Respecting the Medicines: Narrating an Aboriginal Identity." In *Healing Traditions: The Mental Health of Aboriginal Peoples of Canada*, edited by L. J. Kirkmayer and G. Guthrie Valaskaskis, 337–354. Vancouver: UBC Press.

Camilleri-Cassar, F. 2014. "Education Strategies for Social Inclusion or Marginalizing the Marginalized." *Journal of Youth Studies* 17 (2): 252–268. doi:10.1080/13676261.2013.834312.

Clandinin, D. J. 2013. *Engaging in Narrative Inquiry*. San Francisco, CA: Left Coast Press.

Clandinin, D. J., and V. Caine. 2008. "Narrative Inquiry." In *Encyclopedia of Qualitative Research*, edited by L. Given, 541–544. Thousand Oaks, CA: Sage.

Clandinin, D. J., and F. M. Connelly. 1992. "Teacher as Curriculum Maker." In *Handbook of Research on Curriculum*, edited by P. W. Jackson, 363–401. New York: Macmillan.

Clandinin, D. J., and F. M. Connelly. 1995. *Teachers' Professional Knowledge Landscapes*. New York: Teachers College Press.

Clandinin, D. J., and F. M. Connelly. 2000. *Narrative Inquiry: Experience and Story in Qualitative Research*. San Francisco, CA: Jossey-Bass.

Clandinin, D. J., S. Lessard, and V. Caine. 2013. "Reverberations of Narrative Inquiry: How Resonant Echoes of an Inquiry with Early School Leavers Shaped Further Inquiries." *Educação, Sociedade and Culturas* 36: 7–24.

Clandinin, D. J., and J. Rosiek. 2007. "Mapping a Landscape of Narrative Inquiry: Borderland Spaces and Tensions." In *Handbook of Narrative Inquiry: Mapping a Methodology*, edited by D. J. Clandinin, 35–75. Thousand Oaks, CA: Sage.

Clandinin, D. J., P. Steeves, and V. Caine, eds. 2013. *Composing Lives in Transition: A Narrative Inquiry into the Experiences of Early School Leavers*. London: Emerald.

Connelly, F. M., and D. J. Clandinin. 1988. *Teachers as Curriculum Planners: Narratives of Experience*. New York: Teachers College Press.

Connelly, F. M., and D. J. Clandinin. 1999. *Shaping a Professional Identity: Stories of Educational Practice*. New York: Teachers College Press.

Connelly, F. M., and D. J. Clandinin. 2006. "Narrative Inquiry." In *Handbook of Complementary Methods in Education Research*. 3rd ed., edited by J. Green, G. Camilli, and P. Elmore, 477–487. Mahwah, NJ: Lawrence Erlbaum.

EPS (Edmonton Public School). 2009. *Aboriginal Education*. Accessed July 31. http://Aboriginaleducation.epsb.ca/.

Friedel, T. L. 1999. "The Role of Aboriginal Parents in Public Education: Barriers to Change in an Urban Setting." *Canadian Journal of Native Education* 23 (2): 5–34.

Friedel, T. L. 2010. "The More Things Change, the More They Stay the Same: The Challenge of Identity for Native Students in Canada." *Cultural and Pedagogical Inquiry* 1 (2): 22–45.

Greene, M. 1993. "Diversity and Inclusion: Toward a Curriculum for Human Beings." *Teachers College Record* 95 (2): 211–221.

Hollands, R. 2004. "'Rappin' on the Reservation: Canadian Mohawk Youth's Hybrid Cultural Identities." *Sociological Research Online* 9 (3). doi:10.5153/sro.953.

Huber, J., M. S. Murphy, and D. J. Clandinin. 2011. *Places of Curriculum Making*. London: Emerald Press.

Kirmayer, L. J., C. L. Tait, and C. Simpson. 2009. "The Mental Health of Aboriginal Peoples in Canada: Transformations of Identity and Community." In *Healing Traditions. The Mental Health of Aboriginal Peoples of Canada*, edited by L. J. Kirkmayer and G. Guthrie Valaskaskis, 3–35. Vancouver: UBC Press.

LaFromboise, T., J. Trimble, and G. Mohatt. 1990. "Counseling Intervention and American Indian Tradition: An Integrative Approach." *Counseling Psychologist* 18 (4): 628–654. doi:10.1177/ 0011000090184006.

Lessard, S. 2014. "Red Worn Runners. A Narrative Inquiry into the Stories of Aboriginal Youth and Families in Urban Settings." Unpublished Doctoral diss., University of Alberta.

Lugones, M. 1987. "Playfulness, "World"-Travelling, and Loving Perception." *Hypatia* 2 (2): 3–19. doi:10.1111/j.1527–2001.1987.tb01062.x.

NAHO (National Aboriginal Health Organization) 2007. *Broader Determinants of Health in an Aboriginal Context*. Accessed August 1. www.naho.ca/documents/naho/publications/determinants.pdf.

Pless, M. 2014. "Stories from the Margins of the Educational System." *Journal of Youth Studies* 17 (2): 236–251. doi:10.1080/13676261.2013.815700.

Restoule, J. P. 2008. "The Values Carry on: Aboriginal Identity Formation of the Urban-raised Generation." *Canadian Journal of Native Education* 31 (2): 15–33.

Riecken, T., F. Conibear, C. Michel, J. Lyall, T. Scott, M. Tanaka, S. Stewart, J. Riecken, and T. Strong-Wilson. 2006. "Resistance through Re-presenting Culture: Aboriginal Student Film-makers and a Participatory Action Research Project on Health and Wellness." *Canadian Journal of Education* 29 (1): 265–286. doi:10.2307/20054156.

Royal Commission on Aboriginal Peoples. 1996. *Report of the Royal Commission on Aboriginal Peoples*. Ottawa: Canada Communication Group.

Smyth, J., J. Robinson, and P. McInery. 2014. "It's Our Turn – Young People 'Tilting' the Neoliberal Turn." *Journal of Youth Studies* 17 (4): 92–509. doi:10.1080/13676261.2013.830705.

Wilson, K., and E. J. Peters. 2005. "'You Can Make a Place for It': Remapping Urban First Nations Spaces of Identity." *Society and Space* 23: 395–413. http://dx.doi.org/10.1068/d390.

Young, M. 2005. *Pimatisiwin, Walking in a Good Way: A Narrative Inquiry into Language as Identity*. Winnipeg: Pemmican.

12

CURRICULUM AND TEACHER DEVELOPMENT

Jerry Rosiek and D. Jean Clandinin

The word 'curriculum' is a contested term. It is less a word that refers to a single thing, and more a textual Rorschach test upon which teachers, policymakers and scholars project their own values and ideologies. Failure to acknowledge these differences in definition account for the way people seem to talk past one another in conversations about appropriate educational goals and outcomes. Some curriculum theorists focus on narrow cognitive learning outcomes, others focus on ethical and political lessons we teach children, still others focus on holistic habits of being – personal, interpersonal, social, aesthetic, intellectual – that we instil in children. Therefore, before we begin a discussion of the parts that teachers play in the creation of curriculum, we need to circumscribe what we mean by the term 'curriculum'.

'Curriculum' is most commonly used as a noun signifying a course of study prescribed through policy-making processes. Curriculum in this sense is provided to teachers, who in turn deliver it to students through a variety of pedagogical methods. This view presumes curriculum is a kind of object – either a set of books, scope and sequence materials, or a list of content standards. It also presumes a hierarchical relation in which some external authority (usually the state) establishes the curriculum, teachers transmit it with minimal modification, and students are located as passive recipients at the end of a curricular delivery process. This sense of the term is so pervasive it often functions as common sense, making it difficult for listeners to hear 'curriculum' in other ways. Worse, it can function as part of a hegemonic view of education, in which other conceptions of curriculum are ridiculed, deflected with awkward silence, or actively suppressed as subversive.

In communities where more pluralistic conceptions of curriculum are honoured and discussed, this hierarchical view of curriculum is usually described as the mandated curriculum. The addition of the adjective 'mandated' to the term curriculum serves an important function. It rhetorically interrupts the narrow constraints hegemonic ideologies put on the concept by framing a common sense understanding of curriculum as one of many ways of thinking about curricula. In other words, it invites a conversation about what other types of curriculum there might be.

Reprinted with permission of Sage Publications. Acknowledgement; Rosiek, J., & Clandinin, D. J. (2016). Curriculum and teacher development. In D. Wyse, L. Hayward, & J. Pandya (Eds.), *Sage handbook of curriculum, pedagogy, and assessment.* London: Sage.

Beyond mandated curriculum

Once we begin looking beyond the mandated curriculum – beyond textbooks and national, state, and provincial standards – for things that children are taught in schools, a myriad of educational effects come into view. Ideas about curriculum considered in this broader sense are as numerous and varied as ideas about the nature of human minds, society and knowledge. Almost every academic discipline has made its influence felt in the field of curriculum studies, from behaviourist psychology to Marxist sociology, from Aristotelian philosophy to functionalist anthropology, from phenomenology to feminist ethics, from poststructuralist theories of the subject to Critical Race theories about voices from the margins, from STEM professors advocating for inquiry-based curriculum to business leaders making arguments about the importance of good education for economic competitiveness.

This literature provides a variety of other adjectives to describe curriculum, each of which opens up new regions of schooling experience for inquiry and consideration by scholars and policymakers. These include, but are not limited to:

- Planned Curriculum: the outcomes and understandings teachers explicitly seek to achieve with students.

  (Porter, 2006)

- Enacted Curriculum: the outcomes and understandings that are enacted or lived in classrooms.

  (Snyder et al., 1992)

- Assessed Curriculum: the portion of the outcomes and understandings registered by learning assessment practices.

  (Porter, 2006)

- Learned Curriculum: the portion of the planned curriculum that students actually take away from their educational experiences.

  (Porter, 2006)

- Lived Curriculum: the complicated and unexpected ways a planned curriculum unfolds in a classroom.

  (Aoki et al., 2005)

- Hidden Curriculum: the implicit lessons taught by the routines of school life, unacknowledged assumptions organizing subject matter content, tracking systems, and community discourse about schools.

  (Jackson, 1990; Willis, 1997)

- Null Curriculum: the messages conveyed when the explicit school curriculum is silent on a significant topic.

  (Flinders et al., 1986)

- Experienced Curriculum: the holistic learning a student takes away from the events, people, materials, institutional arrangements, social interactions and emotional climate they experience in a course of study.

  (Bobbit, 1918; Connelly and Clandinin, 1988; Dewey, 1902, 1938)

In this chapter, we highlight understandings of curriculum that help us identify the fullest range of teachers' contributions to children's education.

Teachers often begin with a mandated curriculum. Local or federal policymakers provide content standards in the mandated subject matter areas, require the use of certain textbooks or course materials and implement mandatory standardized tests intended to drive teacher curricular decisions. These provide both the resources and constraints within which teachers work. Working within these parameters, however, teachers still need to plan daily, monthly and yearly lessons. This planning process is one of the first places that teachers work as co-creators/co-makers of the curriculum. Dependent upon teachers' work contexts, they may regularly decide what to emphasize, how to represent the content to students, how much time to dedicate to specific content, what activities to set up and how to integrate content in one area with content in another area. These decisions profoundly influence students' experience of the curriculum.

A thoughtful teacher will also attend to the hidden curriculum within the mandated curricula. For example, a biology textbook might describe sperm and egg cells with gender stereotypical adjectives implying that one is active and the other passive in the reproductive process. The teacher could plan to highlight this bias for students, correct the misrepresentation and use it as an opportunity to highlight how sexist assumptions can get in the way of accurate scientific description. Thoughtful teachers will also plan to address the null curriculum within state mandated curricula. For example, a social studies textbook on civil rights struggles might leave out the history of activism for Lesbian, Gay, Bisexual, Transgender and Queer (LGBTQ) rights in a nation. The teacher could plan to include supplementary material on this topic. She might also engage students in a discussion of why this topic is excluded in the textbook and state curricular standards. In this way, the course materials become an illustration of the need for continued struggle for justice and inclusion in our communities.

Once a curriculum is planned, teachers put it into practice and it becomes a lived curriculum or experienced curriculum. It is more accurate to refer to this as curricula because each child and each teacher experiences or lives a different curriculum. Just as the mandated curriculum cannot anticipate or prescribe all the things a teacher needs to plan for a lesson, neither can a teacher's plan anticipate and predict everything that will happen with students in the course of teaching a lesson. Unexpected student responses or other classroom or school events can distract from teaching goals or present opportunities for more profound learning. These unexpected developments require that teachers make improvisational decisions that shape the lived curriculum in their classrooms.

For example, a language arts lesson involving writing about seasons could lead to a question about why leaves change colours. The teacher engages students in a discussion about the possible reasons leaves change colour in the autumn. She along with several students believes this is triggered by changes in temperature, but upon assigning a student the task of researching the question, finds out that it is the shortening length of the day that is the primary trigger for leaf change. In this way a writing lesson evolved into a science lesson in an unplanned way. It also provided the teacher with an opportunity to change her mind based on the evidence gathered by a student.

Teachers also make other less content-specific contributions to the lived curriculum or experienced curriculum (Connelly and Clandinin, 1988). Teacher – student interactions provide opportunities for nuanced influence on student learning. Choice of tone in a response, the way praise is offered, or deciding to withhold direct answers to questions so students can wrestle with uncertainty about a topic, all substantively influence what students learn. Providing scaffolding that helps a student understand their uncertainty as natural, or strategically looking away so a student experiences their inquiry as their own, are also examples of the improvisational contributions teachers make to the lived curriculum. To this we add the inclusion of humour in class, expressing concerns about a sick parent, asking about a volleyball game the previous evening – actions that are not directly related to the planned curriculum but which build personal relationships with students which, in turn, colour the entire experience of schooling for students. The ways that teachers establish the physical environment in the classroom by choices of furniture and arrangement and how each teacher positions him or herself and positions the students in relation to him/her and each other also creates or makes part of the experienced curriculum (Connelly and Clandinin, 1988).

Taken together, these more complex ideas of curriculum make clear the inadequacy of a view of curriculum as something fixed, that is, a discrete object to be delivered by teachers and consumed by students. Curriculum, considered through these multiple lenses, is revealed as an experiential process. It is made or co-constructed as teachers, learners, subject matter and milieu interact in schools and classrooms (Aoki, 1993; Clandinin and Connelly, 1992; Connelly and Clandinin, 1988; Oyler, 2012).

An epistemology and ontology of curriculum making

Practitioners and scholars readily acknowledge that there is much more going on in classrooms than is specified in mandated curricula; however, common sense ideas about curriculum as a package that can be delivered by teachers to their students like a bulk postal mailing remain difficult to dispel. Common sense ideas about the relationship between knowledge, reality and the purpose of learning contribute to this difficulty; therefore, developing educational policy and practice that substantively addresses all levels of curricular content will require some reflection on the epistemologies and ontologies underlying contemporary curricular debates.

Knowledge is framed in popular culture (and in some academic disciplines) as a set of exclusively accurate representations of an independent reality. This conception of knowledge is based on a dualistic ontology that sees the world of objects and the world of ideas as fundamentally separate. Learning, consequently, is the process of sorting through ideas to identify the ones that actually match the world of real objects. This, in turn, informs a conception of education in which teachers' mediating activity and students' interpretative activity are a means to learning, but do not contribute to the content of the curriculum. All that ultimately matters is the match between a child's ideas and an external objective world. This matching process is assumed to be identical for all students, and this view implies nothing else of significance is, or should be, learned in the educational process.

It is this common sense conception of knowledge and education that makes the use of mandatory high stakes standardized testing as a primary driver of education practice seem reasonable. If all students need to learn the same things, then applying a standardized assessment instrument to all students can let us know if we are accomplishing our learning goals. If there is no other more context-dependent learning going on – no enacted, lived, hidden, null or experienced curriculum – then we need not worry about the unintended consequences of the imposition of standardized tests on all schools.

This naïve epistemology and corresponding dualistic ontology, however, does not stand up to critical scrutiny. Critiques of such views by philosophers are myriad. Hermeneuticists since Dilthey in the nineteenth century have argued that all knowledge is context dependent (Dilthey and Rickman, 1979). Marxists and critical theorists for the past 150 years have documented the way economic interests distort claims of objectivity and empirical knowledge (Adorno, 2013; Horkheimer, 2012). Existentialists like Heidegger (1977, 2008) historicize the practice of treating knowledge as if it is a picture of the world, identifying it as a recent modern development that generates a peculiar way of being in the world. Cultural anthropologists have documented the way 'knowledge' is understood and operates differently across different cultures (Gross, 2014; Rabinow et al., 2008). Historians of science have shown how even within the same culture – in this case Western culture – conceptions of what counts as scientific knowledge have changed in response to social and political contexts (Kuhn, 1970; Livingstone, 2003). Sociologists of knowledge have documented how this happens in contemporary disciplines, in macro social and micro social ways (Foucault, 1982; Latour, 2007). Post-structuralists have raised profound questions about the semiotic processes involved in representations of knowledge, highlighting how we never have unmediated access to an independent world (Butler, 2006, 2015; Lather, 2010). Everything we experience is always already mediated. Recently feminist materialists have questioned the idea that we live in a passive world awaiting a single perfect representation of it (Alaimo and Hekman, 2008; Barad, 2007). They offer instead that it is more accurate and ethically sound to think of ways of knowing as the means by which we establish possible ontological intra-actions with a variety of non-human agents. Educational scholars have taken up all of these philosophies and applied their angles of critique to curriculum theorizing, which add to understandings of curriculum making.

For our purposes, classic and contemporary pragmatist philosophy provides the most useful alternative framework for thinking about teachers' work as curriculum makers. Pragmatism has features that make it particularly well suited for thinking about teachers' contribution to curriculum making. First, it affirms that ordinary experience – in this case the ordinary experience of teachers – can be an important source of unique knowledge and insight. According to Dewey (1988), the problem with academic claims to have a monopoly on valid forms of knowledge 'is that in casting aspersion upon the events and objects of experience, they deny the power of common life to develop its own regulative methods and to furnish from within itself adequate goals, ideals, and criteria' (1988: 392). Applied to the field of curriculum theory, this view of knowledge implies that curriculum scholars – whether they are positivists producing curriculum knowledge based on experimental trials or critical theorists producing curriculum knowledge informed by ideological critique – do not have a corner on important curricular insight. It affirms the likelihood that there is content in teaching experience that, if paid attention to, could open unique possibilities of thought and pedagogical action.

Second, pragmatism emphasizes the inclusiveness and continuity of experience. Experience is a fundamental non-dualistic ontological substance for pragmatists (Sorrell, 2004). Experience includes objects as well as our patterns of attention; it is all we have. Epistemology for the pragmatist therefore becomes a form of ontology. Knowledge is not a representation that stands apart from our experience and needs to be matched to it; instead, knowing or composing knowledge is one more form of experience, a mode or habit of being, integrated with other habits of being. The merit of these habits cannot ultimately be measured by how well they conform to some external standard, rather they must be judged by the quality of the transformation it works in the overall continuing stream of a person's experience.

Curriculum, according to this view, is far more than a set of ideas that we pour into students' empty minds. Curriculum, instead, involves assisting students to acquire new habits of being in the world – not just what we narrowly call knowledge, but also temperament, disposition, aesthetic appreciation, enthusiasm for specific topics, emotional intelligence, ethics, compassion, etc. Because everything happening in students' schooling experience potentially contributes to their habits of being, a school's curriculum is essentially everything that happens at school. The ultimate measure of the value of this curriculum is the quality of the overall transformation it works in the life of each child.

Here we begin to see the *necessity* of considering teachers as curriculum makers. Teachers are in the best position to see the full range of curricula that students experience at school and to gauge their effects. Subject matter experts operating outside classrooms might be able to generate lists of concepts or 'standards' they would like to see included in mandated curricula, but those lists can never account for all, or even most, of the learning happening in schools. Accountability policies, which treat everything not on these lists of standards as distractions that can be ignored, are enforcing a lack of accountability for the full range of learning that can and does happen at schools. Taking responsibility for this full range of curricular effects requires preparing, supporting and trusting teachers as curriculum-constituting agents or, in our terms, curriculum makers.

Third, pragmatism includes a politics that is grounded in respecting and listening to others as centres of experience (Dewey, 1916, 1988). To curriculum scholars whose primary influences are critical theory or post-structuralist sociology, pragmatism's emphasis on an ontology of experience may seem to risk acquiescence to dangerous forms of provincialism (Rosiek, 2013). Ideologies and discourses can operate at such a large scale that we do not notice their influence on us; therefore, the claim is made that there are no resources within our experience that permit us to recognize our own complicity with various systems of oppression. This concern is particularly relevant to the practice of curriculum making, wherein educators' cultural and ideological limitations have inflicted all manner of violence on the students in their care (Ferguson, 2001; Pascoe, 2011; Rosiek, forthcoming).

These risks, however, are an existentially inescapable condition for all human inquiry according to pragmatists. Positivists, Marxists and post-structuralists are not exempt from the risk of ignoring salient elements of the experience of others in the pursuit of their favoured analytic approaches (Clandinin and Rosiek, 2007). The most serious obstruction to establishing just and inclusive communities, according to the pragmatist, is the delusion that we can escape provincialism through some appeal to a single onto-epistemic practice of relation – be it totalizing scientific knowledge, a totalizing Marxist historical critique, or a universalized postmodern irony – that transcends all time and context. Any claim to have a transcendental vantage point that reveals what matters most, be it critical or empirical, involves a corresponding claim about whose experience matters less. Such hubris was historically at the heart of settler-society colonialism that dismisses the experiences of indigenous peoples as morally and intellectually primitive, white supremacy that dehumanizes everyone by reducing them to racial signifiers, patriarchal oppression that dismisses the experience of women as irrational and unintelligent, and programs of liberation that ignore the concerns of those being liberated as the products of false consciousness or internalized oppression. Avoiding these excesses, according to pragmatists, requires recognizing that we cannot escape our skins, our location, or our contingent place in history. Such recognition removes an enabling condition of patronizing foundationalism and gives us a chance to begin the work of listening and building community with others (McKenna and Pratt, 2015; West, 2000).

Once we relinquish the enlightenment dream of a totalizing onto-epistemic practice that will underwrite our construction of just communities, what guidance is left for generous cooperation among people? According to the pragmatist, the project of ameliorative social transformation relies on a practice of imagining real finite future possibilities. Our inquiries are transactions between the present and these material futures always coming into view. According to contemporary pragmatist Colapietro (2011):

> 'We do not use the present to control the future. We use the foresight of the future to refine and expand present activity' (Dewey, 2008: 215). But insofar as we do refine and enlarge such activity, we ineluctably reshape the future. Thus, the most compelling reason to imagine the future is to reimagine and, thereby, to mobilize the resources requisite for remaking the present.
>
> *(2011: 161)*

Again, we see the pragmatic principle of the continuity of experience at work. The effort to work towards a better future always involves acknowledging the history that brought us to our present state of relations – global, local and personal histories. It involves creatively working to transform our present relational habits, including epistemic habits, that have a chance of carrying us to a better future. Applied to processes of developing socially transformative curriculum, this means it will not be enough to teach students the general conceptual content of history, or general principles of democratic interaction, or even general mathematical or scientific concepts. Students will need an education that invites them to see the local and personal implications of bodies of general knowledge, and an education that helps establish habits of thought, feeling and sociality that permits amelioration of the conditions of living on this planet.

Making curriculum cannot be a generalized process because students come to learning with different local and personal histories. Although there are general patterns therein that must be addressed within the learning process, students need to be guided from where they are. They also need to be educated to appreciate – not erase – the different histories and experiences of others in the process of learning more general truths. Otherwise, the hidden curriculum of schooling becomes one of suppressing and erasing difference – usually the different histories and ways of knowing of those already at the receiving end of various forms of oppression and erasure.

It is the teacher, if she/he is prepared to listen, who is in the position to understand the different histories that children bring into the room, to see the possibilities latent in the connections that can be made between those personal histories, the local context, and the global settings in which we live and learn. The continuing challenge for the field of curriculum theory is to provide visions of what such teacher preparation might look like.

Theorizing teachers as curriculum makers

The idea of seeing teachers as curriculum makers began to enter the curriculum literature in the 1980s with the work of Snyder, Bolin, Zumwalt, Aoki, Clandinin and Connelly. With the inclusion of the concept of teachers as curriculum makers in the 1992 *Handbook of Research on Curriculum* (Jackson, 1992), the concept entered the curriculum studies canon and gained more scholarly recognition. The idea that teachers were composers, creators or makers of curriculum emerged from three different theory frameworks: curriculum-as-enacted, curriculum-as-lived, and curriculum-as-experienced.

Those who worked with the idea of curriculum enactment (Snyder et al., 1992) argued that curriculum materials may be provided or even mandated, but teachers and students inevitably adapt them to their needs and context. This adaptation is intellectual work and ultimately it is the enacted lessons that constitute the curriculum that students experience.

Similarly, Aoki (1993) explored ways of thinking about curriculum as something made and experienced in situations, in the negotiations between teachers and children. He focused not only on adaptation of externally provided materials, but also on the improvisational moves teachers make in the spaces between curriculum-as-planned and curriculum-as-lived, spaces between the teacher and each child, spaces between the dominant institutional narratives shaping classrooms and school contexts and the 'everyday narratives' lived and told by teachers and children.

Connelly and Clandinin brought their understandings of teachers' knowledge as embodied, temporal, relational, contextual, and as shaped and reshaped in present situations by past experience and future plans (Clandinin, 1985; Connelly and Clandinin, 1988) to a narrative exploration of a 'curriculum of life' as 'something experienced in situations' (p. 6), shaped by 'teachers' and students' lives together in schools and classrooms' (Clandinin and Connelly, 1992: 32). Naming teachers as 'curriculum makers' and drawing on Schwab's (1978) curriculum commonplaces – teacher, learner, subject matter, milieu – they conceptualized curriculum as experience, and curriculum making as the meeting of the diverse lives of teachers, children and families.

In addition to adaptations of received curriculum materials, and in addition to the improvisational moves teachers make in the liminal spaces of teaching, Connelly and Clandinin (1988) drew attention to how teachers' autobiographies and identities were always a part of the context of teaching. Changing the curriculum, therefore, was not just a technical, conceptual or ideological enterprise, it also involved existential transformations of teaching selves. These transformations could be minor or grand, but the work of teaching involved teachers as whole persons.

In these theories, we see the centrality of the inclusive ontological concept of experience – specifically the experience of teachers and students – as the beginning and ending point of curriculum inquiry. We also see that teachers' work of curriculum making happens at many levels and draws upon many resources.

Resources for teachers' curriculum making

Given the wide variety of nested influences on children's educational experiences and the fact that all of these influences contribute in some way to what children learn, narrow definitions of the term 'curriculum' only serve as obstructions to clear dialogue about curricular priorities. We offer, instead, that the term 'curriculum' is best reserved to refer to the full range of things learned by children in schools and other educational settings. In short, curriculum is the experienced curriculum, and each child experiences a different curriculum, even though she/he may be in the same classroom with the same resources at the same time. Where finer grained distinctions are needed, the phrase 'curriculum resources' is both more accurate and appropriate.

Framed as such, teachers are the professionals in schools who are ultimately responsible for curriculum making. Teachers stand at the intersection of all these curricular influences and help guide students to productive engagements with the experienced curriculum. All curricular input – from legislative committees, panels of subject matter experts, publishers, student creativity, parent advocacy, local experts, etc. – constitute different forms of 'curricular resources'.

At their best, curricular resources are flexibly designed to help teachers in this work of integrating with other kinds of influence on student learning. Fortunately, there are many exceptionally well-designed curricular resources available to educators. At their worst, however, curriculum resources are marketed as panaceas and enforced as procrustean displacements of all other influences on children's experience.

To mistake a curricular resource for the curriculum itself constitutes a retreat from the reality of educational processes. The reality of the multiple contextual influences on the content of learning is intrinsic to educational experience and cannot be erased. The effort to do so does not bring improvement, but instead results in deprofessionalization of teaching and deracination of children's educational experience.

Preparing teachers as curriculum makers therefore requires preparing them to be improvisational thinkers, sensitized to the many levels of nested influence on students' experiences, and informed about the many curricular resources available to themselves and students. These curricular resources include (but are not limited to) the following areas.

Mandated curriculum resources

In contexts where there are mandated curricula, one of the sources that teachers look to are the outcomes, aims, purposes and approved materials, such as packaged curriculum materials, textbooks, lab guides, novels, etc. that are approved by the governing bodies. Publishers' materials provided by school districts and schools or that teachers acquire on their own are important resources in the curriculum making processes.

Supplemental curriculum resources

Another source of externally created curriculum materials are materials developed by non-governmental, non-profit and for-profit agencies, such as the Legacy of Hope materials developed by the Aboriginal Healing Foundation in Canada, the Rethinking Schools Publishing group, Teaching for Tolerance, teacherspayteachers.com and various other issue-driven organizations that produce documentaries, websites and paper resources for teachers.

Local curriculum resources

Another source are the materials that are provided by local contexts, such as the local geography, history and people who live in an area. Some of these resources are available in local museums and parks and are increasingly available through social media.

Children's input as curriculum resources

Children's experiences are also curriculum resources when their place as co-constructors of curriculum (that is, as curriculum makers) is acknowledged (He et al., 2008; Huber et al., 2005). Teachers invite children in more or less central ways into classroom curriculum making. We see this, for example, in Oyler's (2012) case studies and in other studies where children and youth become centrally involved in curriculum making.

Families' lives as curriculum resources

Students' families, defined broadly within temporal span, geographic location and cultural diversity, offer rich sources of knowledge as curriculum resources. When families' lives are brought into curriculum making, a richness that spans intergenerational time, place and relationships is made visible (Marsh, 2003; Miller Marsh and Turner-Vorbeck, 2009).

Colleagues' input as curriculum resources

Colleagues' curriculum making in schools, past and present, is an important curriculum resource. In schools where there are teachers committed to inquiry-based learning or attention to social justice practices, teachers shape one another's practices through their classroom visits, through the stories that shape the knowledge landscape in a school or in the stories that children and parents bring to each teacher's curriculum making. Extending this idea backward in time, where a teacher has taught in the past, influences their current curriculum making.

Teacher's personal practical knowledge as curriculum resource

The most important resource in understanding the experienced curricula in classrooms, however, is the teachers' personal practical knowledge as she/he draws forward curriculum resources seen to be relevant. Teacher knowledge, conceptualized as personal practical knowledge, is knowledge 'imbued with all the experiences that make up a person's being. Its meaning is derived from, and understood in terms of a person's experiential history, both professional and personal' (Clandinin, 1985: 362). Teacher knowledge is shaped by what Clandinin and Connelly (1995) called a professional knowledge landscape, a way of thinking of school contexts in order to attend to relationships amongst people, places and things, and to both the moral and intellectual qualities of school contexts. A school's professional knowledge landscape is composed of in- and out-of-classroom places and off landscape places. Off the professional knowledge landscape for each teacher is seen as a personal knowledge landscape (Clandinin et al., 2014). Professional and personal knowledge landscapes are always shifting and changing. Within such a view it is possible to see that each teacher's experiential knowledge from his/her own schooling, his/her life outside of schools, experiences in his/her early life all play a part in shaping how they compose curriculum in the classroom.

Teachers as remixers of curriculum resources

What we have made explicit in this chapter is a conception of curriculum that positions the teacher in a central place in curriculum making. When we position the teacher as a maker (and hence as a person with agency to draw upon various resources), his/her teacher knowledge is a central consideration (Clandinin and Connelly, 1992).

Identifying the teacher as the central mediator of many different curriculum resources brings to mind the image of a music producer who remixes different digital audio files in the process of composing music. Similarly, a teacher draws from a multiplicity of curriculum resources and remixes them to make curriculum in their classrooms. Choice of resources, timing and levels of emphasis all contribute to the overall curricular composition. Ultimately such curriculum remixing depends upon the teacher's knowledge, including what the teacher knows about a particular subject matter, but also their personal experience with the subject matter, their knowledge of the local area and their knowledge of students. Take, for example, the earlier example about the changing colours of the leaves in the autumn. A teacher's knowledge of photosynthetic chemistry makes a difference, as does the availability of curriculum materials on this topic and the teacher's knowledge about local flora. The remixing might be quite different depending upon the curricular resources that she/he has, or is awake to having, available.

Teacher preparation for curriculum making, therefore, requires that careful attention be paid to a teacher's repertoire of curriculum resources. It is not enough to rely on mandated curriculum or on personal experiences. Knowledge of local resources and of the lives and of students' experiences is also essential, as is the understanding of the contradictions that often exist between the different curricular resources. For example, when teaching a history lesson, it matters a great deal whether a teacher draws upon local curriculum resources, such as knowledge of the particular history of a community or on published materials about a particular cultural group. If the teacher relies on a multinational publisher's kit on the history of Aboriginal peoples in Canada, children are invited into a certain kind of understanding and relation to one another. However, if she/he draws upon materials from the Legacy of Hope materials made by an Aboriginal non-profit organization, children are invited into a very different kind of understanding and relation to one another. If she/he relies on her/his own experiences of growing up in the late 1990s in western Canada, depending upon her/his life stories, children are invited yet another very different kind of understanding and relation to one another. We can see that a great deal is at stake in the processes of remixing as the teacher weaves together curriculum resources in ways that make sense to them. This example illustrates the way colonialist ideologies operate or are resisted, not only in curriculum resource production, but also in classroom curriculum making (Lessard, 2014).

Understanding curriculum making in this way draws attention to the need for time and support for teachers' inquiries into multiple ways of remixing curriculum resources. In comparing various remixing strategies, teachers can become better at thinking through the multiple implications of their curricular decisions. Without such future oriented thinking, fostering respect for difference, social justice and democratic ideals in their classrooms is not substantively possible. This highlights the need for reimagining teacher education, both pre- and in-service, in ways that are seen less as monitoring performance or outcomes and more as creating inquiry spaces for teachers (Zeichner, 2010).

Creating curriculum in a variety of contexts

We have highlighted the ways that teachers draw forward different curriculum resources and remix them in ways that are congruent with each teacher's knowledge.

The picture we created was one with a great deal of teacher autonomy; however, we need to make explicit that teachers do not work in isolation, nor do they work in contexts of their own choosing.

The curriculum that is being made at the intersection of children's and teachers' lives in relation to subject matter also depends upon attending to the places within which curriculum is made. What curriculum is made depends upon the particular place nested within larger places in which each teacher works. For example, place would certainly make a difference for the curriculum making about the civil rights struggle for LGBTQ rights in a nation. Both time and place would influence the likely reception of such lessons. Some years ago in Canada and the US, most policymakers would not have seen the oppression of LGBTQ persons and families as a civil rights or human rights issue, which would have made teaching such a lesson more difficult and even professionally risky; however, LGBTQ rights are increasingly codified in Canadian and US society. This normalizes teaching about the subject and permitting more informed and receptive discussions of the topic. These differences in context influence curriculum making in profound ways.

In an international handbook such as this we need to be attentive to the complexity of what we mean by place, that is, place in the sense of particular geographies and natural and man-made architectures but also place in the sense of particular governments and policies. State education policies shape teacher autonomy and professionalism almost everywhere that formal teaching is occurring. National contexts, such as the one currently shaping the curriculum making in Finland's schools, come to mind. In Finnish schools, there is a great deal of respect for teachers as curriculum makers. As the research literature indicates (Sahlberg, 2011), curriculum making in Finland relies heavily upon teacher knowledge because teachers come together in collaborative ways to create curriculum in schools. However, it is important to note that even within a particular place, particular knowledge landscapes also shape the curriculum making that occurs, that is, it matters where the school is locate (in urban, rural or suburban places) and whether the school is in the north of Finland or in the more urban south. It also matters what particular cultures or narratives shape the knowledge landscapes in particular schools. In other places, such as the US, where there is less emphasis on teacher autonomy and teacher professionalism, curriculum making occurs in different ways because mandated curriculum with attendant standardized testing shapes what is possible for teachers to compose in their classrooms with students.

Contexts also include the cultural values and traditions that shape parent – teacher relationships. There are some places where there are robust parent – teacher collaborative cultures, that is, places structured in ways that see parents and teachers as engaging together to create educative experiences for children. In such places there is a sense that the voices and experiences of both teachers and parents/families are respected and heard. In other places parents do not work from a position of respecting teachers as holders of knowledge, and teachers do not value and access parent knowledge in their curriculum making. These differences in context can easily change the educational character of places to ones where mutuality and respect are not visible (Ayers, 1989; Goldstein, 1998).

Other contextual influences include the way schooling is shaped by stratified educational opportunity and oppressive hidden curricula. These places can be ones where some children and families have access to more and richer resources than are available to other children and families. We see this in evidence in some school settings where children are marked as different either in intellectual and physical abilities, cultural and economic status, or in other ways (Chan, 2006; Chang and Rosiek, 2003; Goldstein, 1998; Rosiek and Heffernan, 2014).

The important thing to acknowledge here is that teachers are always making curriculum with their students even when they work in policy contexts that do not see them as curriculum makers. In such situations teachers often have to work against dominant discourses that ignore or suppress their contributions to curriculum making (Miller, 2005). For example, there are many contexts that are shaped by nationalized curricular movements. These nationalized curricula movements, such as the maths and science curricular reforms of the 1960s in the US, strongly shaped teachers' work. Mandated curriculum resources were prescribed in order to increase students' knowledge of mathematics and sciences. There have been other nationalized curricular movements, such as the communicative language mandates in China or the balanced literacy movements in Canada.

In recent years we have noticed a wave of mandated assessments being used to enforce nationally mandated curricula in many countries. Pushed by concern about rankings on the Programme for International Student Assessment (PISA) tests, many countries are now developing their own testing regimes in order to monitor how students and the teachers of students perform in the tests. Many of these testing programs are built using either an implicitly or explicitly teacher-proof view of curriculum, that is, the mandated resources are designed to ensure teachers will deliver the curriculum in a narrowly prescribed manner. As we have seen, this is not an adequate view of curriculum making that acknowledges the complex processes of the experienced or lived curriculum. Neither is it an adequate view of assessment. Nonetheless, this narrow view of teaching and learning is currently at work in many schools in different nations.

Although contexts influence the possibilities of what curricula are made, it does not change the fact that curricula are being made and remade by teachers. Whether the teacher works in a suburban context in Canada or the US or in a rural context in China, the teacher is a central actor in the curriculum making process. Similarly whether the teacher is teaching a prescribed curriculum resource that is designed to be teacher proof or if she/he is remixing curriculum materials from the community, she/he is still a central actor in the process. For us, what is of central importance is that each teacher understands and is critically reflective about who she/he is as a curriculum maker (Connelly and Clandinin, 1988).

How to prepare teachers as curriculum makers

Our starting point therefore as teacher educators is to work with teachers and prospective teachers to help them recognize their role as curricular agents. There are several possible starting points to help them begin to see themselves as central in curriculum making. We can begin by engaging ourselves as teacher educators and those who we teach in autobiographical inquiry, such as described by Connelly and Clandinin (1988), Grumet (1987), Pinar (1994) and others. It is important that these inquiry processes begin not with a narrow view of the teacher but with understandings that we are in the processes of becoming teachers and people, shaped by multiple contexts over time, place and relationships, and that different situations draw different responses from each of us. Context does make a difference.

As we engage teachers in these autobiographical inquiries it is important that we engage with them in multiple contexts, in and out of schools, and that we ask them to attend closely to what they learn about themselves as they engage with diverse children and youth on a range of subject matters. For example, we might ask them to work with children and youth in urban communities in settings such as Boys and Girls clubs (Desrochers, 2006) or in summer technology education enrichment programs in wealthy suburbs. These experiences, properly facilitated, can help them learn what such situations call forth from their personal history and knowledge. Similarly, we can ask them to inquire into what viewing books, movies and other media and artworks demands from them, not to engage in a therapeutic process but to surface the multiplicity of stories they tell of who they are and who they are becoming (Seiki, 2014).

As teacher educators, part of the work we engage in with teachers involves providing spaces where they can begin these autobiographical inquiries that can enable them to question, affirm and/or change how they know and what they know. These autobiographical inquiries are starting points for building an understanding of what curricular resources we each draw upon and how we remix them when we engage with children and youth in curriculum making situations (Gomez, 2014).

Our task as teacher educators is to help prepare teachers to organize and select materials with attentiveness to the broad range of learning they can foster through their remixing. We also need to help them prepare to influence the contexts in which they work, whether these contexts are at the school level, the community level or the district and state/provincial levels (Craig, 2012). In part this requires encouraging teachers to see their work as influencing not only the students in their classrooms, but also understanding that they are agents who can shape the broader milieus or contexts within which they work (Rodgers, 2002).

This work requires of teacher educators what we ask of teachers: that we pay close attention to teachers in their curriculum making process, working and thinking alongside them, and helping them be awake to, but not overwhelmed by, the responsibility they face. As teacher educators, we have heard young teachers who aspire to be curriculum makers describe themselves as failures because they have found themselves using packaged curricular materials. This either/or logic is neither helpful nor is it accurate. It is based on the oversimplified view that the published form of curriculum, rather than curriculum experienced by students, is the crucial issue. Packaged curriculum materials can be of value, but only if we use the materials in ways that create educative situations for the children and youth with whom we are engaged. Of course some curricular materials have more curriculum potential (Ben-Peretz, 1990) than others.

Although teachers cannot always control the material and institutional context in which they work, they can, to a great degree, control the way they think about students and imagine their possibilities. A sense of responsibility for this, rather than curricular form, is what teacher educators should foster. Teachers need to be attentive to how their gaze constructs their students' experienced curriculum. For example, it is well established (Lessard et al., 2015) that if my gaze, as a curriculum maker, on a child frames the student in terms of their deficits as opposed to their resiliency and strength, this harms students. If my gaze as a curriculum maker is only grounded in a particular disciplinary knowledge without an understanding of the life of a young person, it has profound impact on the experienced curriculum of that child. If my gaze as a curriculum maker fails to notice and respond to students' excitement about a particular topic, opportunities are missed that have a profound impact on the experienced curriculum of that child or youth. As teacher educators we need to find ways to ensure that teachers understand the impact they have on the curriculum that they are making with children and youth. Without that starting point, curriculum is reduced to the unmanaged consequence of students encountering resource materials. All the learning made possible by thoughtful teacher mediation of those materials is lost.

Conclusion

Our task as teacher educators is to work in experiential ways with teachers and prospective teachers to help them claim their places as curriculum makers with children and families. Greene (1993) reminds us to work alongside teachers as curriculum makers to awaken them to 'the contradictions, the instances of savagery, the neglect, and the possibility of care' (1993: 220) that we meet in classrooms. We must work alongside teachers to face ourselves, and how we – and they – are complicit in curriculum making. Our task is not only one of showing them what is, but also to help them imagine otherwise – to be wide awake enough to sense when they could work with children to co-construct curricula of possibility, curricula that are not yet but which could be. Our work as teacher educators is to ignite imaginative possibilities (Eisner, 1985). Being able to imagine otherwise is one of the most important skills that we can develop in ourselves as curriculum makers and in the teachers with whom we work.

References

Adorno, T. W. (2013) *Against Epistemology: A Metacritique: Studies in Husserl and the Phenomenological Antinomies* [W. Domingo, trans.]. Malden, MA: Polity Press.

Alaimo, S., and Hekman, S. J. (eds.) (2008) *Material Feminisms*. Bloomington, IN: Indiana University Press.

Aoki, T. (1993) 'Legitimating lived curriculum: towards a curricular landscape of multiplicity', *Journal of Curriculum and Supervision*, 8(3): 255–68.

Aoki, T., Pinar, W. and Irwin, R. (eds.) (2005) *Curriculum in a New Key: The Collected Works of Ted T. Aoki*. Mahwah, NJ: Erlbaum Associates.

Ayers, W. (1989) *The Good Preschool Teacher: Six Teachers Reflect on Their Lives* New York, NY: Teachers College Press.

Barad, K. M. (2007) *Meeting the Universe Halfway: Quantum Physics and the Entanglement of Matter and Meaning*. Durham, NC: Duke University Press.

Ben-Peretz, M. (1990) *The Teacher–Curriculum Encounter: Freeing Teachers From the Tyranny of Texts*. Albany, NY: State University of New York Press.

Bobbitt, F. (1918) *The Curriculum*. Boston, MA: Houghton Mifflin.

Butler, J. (2006) *Gender Trouble: Feminism and the Subversion of Identity*. New York, NY: Routledge.

Butler, J. (2015) *Senses of the Subject*. New York: Fordham Press.

Chan, E. (2006) 'Teacher experiences of culture in the curriculum', *Journal of Curriculum Studies*, 38(2): 161–76.

Chang, P. and Rosiek, J. (2003) 'Anti-colonial antinomies: a case of cultural conflict in the high school biology curriculum', *Curriculum Inquiry*, 33(3): 251–90.

Clandinin, D. J. (1985) 'Personal practical knowledge: a study of teachers' classroom images', *Curriculum Inquiry*, 15(4): 361–85.

Clandinin, D. J. and Connelly, F. M. (1992) 'Teacher as curriculum maker', in P. W. Jackson (ed.), *Handbook of Research on Curriculum*. New York, NY: Macmillan. pp. 363–401.

Clandinin, D. J. and Connelly, F. M. (1995) *Teachers' Professional Knowledge Landscapes*. New York, NY: Teachers College Press.

Clandinin, D. J. and Rosiek, J. L. (2007) 'Mapping the landscape of narrative inquiry: borderland spaces and tensions', in D. J. Clandinin (ed.), *Handbook of Narrative Inquiry: Mapping a Methodology* Thousand Oaks, CA: Sage Publications. pp. 35–76.

Clandinin, D. J., Schaefer, L. and Downey, C. A. (2014) *Narrative Conceptions of Knowledge: Toward Understanding Teacher Attrition*. Bingley, UK: Emerald Group.

Colapietro, V. (2011) 'Customary reflection and innovative habits', *The Journal of Speculative Philosophy*, 25: 161–73.

Connelly, F. M. and Clandinin, D. J. (1988) *Teachers As Curriculum Planners: Narratives of Experience*. New York, NY: Teachers College Press.

Craig, C. (2012) '"Butterfly under a pin": an emergent teacher image amid mandated curriculum reform', *Journal of Educational Research*, 105(2): 90–101.

Desrochers, C. (2006) 'Towards a New Borderland in Teacher Education for Diversity: A Narrative Inquiry Into Preservice Teachers' Shifting Identities Through Service Learning'. Unpublished doctoral dissertation, University of Alberta, Edmonton.

Dewey, J. (1902) *The Child and the Curriculum*. Chicago: University of Chicago Press.

Dewey, J. (1916) *Democracy and Education: An Introduction to the Philosophy of Education*. New York, NY: MacMillan.

Dewey, J. (1938) *Experience and Education*. New York, NY: Simon and Schuster.

Dewey, J. (1988) *The Later Works of John Dewey, Volume 1, 1925–1953: 1925 Experience and Nature*. Carbondale, IL: Southern Illinois University Press.

Dewey, J. (2008) *The Middle Works of John Dewey, Volume 9, 1899–1924: Democracy and Education, 1916*. Carbondale, IL: Southern Illinois University Press.

Dilthey, W. and Rickman, H. P. (1979) *Selected Writings*. Cambridge: Cambridge University Press.

Eisner, E. (1985) *The Educational Imagination: On the Design and Evaluation of School Programs*. New York, NY: Macmillan Publishing.

Ferguson, A. A. (2001) *Bad Boys Public Schools in the Making of Black Masculinity*. Ann Arbor, MI: University of Michigan Press.

Flinders, D. J., Noddings, N. and Thornton, S. J. (1986) 'The null curriculum: its theoretical basis and practical implications', *Curriculum Inquiry*, 16(1): 33. doi:10.2307/1179551

Foucault, M. (1982) *The Archeology of Knowledge*. New York, NY: Pantheon Books.

Goldstein, L. (1998) 'Caught in the middle: tensions and contradiction in enacting the primary grade curriculum', *Curriculum Inquiry*, 28(3): 311–37.

Gomez, M. L. (2014) 'Examining discourses of an aspiring teacher of color in the figured world of schooling', *Teacher Education Quarterly*, 41(1): 45–62.

Greene, M. (1993) 'Diversity and inclusion: toward a curriculum for human beings', *Teachers College Record*, 95(2): 211–21.

Gross, L. W. (2014) *Anishinaabe Ways of Knowing and Being*. Burlington, VT: Ashgate.

Grumet, M. (1987) 'The politics of personal knowledge', *Curriculum Inquiry*, 17(3): 319–29.

He, M. F., Phillion, J., Chan, E. and Xu, S. (2008) 'Immigrant students' experiences of curriculum', in F. M. Connelly, M. F. He and J. Phillion (eds.), *The Sage Handbook of Curriculum and Instruction*. Thousand Oaks, CA: Sage Publications. pp. 219–39.

Heidegger, M. (1977) 'The age of the world picture', in *The Question Concerning Technology, and Other Essays*. New York, NY: Harper and Row. pp. 115–54.

Heidegger, M. (2008) *Being and Time* [Trans. J. Macquarrie and E. Robinson]. New York, NY: HarperPerennial/Modern Thought.

Horkheimer, M. (2012) *Critique of Instrumental Reason* [Trans. M. J. O'Connell]. London; New York, NY: Verso.

Huber, J., Murphy, S. and Clandinin, D. J. (2005) 'Creating communities of cultural imagination: negotiating a curriculum of diversity', in J. Phillion, M. F. He and F. M.

Connelly (eds.), *Narrative and Experience in Multicultural Education*. Thousand Oaks, CA: Sage Publishing. pp. 270–90.
Jackson, P. W. (1990) *Life in Classrooms*. New York, NY: Teachers College Press.
Jackson, P. W. (ed.) (1992) *Handbook of Research on Curriculum: A Project of the American Educational Research Association*. New York, NY: Macmillan.
Kuhn, T. (1970) *The Structure of Scientific Revolutions*. Chicago, IL: University of Chicago Press.
Lather, P. (2010) *Engaging Science Policy: From the Side of the Messy*. New York, NY: Peter Lang.
Latour, B. (2007) *Reassembling the Social: An Introduction to Actor–Network-Theory*. Oxford: Oxford University Press.
Lessard, S. (2014) 'Red Worn Runners. A Narrative Inquiry Into the Stories of Aboriginal Youth and Families in Urban Settings'. Unpublished doctoral dissertation, University of Alberta, Edmonton.
Lessard, S., Caine, V. and Clandinin, D. J. (2015) 'A narrative inquiry into familial and school curriculum making: attending to multiple worlds of aboriginal youth and families', *Journal of Youth Studies*, 18(2): 197–214.
Livingstone, D. N. (2003) *Putting Science in Its Place: Geographies of Scientific Knowledge*. Chicago, IL: University of Chicago Press.
Marsh, J. (2003) 'One-way traffic? Connections between literacy practices at home and in the nursery', *British Educational Research Journal*, 29(3): 369–82.
McKenna, E. and Pratt, S. (2015) *American Philosophy: From Wounded Knee to the Present*. New York, NY: Bloomsbury Academic.
Miller, J. (2005) *The Sounds of Silence Breaking: Women, Autobiography, Curriculum*. New York, NY: Peter Lang.
Miller Marsh, M. and Turner-Vorbeck, T. (2009) *(Mis)Understanding Families: Learning From Real Families in Our Schools*. New York, NY: Teachers College Press.
Oyler, C. (2012) *Actions Speak Louder than Words: Community Activism as Curriculum*. New York, NY: Routledge.
Pascoe, C. J. (2011) *Dude, You're a Fag: Masculinity and Sexuality in High School*. Berkeley, CA: University of California Press.
Pinar, W. (1994) *Autobiography, Politics, and Sexuality: Essays in Curriculum Theory 1972–1992*. New York, NY: Peter Lang.
Porter, A. C. (2006) 'Curriculum assessment', in J. L. Green, G. Camilli, and P. B. Elmore (eds.), *Handbook of Complementary Methods for Research in Education*. 3rd edn. Washington, DC: American Educational Research Association.
Rabinow, P., Marcus, G. E., Faubion, J. D. and Rees, T. (2008) *Designs for an Anthropology of the Contemporary*. Durham, NC: Duke University Press.
Rodgers, C. (2002) 'Redefining reflection: another look at John Dewey and reflective thinking', *Teachers College Record*, 104(4): 842–66.
Rosiek, J. L. (2013) 'Pragmatism and post-qualitative futures', *International Journal of Qualitative Research*.
Rosiek, J. L. (forthcoming) *Resegregation as Curriculum*. New York, NY: Routledge.
Rosiek J. L. and Heffernan, J. (2014) 'Can't code what the community can't see: a case of the erasure of gendered harassment', *Qualitative Inquiry*, 20(7).
Sahlberg, P. (2011) *Finnish Lessons: What Can the World Learn from Educational Change in Finland?* New York, NY: Teachers College Press.
Schwab, J. J. (1978) *Science, Curriculum, and Liberal Education: Selected Essays* (I. Westbury and N. J. Wilkof eds.). Chicago, IL: University of Chicago Press.
Seiki, S. (2014) 'Embodying shared history: narrative inquiry as pedagogy', *Teacher Education Quarterly*, 41(1): 29–44.

Snyder, J., Bolin, F. and Zumwalt, K. (1992) 'Curriculum implementation', in P. Jackson (ed.), *Handbook of Research on Curriculum*. New York, NY: Macmillan. pp. 402–35.

Sorrell, K. S. (2004) *Representative Practices: Peirce, Pragmatism, and Feminist Epistemology*. 1st ed. New York, NY: Fordham University Press.

West, C. (2000) *The Cornel West Reader*. New York, NY: Basic Civitas Books.

Willis, P. (1997) *Learning to Labour*. New York, NY: Colombia University Press.

Zeichner, K. (2010) 'Economic rationalization, increased surveillance, and attacks on diversity: neo-liberalism and the transformation of teacher education in the US', *Teaching and Teacher Education*, 26(8): 1544–52.

SECTION IV

Journeying with narrative ideas

Considerations of the ontological, methodological, ethical, and political

13

NARRATIVE INQUIRY

Both a view of, and a methodology for, studying experience

Introduction

It has been 13 years since Michael Connelly and I wrote *Narrative Inquiry: Experience and Story in Qualitative Research*, and more than 23 years since we wrote the first article (Connelly & Clandinin, 1990) that began to address our understandings of narrative inquiry as both a methodology and a way of understanding experience narratively. Michael Connelly and I began this work on narrative inquiry many years ago, in part because we were trying to give an account of teachers' experiential knowledge. We wanted to find a way to build on what Dewey (1938) wrote of experience, and to use his ideas to think about teacher knowledge as knowledge that was personal, practical, shaped by, and expressed in, practice. Mark Johnson, in the early 1980s, turned our attention to how thinking narratively could help us do the work we were imagining.

In March 1983, we invited Mark Johnson to the Ontario Institute for Studies in Education, University of Toronto to spend time with us on a project focused on how we could understand policy implementation from the perspective of teachers when new policies were implemented at a school district level. We framed the study as a problem in understanding both teacher knowledge, and change in teacher knowledge. We situated it as a reconceptualization of knowledge utilization. We were well into the study in March 1983 when Mark arrived to talk with us. At the time I was struggling to find ways to represent the experiential knowledge of the two participants in my doctoral study. I was concerned that my analysis of what I was calling their images, part of their personal practical knowledge, had resulted in my taking away, or diminishing, the wholeness of their lives. I had, in a way, dissected them. Dissection had not been my intent. Mark talked with me at a local hotel bar after he worked with the research team for the day. As we talked, he suggested that I should read Alasdair MacIntyre's book, *After Virtue* (1981). "Not the whole thing," he said, "Just the chapter on narrative unity." He wrote on the hotel note paper, "So say more about how you see knowledge as embodied, embedded in a culture, and based on narrative unity."

Reprinted with permission. Acknowledgement; Clandinin, D. Jean (2013) Introduction and Chapter One: Living, telling, and retelling: Processes of narrative inquiry. In Clandinin, D. Jean. Engaging in narrative inquiry. London, England: Routledge. Pp 9–31.

With those words, he gave me a way forward to finishing my dissertation. I read the chapter and realized that what I was then calling interpretive accounts were ways to write of the two teachers in the study as people composing, and living, complex lives. I did not yet call these interpretive accounts narrative accounts. Looking back on my much marked-up copy of MacIntyre's book I noted that I underlined the words "a concept of self whose unity resides in the unity of a narrative which links birth to life to death as narrative beginning to middle to end" (p. 191) and

> it is because we all live out narratives in our lives and because we understand our own lives in terms of the narratives that the form of narrative is appropriate for understanding the actions of others. Stories are lived before they are told.
>
> *(p. 197)*

While I marked many other lines, those lines were the introduction of the idea of narrative into the work with which Michael and I were engaged. We began to think narratively about the lives of the teacher participants, about the school, and about the school contexts in which we worked. However, our shift to thinking narratively about lives also brought us into thinking narratively about methodology, and the methods, we used for the study of lives. When we wrote our article for *Educational Researcher* (Connelly & Clandinin, 1990), some 7 years after the completion of my doctoral work (Clandinin, 1983), we made explicit our interest in narrative inquiry as a research methodology. While there were other ways of making the turn to narrative ways of thinking, our turn to narrative came through our interest in understanding experiential knowledge.

A sharp turn to narrative

Since that time there has been an explosion of interest in narrative inquiry. Narrative inquiry is a ubiquitous practice in that

> human beings have lived out and told stories about that living for as long as we could talk. And then we have talked about the stories we tell for almost as long. These lived and told stories and the talk about the stories are one of the ways that we fill our world with meaning and enlist one another's assistance in building lives and communities. What feels new is the emergence of narrative methodologies in the field of social science research.
>
> *(Clandinin & Rosiek, 2007, p. 35)*

Since the late 1980s and early 1990s, research in the social sciences has taken a narrative turn to studying experience (Pinnegar & Daynes, 2007). While there is a history of narrative work within the traditions of narratology (the theory and study of narrative) and narrative research, it was in 1990 that we described this research methodology we were developing as narrative inquiry. While initially we wrote of narrative inquiry as both phenomenon and method, we quickly began to understand it was a research methodology. What was apparent was how interwoven narrative ways of thinking about phenomena are with narrative inquiry as research methodology. It was "the interweaving of narrative views of phenomena and narrative inquiry that marks the emerging field and that draws attention to the need for careful uses and distinctions of terms" (Clandinin & Rosiek, 2007, p. 36).

What we saw as a need for careful attention to terms has led to debates within the emerging methodology. Reissman and Speedy (2007) pointed out that "narrative inquiry in the human sciences is a 20th century development; the field has 'realist', 'postmodern', and constructionist strands, and scholars and practitioners disagree on origin and precise definition" (p. 429). This diversity in the various ways that narrative inquiry is taken up both enriches, and troubles, those of us engaged in narrative inquiry. Without a clear sense of the epistemological and ontological commitments of those who work within the field, much is blurred.

Narrative has, for example, come to refer to almost anything that uses, for example, stories as data, narrative or story as representational form, narrative as content analysis, narrative as structure, and so forth. I had, for example, a well-known editor point out to me that s/he had found many references that I had omitted from a review manuscript on narrative inquiry. When I questioned him/her about what s/he had found, and that I had missed, it turned out that s/he had used the search term "narrative" alone and the search engine reported links to many articles with often tangential links to what we are calling narrative inquiry. What is apparent is that some forms of what is called narrative analysis such as thematic analysis, linguistic analysis, structural analysis, and, more recently, visual analysis, are used as methods within other qualitative research methodologies. While they are all grouped under a label of narrative analysis, what narrative refers to as a descriptor varies widely. Within the field of qualitative research, there are many analytic methods or forms of narrative analysis (Josselson & Lieblich, 1995; Josselson, Lieblich, & McAdams, 2003; Polkinghorne, 1988; Reissman, 2008). Stories or narratives are also used as data in other qualitative methodologies such as phenomenology and case study. Narratives or stories are used as representational forms for results or findings in various qualitative and quantitative methodologies. More recently narratives or stories are used in knowledge translation in health science, education, and other professional disciplines. Questions about just what each of us means by our use of the term narrative is becoming increasingly important.

Narrative inquiry, as its own methodology, has developed important terms and distinctions that have become more apparent and well-recognized as guiding what counts, or what fits, within the field of narrative inquiry or narrative research. There is now a well-established view of narrative inquiry as both methodology and phenomena (Clandinin, 2007).

Dewey's theory of experience (1938) is most often cited as the philosophical underpinning of narrative inquiry (Clandinin & Connelly, 2000). Dewey's two criteria of experience – interaction and continuity enacted in situations – provide the grounding for attending to a narrative conception of experience through the three-dimensional narrative inquiry space with dimensions of temporality, place, and sociality. Paradigmatic and narrative knowing (Bruner, 1986), narrative structure and coherence of lives (Carr, 1986), concepts of continuity and improvisation as a response to the uncertainties in life and life contexts (Bateson, 1989; 1994), and narrative in life and teaching practice (Coles, 1989) also ground our understandings of experience as narratively composed. Drawing on all of these works, Clandinin and Rosiek (2007) point out,

> Framed within this view of experience, the focus of narrative inquiry is not only on individuals' experience but also on the social, cultural, and institutional narratives within which individuals' experiences are constituted, shaped, expressed, and enacted. Narrative inquirers study the individual's experience in the world, an experience that is storied both in the living and telling and

> that can be studied by listening, observing, living alongside another, and writing, and interpreting texts.
>
> *(pp. 42–43)*

Rosiek and I make clear that narrative inquiry, working from a particular ontological and epistemological stance, is a way of understanding and inquiring into experience. It is nothing more and nothing less. Narrative inquiry is situated in relationships and in community, and attends to notions of expertise and knowing in relational and participatory ways.

Ontological and epistemological commitments

Since Michael Connelly and I first began to name our work as narrative inquiry, we have held firm to our view that narrative inquirers study experience. Our argument (Connelly & Clandinin, 1990, 2006) for the development and use of narrative inquiry is inspired by a view of human experience in which humans, individually and socially, lead storied lives:

> People shape their daily lives by stories of who they and others are and as they interpret their past in terms of these stories. Story, in the current idiom, is a portal through which a person enters the world and by which their experience of the world is interpreted and made personally meaningful. Narrative inquiry, the study of experience as story, then, is first and foremost a way of thinking about experience. Narrative inquiry as a methodology entails a view of the phenomenon. To use narrative inquiry methodology is to adopt a particular view of experience as phenomenon under study.
>
> *(Connelly & Clandinin, 2006, p. 375)*

We, and others, have, over many years and many studies, continued to work from a Deweyan-inspired understanding of experience. While we continued our work from that philosophical view of experience, we were always cognizant of other views of experience. In an attempt to make clear our philosophical stance, Jerry Rosiek and I laid our Deweyan-inspired understandings of experience alongside other

> philosophical treatments of the word experience, from Aristotle's dualistic metaphysics in which knowledge of particulars and universals were considered separately, to early empiricist atomistic conceptions of experience, Marxist conceptions of experience distorted by ideology, behaviorist notions of stimulus and response, and post-structuralist assertions that state our experience is the product of discursive practices.
>
> *(2007, p. 37)*

By doing this, we were able to clarify "differences and affinities narrative inquiry has with other areas of scholarship" (Clandinin & Rosiek, 2007, p. 37). Our purpose was to make visible the distinctions among narrative inquiry and other methodologies so that scholars could understand our project as narrative inquirers as distinct from the work of those grounded in other views of experience. While that is not my main purpose here, I pull forward some of those distinctions in order to remind readers of what grounds our work as narrative inquirers.

As we contrasted the underlying view of experience held by narrative inquirers with those held by researchers working from other views of experience, Rosiek and I outlined Dewey's conception, noting that "It does not refer to some precognitive, precultural ground on which our conceptions of the world rest. Instead, it is a changing stream that is characterized by continuous interaction of human thought with our personal, social, and material environment" (Clandinin & Rosiek, 2007, p. 39). Drawing on Dewey's words

> In an experience, things and events belonging to the world, physical and social, are transformed through the human context they enter, while the live creature is changed and developed through its intercourse with things previously external to it.
>
> *(as cited in Boydston, 1981, p. 251)*

We argued (Clandinin and Rosiek, 2007) argued that

> Dewey's ontology is not transcendental, it is transactional. The epistemological implications of this view are nothing short of revolutionary. It implies that the regulative ideal for inquiry is not to generate an exclusively faithful representation of a reality independent of the knower. The regulative ideal for inquiry is to generate a new relation between a human being and her environment – her life, community, world – one that "makes possible a new way of dealing with them, and thus eventually creates a new kind of experienced object, not more real than those which preceded but more significant, and less overwhelming and oppressive" (Dewey, 1981b, p. 175). In this pragmatic view of knowledge, our representations arise from experience and must return to that experience for their validation.
>
> *(p. 39)*

Working within this ontology of experience shapes narrative inquiry in a particular way. By highlighting the temporality of knowledge generation, we draw attention to the understanding that experience "is always more than we can know and represent in a single statement, paragraph, or book. Every representation, therefore, no matter how faithful to that which it tries to depict, involves selective emphasis of our experience" (Clandinin & Rosiek, 2007, p. 39). We used Dewey (1958) to argue "against obscuring the selection process, thus naturalizing the objects of our inquiry and treating them as if they are given" (p. 40). In this way we argued for showing inquiries "as a series of choices, inspired by purposes that are shaped by past experience, undertaken through time, and [that] trace the consequences of these choices in the whole of an individual or community's lived experience" (p. 40). Narrative inquiry comprises a view of experience as composed and lived over time, as studied and understood as a narrative phenomenon, and as represented through narrative forms of representation.

Arguing for narrative inquiry as a way to understand experience, and a way to study experience, sharpened the distinctions between narrative inquiry and the ways that narrative forms of representation are often used in inquiries framed by other philosophical stances. Michael Connelly and I (Connelly & Clandinin, 1990) carefully distinguished the work of narrative inquirers from the work of those who used narrative representational forms but who worked from other philosophical views of experience. As Rosiek and I argued, when narrative forms of representation are taken up from other philosophical frameworks, they are

> almost always regarded as having a degraded epistemic status; if the reality we seek to describe is presumed to be independent of our representations of it, then there is no need to tell the story of how our representation of the world emerged within a stream of experience nor how it returned to that experience.
>
> *(Clandinin & Rosiek, 2007, p. 41)*

As Rosiek and I outlined, the underlying ontological commitments of narrative inquirers are sometimes quite different from the ways that some researchers expect to engage in narrative inquiry. For some, narrative inquiry appears to be a way of only representing data. It is a representational form, one way of representing from a range of representational forms. A lack of clarity around this point leads to the many questions and comments that narrative inquirers receive such as "people tell me that my research will be more compelling if I represent it in a narrative." For us, that is not what we mean by narrative inquiry. Working from the view of experience as laid out above, narrative inquiry is much more than that. Clarifying, and continually working with, and from, a transactional or relational ontology is what is fundamental to narrative inquiry. It is a point I emphasize throughout this book.

This point is closely connected to the next point, that is, that narrative inquirers understand experience as a narratively composed phenomenon. Narrative inquiry is thus methodology and phenomenon. This is also important in understanding what we mean by narrative inquiry. While this is not the main focus of this book, as we (Clandinin & Connelly, 2000; Clandinin & Rosiek, 2007) have argued these points elsewhere, I want to highlight the underlying ontological and epistemological assumptions that undergird narrative inquiry. The differences that result from how one understands their work at a philosophical level leads to very different understandings between narrative inquiry and what others sometimes call narrative analysis or narrative research. While at one point we tended to agree with Mishler (as cited in Clandinin, 2007) that we did not want to police the boundaries of what counts as narrative inquiry, we now see it is important to carefully distinguish our epistemological and ontological assumptions rather than relying on readers to be able to make distinctions. As narrative inquirers, we can now more clearly make distinctions between narrative inquiry and some other forms of narrative analysis and narrative research. And, in part, these distinctions rest on the underlying view of experience.

Working from a Deweyan-inspired view of experience allowed us to attend to continuity, that is,

> the idea that experiences grow out of other experiences, and experiences lead to further experiences. Wherever one positions oneself in that continuum – the imagined now, some imagined past, or some imagined future – each point has a past experiential base and leads to an experiential future.
>
> *(Clandinin & Connelly, 2000, p. 2)*

Narrative inquirers understand continuity as an ontological matter. Experiences are continuous. As we argued, "what you see (and hear, feel, think, love, taste, despise, fear, etc.) is what you get. That is all we ultimately have in which to ground our understanding. And that is all we need" (Clandinin & Rosiek, 2007, p. 41). For narrative inquirers this view of continuity has important implications for the way we think about our inquiries. Inquiry is "within a stream of experience that generates new relations that then become a part of future experience" (p. 41).

It is continuity that helps us understand narrative inquiry as both a relational methodology for studying experience as well as an aspect of experience. The initial parameters for narrative inquiry, we argued, "are themselves a form of relation that can and should be questioned in the course of ongoing research" (Clandinin & Rosiek, 2007, p. 41). We noted that

> Referring to inevitable inferential spillover of our inquiries, Dewey describes experience as having something that "stretches." This stretch is almost "indefinitely elastic" and extends into realms of personal, aesthetic, and social meaning.
>
> *(p. 41)*

A third feature or aspect of our Deweyan-inspired view of experience that underlies narrative inquiry is the emphasis on the social dimension of our inquiries. Narrative inquiries explore the stories people live and tell. As we (Clandinin & Rosiek, 2007) argued,

> These stories are the result of a confluence of social influences on a person's inner life, social influences on their environment, and their unique personal history. These stories are often treated as the epiphenomenal to social inquiry – reflections of important social realities but not realities themselves.
>
> *(p. 41)*

These three aspects of our view of experience – that it is relational, continuous, and social – are fundamental to what we see as narrative inquiry.

A definition of narrative inquiry

Narrative inquiry is an approach to the study of human lives conceived as a way of honoring lived experience as a source of important knowledge and understanding:

> Narrative inquiry is a way of understanding experience. It is collaboration between researcher and participants, over time, in a place or series of places, and in social interaction with milieus. An inquirer enters this matrix in the midst and progresses in the same spirit, concluding the inquiry still in the midst of living and telling, reliving and retelling, the stories of the experiences that made up people's lives, both individual and social.
>
> *(Clandinin & Connelly, 2000, p. 20)*

Narrative inquiry begins and ends with a respect for ordinary lived experience. A Deweyan view of experience allows for the study of experience that acknowledges the embodiment of the person living in the world (Johnson, 1987). However, the focus of narrative inquiry is not only valorizing individuals' experience but is also an exploration of the social, cultural, familial, linguistic, and institutional narratives within which individuals' experiences were, and are, constituted, shaped, expressed, and enacted. Understood in this way, narrative inquiries begin and end in the storied lives of the people involved. Narrative inquirers study the individual's experience in the world, an experience that is storied both in the living and telling, and that can be studied by listening, observing, living alongside an other, and writing and interpreting texts. Through the inquiry, we seek ways of enriching and transforming that experience for themselves and others.

Viewed in this way, narrative inquiry is an approach to research that enacts many, if not all, of the principles of a Deweyan theory of inquiry. Clandinin and Rosiek (2007) offered that narrative inquiry "is a quintessentially pragmatic methodology. What genealogy is to post-structuralist Foucauldian sociology, what critical ethnography is to critical theory, what experiments are to positivism, narrative inquiry is to Deweyan pragmatism" (p. 42).

However, in this book, my intention is to return to the question of what it is that narrative inquirers do, a question that Michael Connelly and I used to frame *Narrative Inquiry*, our 2000 book. In the years since the publication of that book, I have received many requests from researchers to share how to live out narrative inquiry in a research project. Addressing what it means to live in relational ways, ways that allow us to attend to understanding our own and other's experiences through narrative inquiry, is what many people struggle to understand. It is the experiential sense that people most want to understand. In the chapters that follow, I try to give a sense of that. I make clear in the following chapters, rich with illustrations, the ways I work from, and with, my ontological and epistemological commitments. I begin Chapter 2 with a quotation that speaks to me of what I understand it means to live a narrative inquiry as a researcher. I represent it in a poetic form although it was not in such a form when I read it. Written by Ben Okri, someone Thomas King calls a Nigerian storyteller (King, 2003, p. 153), it provides a kind of grounding for what it means to engage and live out a narrative inquiry. Narrative inquiry is relational in all of the ways that our Dewey-inspired view of experience makes visible; that is, it is relational across time, places, relationships.

Chapter 1:
Living, telling, and retelling: processes of narrative inquiry

In a fractured age,
when cynicism is god,
here is a possibly heresy:
we live by stories,
we also live in them.
One way or another we are living the stories
planted in us early or along the way,
or we are also living the stories we planted –
knowingly or unknowingly – in ourselves
We live stories that either give our lives meaning
or negate it with meaninglessness.
If we change the stories we live by,
Quite possibly we change our lives.
(Okri, 1997, p. 46)

"We live by stories." In these words Okri (1997, p. 46) directed my attention to who we are, and who we are becoming, an idea that we (Connelly & Clandinin, 1999) have long thought of as a set of complex relationships among knowledge, contexts, and identities. It is a way of thinking about identities relationally. We (Clandinin et al., 2006; Connelly & Clandinin, 1999) speak of stories to live by or, as Okri would have it, we live by stories.

"We also live in them" (Okri, 1997, p. 46). Living in stories. This idea also shaped my thinking. I think of the interconnected, nested stories in which we live. I live in familial intergenerational stories; stories composed and handed down as Elizabeth Stone (1988) reminded us so many years ago. I live in cultural temporal stories, stories that have shaped each of our cultures whether they are the narratives shaped by cultural plotlines of respect, or cultural plotlines of the connections among all living things, or cultural plotlines of independence and self-reliance. I live in stories, cultural stories.

I also live in institutional stories, stories of school. I live in other institutional stories but the institutional stories of school profoundly shape us all. I know that from our narrative inquiries into the experiences of teachers (Clandinin, 1986; Clandinin & Connelly, 1995; Clandinin, Davies, Hogan, & Kennard, 1993; Connelly & Clandinin, 1999; Huber & Keats Whelan, 2000), children (Murphy, 2004; Pearce, 2005), early school leavers (Clandinin et al., 2010), parents (Houle, 2012), administrators (Rose, 1997), and others. The stories we live by, and the stories we live in, over time, are indelibly marked for all of us by stories of school. Of course teachers, children, and families with children in schools are in the midst of being shaped by their living in stories of school. Stories of school are powerful shapers of these stories we live in and we live by.

I also live in personal stories. "One way or another we are living the stories planted in us early or along the way, or we are also living the stories we planted – knowingly or unknowingly – in ourselves" (Okri, 1997, p. 46). Maxine Greene (1995) reminds us of the shaping power of our early landscapes – what we know first. As we engage in narrative inquiry with ourselves, and with our participants, we need to inquire into all of these kinds of stories, stories that have become intertwined, interwoven into who we are and are becoming. These stories live in us, in our bodies, as we move and live in the world.

These reflections on Okri's words provide a starting point for thinking of narrative inquiry as relational inquiry. These stories we live in, or live by, point toward the relational and how we think of the relational aspects of narrative inquiry. Okri's last two lines, "If we change the stories we live by, quite possibly we change our lives" suggest the possibilities that are created by attending to the relational by thinking narratively about how relationships unfold in inquiry. Okri's words help me think about how thinking narratively about experience illuminates new understandings. His words about changing the stories we live by, changing who we are, also directs my attention to the relational ethics around engaging in narrative inquiry for we might change, not only our own lives and those who live in relation with us, but also the lives of participants and those others who live in relation with them. Thinking narratively is risky business. It calls me to be attentive to my own unfolding, enfolding, storied life, and the lives of those with whom I engage.

Ben Okri, however, is not talking about narrative inquiry. I am the one who calls his words forward to help me think about narrative inquiry, inquiry where lives meet in storied ways, where spaces between open up and create the possibility of world travelling and loving perception that Lugones (1987) speaks of, where being in relation allows us to travel to other worlds and understand what it is to be other and what it is to be ourselves in other's eyes (p. 17).

I speak often of narrative inquiry as a relational methodology and it is important to make clear what I mean by a relational methodology. I sometimes answer in terms of the ontological commitment of narrative inquiry (Clandinin & Murphy, 2009; Clandinin & Rosiek, 2007) in the ways that I laid out above. But there is another way of answering that I want to make clear in what follows, that is, I speak to the conceptual underpinnings of the relational living alongside in narrative inquiry.

Working from the definition of narrative inquiry quoted in the Preface, I note how this simple definition, in many ways, assumes the relational – the relational between the person and his/her world; a temporal understanding of the relational between the past, present, and future, including the relational in the intergenerational; the relational between person and place; the relational between events and feelings; the relational between us as people; the relational between the physical world and people; the relational in our cultural, institutional, linguistic, and familial narratives; and so on. Thinking relationally is, then, part of thinking narratively, and of thinking narratively as a narrative inquirer. In other places, we have written that narrative inquiry is people in relation studying people in relation.

In narrative inquiry, we intentionally come into relation with participants and we, as inquirers, think narratively about our own experiences, about our participants' experiences, and about those experiences that become visible as we live alongside, telling our own stories, hearing an other's stories, moving in, acting in, the places, the contexts in which our lives meet. We intentionally put our lives alongside an other's life. In that intentionality we are attending in relation to our own life, to others' lives, to the present time and to other times, and to this place where we meet, and to other places. As narrative inquirers, our lived and told stories are always in relation to, or with, those of participants and with their, and our, landscapes (Clandinin & Connelly, 1995). As we tell our stories and listen to participants tell their stories in the inquiry, we, as inquirers, need to pay close attention to who we are in the inquiry and to understand that we, ourselves, are part of the storied landscapes we are studying. Thus, as inquirers, we are part of the present landscape and the past landscape, and we acknowledge that we helped make the world in which we find ourselves. As narrative inquirers, we become part of participants' lives and they part of ours. Therefore, our lives, and who we are and are becoming on our, and their, landscapes, is also under study. We are not objective inquirers. We are relational inquirers, attentive to the intersubjective, to the relational, embedded spaces in which lives are lived out. We do not stand metaphorically outside the inquiry but are part of the phenomenon under study.

This is a partial account of the relational in narrative inquiry.

However, in what I have just said, there is another way in which narrative inquiry is relational inquiry. The stories lived and told in a narrative inquiry relationship are always a co-composition, an intentional co-composition. The stories are co-composed in the spaces between us as inquirers and participants.

To illustrate this, I draw on a narrative inquiry into the curriculum making experiences of children, teachers, and families (Huber, Murphy, & Clandinin, 2011). We are interested in the storied experiences of children, teachers, and families in the curriculum making that happens as lives meet in classrooms, schools, homes, and communities. That sets the research context and research puzzle. I decided to linger with my experiences in this study to further understand what I mean by the relational in narrative inquiry. I draw on my experience as a source for illustrating what I mean, and as a way to capture your imagination so that you might come alongside me in my wonderings.

I remember my first day in the Grade 3 classroom situated in a suburban school where Song Lee taught and where I spent Wednesday afternoons for almost a year as part of the narrative inquiry. It was my first day in the classroom and it was a rainy September day. Shortly before recess, the principal's voice came over the intercom system advising that there would be indoor recess. "Oh great," I thought. I had hoped to have a chat with Song Lee while the children were out on the playground. I wanted to know more about the stories of school in which she and the children and the families were situated and about the context of her classroom.

Song Lee came over and asked if she could go to the workroom to pick up some supplies. She had just told the children to select games, puzzles, or books, and to play quietly for the indoor recess period.

"Are you all right alone with the kids?" she asked.

"Sure," I said cautiously, looking around and wondering if I remembered any of the children's names. As a narrative inquirer just beginning to work in this new classroom, I did want to get to know the children but I had hoped for a bit of time before I was alone with all of them. Old memories of children becoming loud and aggressive when kept inside during recess drifted through my mind.

Song Lee left the room and the children selected books to read at their desks, or games to play in small groups. A few children pulled out their hand-held computer games. There was no visible change in the classroom when Song Lee left.

Almost immediately, a girl, who I later learned was Lilly, appeared at my side and asked, "Ms. Jean, would you like to play a game with us?"

In that moment, a space appeared between Lilly and I, a space filled with both the stories we lived by and composed, in part, by the stories we lived within. What made this girl child of 8 years of age come to invite me to play? Had she recognized that somehow I needed a space in this classroom too?

Now sliding backward and forward in time, in and out of places, and attending to all we came to know about each other in our various relationships that year, I try to give an account of the relational in narrative inquiry. Of course, I know I cannot even begin to represent the complexity of Lilly's stories. Nor, I suppose, can I begin to represent the complexity of mine. What I hope I can do here is draw on my experiences with Lilly as she engaged in a year-long narrative inquiry alongside me, Song Lee, and Simmee Chung, a graduate student, to provide a sense of the relational as situated in a narrative inquiry in the midst of a busy classroom.

First, to the institutional stories of school that shaped the space between Lilly and I, the space which allowed me to attend to the relational of narrative inquiry, but also allowed Lilly and I to co-compose a relationship within that space. It was September and school had only been in session for a week or so when Lilly offered her invitation to me. Lilly was not new to the school. She had attended the school since kindergarten. Later, as we came to know more of her, she spoke knowledgeably about her former teachers and classmates in the school. Her brother, Cole, also attended, as well as her best friend, Ella. Her family also storied Streamside School as a place like home, often situating Lilly's stories of school within her friendship with Ella and their friendship with Ella's family. This was the start of Lilly's fourth year at Streamside School. I was new to the school, having only visited once before. We were both new to the classroom. I did know Song Lee from our work together at the university, but I did not know her in the context of her classroom and school.

And let me, for a moment, draw forward those storied pasts that lived in us and that shaped that invitation to play. I have taught in schools, worked in schools, and researched in schools for many years. I am a teacher and have taught many teachers. My knowing is deeply shaped by knowing schools, first as a student, then a teacher, then a teacher educator, and now a researcher of teaching. Lilly is much newer to schools. In this moment she is beginning her fourth year in this particular school and, as she told me at one point, she felt at home in the school.

My stories of school as a child were less comfortable. A rural student, I was bussed into a small town to attend schools, and school was never a familiar place to me. In the stories I tell myself, I always felt somewhat outside, a visitor, a stranger to the school which was "in town," and which I was always conscious of needing to get to and to get from. Even though I did well in schools, I always felt somewhat situated on the edge, waiting for the bus to take me "home," away from there.

I had learned to be a bit more comfortable in schools as a teacher, a school counselor, and a psychologist. Even as I write this, I realize that I always kept myself on the edges of the dominant stories of school: teaching part time, in portable classrooms, as a support person in the roles of counselor and psychologist. Schools were never easy places for me and I wonder once again about why I keep attending to lives there. I do however "know" schools: the rhythms of the year, the furniture, the physical and emotional places, the subject matters, the uneasy relationships, the report cards, and so on. My sense of being from away, and always on my way "away" from schools, was part of what shaped my experiences in those early landscapes.

Lilly also knew about being from away, and, as I lived alongside her over the school year, she shared that she was an immigrant child, someone born in another country, someone whose parents were migrants from one country to another country to another country. Lilly loved one of the books we read in the classroom, a children's book titled *What You Know First* (MacLachlan, 1995). It was a book I had long been drawn to for it spoke of rural life, family, and transitions. But I knew nothing of Lilly on that first afternoon recess.

In that moment of invitation, did Lilly see me as someone not quite sure of who she was in this urban affluent school? Did she sense my unease of not knowing people? Did she want to help me feel part of the class? What brought her to invite me "to play"? I came to know that Lilly lived by stories of inviting people to play and hoping that when someone was from *away* they would be invited in. When one of the students left the classroom, and Streamside School, mid-year, Lilly wrote a letter to him sharing her hope that he would make friends in his new class. She wrote that she knew school was sometimes not an easy place to be when you did not know anyone.

There were other stories in that space between us that morning, stories that we each lived by and lived within. We both felt resonance with the teacher. Lilly often shared that Song Lee was like her and, indeed, physically there was a kind of resonance. They were both small and of Chinese heritage. They both had long dark hair and beautiful brown skin. But I too felt a resonance with Song Lee. We had worked together at the university and she was my connection to the school. I knew she was a researcher in the making as we had written and talked and shared ideas together. Both Lilly and I felt comfortable with Song Lee. My comfort with Song Lee came from knowing her outside her classroom and Lilly's knowing was situated within the classroom.

My stories lived in me, and I lived by those stories. Song Lee's stories lived in her, and she lived by those stories. We were also living in stories, our family stories, our stories shaped in early landscapes, our cultural stories, and our stories of school. There, on that rainy September morning, staying indoors for recess, another school story in western Canada where we live, we were living within an institutional story, a story of school. And I was intentionally engaging in a narrative inquiry, and Lilly had invited herself into my story as she invited me to play. There was intentionality in Lilly's actions as well as she sought to invite me into her, and what she hoped would become our, community.

Of course we were not awake to each other's complex stories at that moment of the invitation, and we only came to know something of each other's stories as they were being lived out, composed, told, and retold, and then relived as we worked alongside each other over the school year. It is interesting that Lilly seemed to hold open that space, that invitation to belong alongside her, throughout the year.

I turn to two other moments in all the moments in the narrative inquiry when Lilly and I shared a space between. This again, I hope, shows something of what the relational means in narrative inquiry. What I hope is becoming apparent is the mutuality and reciprocity in the living spaces between Lilly and I.

As part of our narrative inquiry, the children, Song Lee, Simmee Chung, and I engaged in co-composing field texts. The children took photographs of their belonging places in the classroom, in their homes, and in their communities, and together, over many months, they shared them with each other and with us, telling and retelling stories of their experiences of belonging. As one of the tasks in the belonging project, Song Lee and Simmee asked the children to take photographs that represented a metaphor of their belonging. Lilly took a photograph of a brick of butter. The story she told was remarkable. Telling of her best friend Ella's journey to visit her extended family in her homeland and an absence from school of several weeks, Lilly likened friendship and belonging to butter. "If you do not attend to your friends, then like butter left on the counter, it may possibly melt away." As Lilly explained her metaphor of friendships and belonging to her classmates and us, she explained that butter, when melted and then cooled, changes shape and texture. It will never be the same again. As she continued, Lilly explained that, like butter, if you don't pay attention to someone, they might feel ignored and not return to the relationship in the same way.

The children responded to Lilly's photograph and clearly resonated with her metaphor for belonging. Carter responded saying, "I liked the picture of the butter because it reminded me of friendship because when Nolan went to Calgary, I felt like I was melting away too" (May 7, 2007).

Ji-Sook said to Lilly, "I like the way you wrote about the butter because when I was coming to Canada my friends were like butter because I was far, far away and if I think of them they look small like ants." What seemed remarkable to me is that the other children recognized Lilly's stories to live by and her knowledge in context as they responded to her and resonated with her metaphor. Response is a concept frequently used in narrative inquiry. Taken from the same root as responsibility, it signals the importance of making spaces for telling and listening to stories as well as the responsibilities for sustaining each other (Lopez, 1990; Schultz, 1997).

As Lilly shared her photographs, both metaphorically and relationally, she again created a space between, a space that invited me to consider what it means to engage in inquiry relationally. This metaphor became a kind of relational space, which, when she made it visible, allowed others to come to understand who they might be in her stories, and who she might be in theirs.

Ten months after our first day together, Lilly stood beside me on a day when all class members were preparing to celebrate traditions in their family stories with each other. The idea of devoting the last day in the classroom together to a sharing of traditions came forward in mid-June as the children proposed this idea to Song Lee, Simmee Chung, and I. The idea of traditions had bubbled to the surface in many of the responses written after the sharing of the photographs and collages. At first traditions were only spoken of in relation to "foreign countries" but gradually Song Lee, Simmee, and I were helping all of the children make visible their traditions.

Spending the day telling stories of their living traditions was something we all looked forward to. We were preparing to serve ice cream, my family tradition, to the class. It was once again recess time and Lilly and I were talking. She reminded me of my first day in the class and of her invitation to join her.

> "Do you remember Ms. Jean?"
> "I do remember, Lilly."
> "We didn't finish our game."
> "I know," I said and we gave each other a hug.
> *(Field notes, June 2008)*

This day was also a day that caused me to think about the relational in narrative inquiry. The year-long narrative inquiry allowed me to consider more deeply, and in an embodied way, what it means to live relationally, to know that in the inquiry both the storied experiences of researcher and participants are open to the inquiry.

Thinking about stories as distinct from thinking with stories

David Morris, in a chapter in Charon and Montello's (2002) book, makes the distinction that in our Western society we mostly think *about* stories and that we no longer think *with* stories.

> The concept of thinking with stories is meant to oppose and modify (not replace) the institutionalized Western practice of thinking about stories. Thinking about stories conceives of narrative as an object. Thinking with stories is a process in which we as thinkers do not so much work on narrative as of allowing narrative to work on us.
>
> *(Morris, 2002, p. 196)*

While we can think with stories both in and outside of narrative inquiry, thinking with stories is primarily thinking relationally. By this I draw attention to thinking about the other's experience, to thinking of the narratives that shape each person in her contexts, in her unfolding life, in that moment which comes out of all the other moments and points toward a future. When we begin to engage in narrative inquiry, we need to be attentive to thinking with stories in multiple ways, toward our stories, toward the other's stories, toward all the narratives in which we are embedded as well as toward what begins to emerge in our shared lived and told stories. It was this that I attempted to show in the narrative inquiry with Lilly.

"Do you remember, Ms. Jean," Lilly reminded me as she took me back to our first encounter. Our stories are always in relation, always composed in between, in those spaces between time and people and generations and places. As we tell our stories and listen to participants tell their stories in the inquiry, we, as inquirers, need to pay close attention to who we are in the inquiry and to understand that we, ourselves, are part of the storied landscapes we are studying.

As narrative inquirers, we become part of participants' lives and they part of ours. Therefore, our lives, and who we are, and are becoming, on our and their landscapes, is also under study.

Narrative inquiry is a deeply ethical project. Narrative inquiry understood as ethical work means we cannot separate the ethical out as separate from the living out of narrative inquiry. Relational ethics live at the very heart, perhaps is the very heart, of our work as narrative inquirers. Relational ethics are founded in an ethics of care (Noddings, 1984) and are the starting point and stance that narrative inquirers take throughout a narrative inquiry. A commitment to relationships, that is, to live in collaborative ways, allows us to re-compose and negotiate stories. Relational ethics calls us to social responsibilities, to how we live in relation with others and with our worlds.

Morris also writes of the ethical heart of narrative inquiry as he writes about living alongside in the living and telling of stories. He writes one Apache male describes how such tales, "when retold in the context of moral misconduct, have a way of almost literally getting under your skin: That story is working on you now. You keep thinking about it. That story is changing you now, making you want to live right. That story is making you want to replace yourself" (Morris, 2002, p. 197).

As I reflect back on my time alongside Lilly, I know that the experience has changed me. I cannot say if Lilly's experience changed her. I know the stories Lilly co-composed with me are working on me now, making me want to replace myself. This chapter is one way of living alongside as we engage in the relational methodology of narrative inquiry.

References

Basso, K. (2002). *Wisdom sits in places. Landscape and language among the western Apache.* Albuquerque, NM: University of New Mexico Press.

Bateson, M. C. (1989). *Composing a life.* New York: Atlantic Monthly Press.

Bateson, M. C. (1994). *Peripheral visions: Learning along the way.* New York: HarperCollins.

Boydston, J. A. (1981). *The later works, 1925-1953: John Dewey, volume 1, 1925, experience and nature.* Carbondale, IL: Southern Illinois University Press.

Bruner, J. (1986). *Actual minds, possible worlds.* Cambridge, MA: Harvard University Press.

Carr, D. (1986). *Time, narrative, and history.* Bloomington, IN: Indiana University Press.

Clandinin, D. J. (1983). *A conceptualization of image as a component of teacher personal practical knowledge in primary school teachers' reading and language programs.* Unpublished doctoral dissertation, University of Toronto.

Clandinin, D. J. (1986). *Classroom practice: Teacher images in action.* London/Philadelphia, PA: Falmer Press.

Clandinin, D. J. (Ed.). (2007). *Handbook of narrative inquiry: Mapping a methodology.* Thousand Oaks, CA: Sage Publications.

Clandinin, D. J., & Connelly, F. M. (1995). *Teachers' professional knowledge landscapes.* New York: Teachers College Press.

Clandinin, D. J., & Connelly, F. M. (2000). *Narrative inquiry: Experience and story in qualitative research.* San Francisco, CA: Jossey-Bass.

Clandinin, D. J., Davies, A., Hogan, P., & Kennard, B. (1993). *Learning to teach: Teaching to learn. Stories of collaboration in teacher education.* New York: Teachers College Press.

Clandinin, D. J., Huber, J., Huber, M., Murphy, M. S., Murray Orr, A., Pearce, M., & Steeves, P. (2006). *Composing diverse identities: Narrative inquiries into the interwoven lives of children and teachers.* London/New York: Routledge.

Clandinin, D. J., & Murphy, M. S. (2009). Relational ontological commitments in narrative research, *Educational Researcher, 38*(8), 598–602.

Clandinin, D. J., & Rosiek, J. (2007). Mapping a landscape of narrative inquiry: Borderland spaces and tensions. In D. J. Clandinin (Ed.), *Handbook of narrative inquiry: Mapping a methodology* (pp. 35–75). Thousand Oaks, CA: Sage.

Clandinin, D. J., Steeves, P., Li, Y., Mickelson, R., Buck, G., Pearce, M. . . . & Huber, M. (2010). *Composing lives: A narrative inquiry into the experiences of youth who left school early.* Edmonton: Alberta Centre for Child, Family, & Community Research.

Coles, R. (1989). *The call of stories: Teaching and the moral imagination*. Boston, MA: Houghton Mifflin.

Connelly, F. M. & Clandinin, D. J. (1999). *Shaping a professional identity: Stories of educational practice*. New York: Teachers College Press.

Connelly, F. M., & Clandinin, D. J. (1990). *Stories of experience and narrative inquiry. Educational Researcher, 19*(5), 2–14.

Connelly, F. M., & Clandinin, D. J. (2006). Narrative inquiry. In J. Green, G. Camilli, & P. Elmore (Eds.), *Handbook of complementary methods in education research* (3rd ed., pp. 477–487). Mahwah, NJ: Lawrence Erlbaum.

Dewey, J. (1938). *Experience and education*. New York: Collier Books.

Dewey, J. (1958). *Experience and nature*. New York: Dover.

Greene, M. (1995). *Releasing the imagination: Essays on education, the arts, and social change*. San Francisco, CA: Jossey-Bass Publishers.

Houle, S. (2012). *A narrative inquiry into the lived curriculum of grade 1 children identified as struggling readers: Experiences of children, parents, and teachers*. Unpublished doctoral dissertation. University of Alberta, Edmonton, Canada.

Huber, J., & Keats Whelan, K. (2000). *Stories within and between selves: Identities in relation on the professional knowledge landscape*. Unpublished doctoral dissertation. University of Alberta, Edmonton, Canada.

Huber, J., Murphy, M. S., & Clandinin, D. J. (2011). *Places of curriculum making: Narrative inquiries into children's lives in motion*. London: Emerald.

Josselson, R., & Lieblich, A. (Eds.) (1995). *Interpreting experience: The narrative study of lives* (Vol. 3). Thousand Oaks, CA: Sage Publications.

Josselson, R., Lieblich, A., & McAdams, D. P. (Eds.) (2003). *Up close and personal: The teaching and learning of narrative research*. Washington, DC: American Psychological Association.

King, T. (2003). *The truth about stories: A native narrative*. Toronto: House of Anansi Press.

Lopez, B. (1990). *Crow and weasel*. New York: North Point Press.

Lugones, M. (1987). Playfulness, "world"-travelling, and loving perception. *Hypatia, 2*(2), 3–19. doi:10.1111/j.1527-2001.1987.tb01062.x

MacLachlan, P. (1995) *What you know first*. New York: HarperCollins.

Maclntyre, A. C. (1981). *After virtue: A study in moral theory*. Notre Dame, IN: University of Notre Dame Press.

Morris, D. B. (2002). Narrative, ethics, and pain. Thinking with stories. In R. Charon & M. Montello (Eds.), *Stories matter: The role of narratives in medical ethics* (pp. 196–218) New York: Routledge.

Murphy, M. S. (2004). *Understanding children's knowledge: A narrative inquiry into school experiences*. Unpublished doctoral dissertation. University of Alberta, Edmonton, Canada.

Noddings, N. (1984). *Caring: A feminine approach to ethics and moral education*. Berkeley and Los Angeles, CA: University of California Press.

Okri, B. (1997). *A way of being free*. London: Phoenix House.

Pearce, M. (2005). *Community as relationship: A narrative inquiry into the school experiences of two children*. Unpublished doctoral dissertation. University of Alberta, Edmonton, Canada.

Pinnegar, S., & Daynes, J. G. (2007). Locating narrative inquiry historically: Thematics in a turn to narrative. In D. J. Clandinin (Ed.), *Handbook of narrative inquiry: Mapping a methodology* (pp. 3–34). Thousand Oaks, CA: Sage Publications.

Polkinghorne, D. E. (1988). *Narrative knowing and the human sciences*. New York: State University of New York Press.

Reissman, C. K. (2008). *Narrative methods for the human sciences*. Thousand Oaks, CA: Sage Publications.

Reissman, C. K., & Speedy, J. (2007). Narrative inquiry in the psychotherapy professions: A critical review. In D. J. Clandinin (Ed.), *Handbook of narrative inquiry: Mapping a methodology* (pp. 426–456). Thousand Oaks, CA: Sage Publications.

Rose, C. (1997). *Stories of teacher practice: Exploring the professional knowledge landscape.* Unpublished doctoral dissertation. University of Alberta, Edmonton, Canada.

Schultz, R. (1997). *Interpreting teacher practice: Two continuing stories.* New York: Teachers College Press.

14

MAPPING A LANDSCAPE OF NARRATIVE INQUIRY

Borderland spaces and tensions

D. Jean Clandinin and Jerry Rosiek

> *Epistemic agents may no longer claim merely to find the world and so thereby shirk responsibility not only for what they find, but also for the nature of what is found. These objects, these substances of the world, are so often not just epistemic constructions but rather ontological artifacts of our own making and doing . . . practices of representation are peculiarly situated in this process, for representation is itself a mode of intervention.*
>
> –*Kory Sorrell (2004)*

> *The only thing that keeps us from floating off with the wind is our stories. They give us a name and put us in a place, allow us to keep on touching.*
>
> – *Tom Spanbauer (1992)*

Narrative inquiry is an old practice that may feel new to us for a variety of reasons. Human beings have lived out and told stories about that living for as long as we could talk. And then we have talked about the stories we tell for almost as long. These lived and told stories and the talk about the stories are one of the ways that we fill our world with meaning and enlist one another's assistance in building lives and communities. What feels new is the emergence of narrative methodologies in the field of social science research. With this emergence has come intensified talk about our stories, their function in our lives, and their place in composing our collective affairs. This development has required greater philosophical precision in our use of the terms *narrative* and *narrative inquiry*, classification schemes that respectfully acknowledge the diversity of lived and told stories and story talk, and an examination of the boundaries with other traditions of research.

As seen in Chapter 1, each of the various approaches to the use of narrative inquiry has a history, a history that is itself becoming a topic of scholarly discussion. Leiblich, Tuval-Mashiach, and Zilber (1998, p. 1) referred to a "narrative revolution" that was made possible by the decline of an exclusively positivist paradigm for social

Reprinted with permission of Sage. Acknowledgement; Clandinin, D. Jean and Rosiek, J. (2007) *Mapping a landscape of narrative inquiry: Borderland spaces and tensions.* In Clandinin, D. J. (Ed.) *Handbook of Narrative Inquiry: Mapping a methodology* (pp 35–75). Thousand Oaks, CA: Sage.

science research. Also commenting on this revolution some years earlier, Connelly and Clandinin (1990) wrote that although the idea of narrative inquiry as research methodology is new to the social sciences, it has intellectual roots in the humanities and other fields under the broad heading of narratology. Hurwitz, Greenhalgh, and Skultans (2004) trace the emergence of narrative research in the field of medicine as a response to ethical scandals in medical research of the 20th century and the adversarial relationship it precipitated between patients and doctors. Narrative inquiry, they argue, can help heal that relationship. Writing in the field of women's studies, Vaz (1997) locates the inspiration for the use of oral narrative research in a history of Africana women struggling against patriarchy and colonialism.

What becomes apparent in this brief historical tracing is how interwoven narrative ways of thinking about phenomena are with the ways that narrative methodologies are emerging. For example, we hear Bruner speaking of narrative ways of knowing when he says, "Telling stories is an astonishing thing. We are a species whose main purpose is to tell each other about the expected and the surprises that upset the expected, and we do that through the stories we tell" (Bruner, cited in Charon, 2002, p. 8). While Bruner points us toward narrative as a mode of knowing, Lieblich, Tuval-Mashiach, and Zilber (1998) point us toward the need for narrative inquiry as a methodological response to the positivist paradigms. Connelly and Clandinin (1990) link the research methodological turn to the alternative ways of thinking about experience. The need for both narrative ways of thinking about experience and new narrative methodologies becomes apparent in the works of Hurwitz et al. (2004) and Vaz (1997). It is this interweaving of narrative views of phenomena and narrative inquiry that marks the emerging field and that draws attention to the need for careful uses and distinctions of terms. The ways that scholars in many fields have taken this narrative turn both in thinking about the phenomenon of experience and in thinking about research methodologies makes the situation even more complex.

Reissman and Speedy (this volume) hint at this complexity when they note,

> Beginning in the late 1960s and continuing at a hectic pace, the idea of narrative has penetrated almost every discipline and school. No longer the sole province of literary scholarship, narrative study is now cross-disciplinary, not fitting within the boundaries of any single scholarly field.

Furthermore, they note that while "narrative inquiry in the human sciences is a 20th-century development, the field has 'realist,' 'modernist,' 'post-modern,' and 'constructionist' strands, and scholars disagree on origins and precise definition" (Reissman and Speedy, this volume). Sconiers and Rosiek (2000) note similar divergences within the field, citing phenomenological, post-modern, and performative approaches to narrative research. From these different standpoints, we want to draw attention to the narrative turn, a turn that is remarkable in the intensity and enthusiasm with which it has shifted research methodological undertakings.

Any attempt to organize these divergent views into a summary representation inevitably risks shortchanging one view in favor of the priorities of another. There are, however, real differences of opinion on the epistemological, ideological, and ontological commitments of narrative inquirers as well as real differences with those who do not identify as narrative inquirers. These differences, we believe, require careful attention and discussion if the field of narrative inquiry is to realize its potential for making a contribution to the study of human experience and lives. It is the project of this chapter to help clarify these discussions by mapping some of those differences.

Our approach to this conceptual cartography will not be naively objectivist. We do not assume we have access to a stance outside of the history of the field, from which to impartially document all its parts. We are, after all, among those whose work is part of what is being mapped. Leslie Marmon Silko (1997) describes the problem with the metaphor of mapping:

> "A portion of territory the eye can comprehend in a single view" does not correctly describe the relationship between the human being and his or her surroundings. This assumes the viewer is somehow outside or separate from the territory she or he surveys. Viewers are as much a part of the landscape as the boulders they stand on.
>
> *(p. 27)*

Following Piles and Thrift (1995), authors of *Mapping the Subject*, we therefore employ the metaphor of mapping with a cognizance that all representations are partial and involve trade-offs between distortions and instrumental ends.[1] We will offer a representation of the field of narrative inquiry that holds one aspect of narrative inquiry constant and uses this as a point of reference from which to examine the internal and external borders of this area of scholarship. The map we construct, with its borders and borderlands, allows researchers to locate themselves on the landscape of narrative inquiry methodologies.

The point of constancy we take as our point of departure is the observation that narrative inquirers study experience. Connelly and Clandinin (1990, 2006) observed that arguments for the development and use of narrative inquiry are inspired by a view of human experience in which humans, individually and socially, lead storied lives:

> People shape their daily lives by stories of who they and others are and as they interpret their past in terms of these stories. Story, in the current idiom, is a portal through which a person enters the world and by which their experience of the world is interpreted and made personally meaningful. Narrative inquiry, the study of experience as story, then, is first and foremost a way of thinking about experience. Narrative inquiry as a methodology entails a view of the phenomenon. To use narrative inquiry methodology is to adopt a particular view of experience as phenomenon under study.
>
> *(Connelly & Clandinin, 2006, p. 375)*

There are many philosophical treatments of the word *experience*, from Aristotle's dualistic metaphysics in which knowledge of particulars and universals were considered separately, to early empiricist atomistic conceptions of experience, Marxist conceptions of experience distorted by ideology, behaviorist notions of stimulus and response, and post-structuralist assertions that state our experience is the product of discursive practices. The view of experience to which Clandinin and Connelly refer, and which will serve as the cornerstone of our analysis, has its roots in John Dewey's (1938) pragmatic philosophy.

By situating the philosophical foundation of narrative inquiry within a Deweyan theory of experience, we intend to work toward clarifying differences and affinities narrative inquiry has with other areas of scholarship. Our intent in claiming a

Deweyan theory of experience as central to the epistemology and ontology of narrative inquiry allows us to sharpen distinctions between both narrative inquiry and other scholarly traditions as well as to sharpen distinctions within the field of narrative inquiry. Through highlighting the tensions at the borders with other areas of scholarship, we bring into sharper relief the differences with other areas of scholarship. However, as we bring into sharper relief the distinctions, we also highlight the affinities among narrative inquiry and other forms of scholarship.

Deweyan theory of experience[2]

For the purposes of our discussion, there are two particularly salient features of Dewey's (1976) conception of experience. The first is that experience is the fundamental ontological category from which all inquiry – narrative or otherwise – proceeds:

> The importance attached to the word "experience," then . . . is to be understood as an invitation to employ thought and discriminative knowledge as a means of plunging into something which no argument and no term can express; or rather as an invitation to note the fact that no plunge is needed, since one's own thinking and explicit knowledge are already constituted by and within something which does not need to be expressed or made explicit. . . . The word "experience" is, I repeat, a notation of an inexpressible as that which decides the ultimate status of all which is expressed; inexpressible not because it is so remote and transcendent, but because it is so immediately engrossing and matter of course.
>
> *(p. 325, footnote 1)*

The last line here is important, because it points us to the aspect of pragmatism that makes it unique in the Western philosophical tradition as well as particularly germane to narrative inquiry. Dewey says experience is "a notation of an inexpressible." Other philosophers have made similar claims. Kant spoke of the ding an sich or "thing-in-itself," an idea necessary for a coherent theory of knowledge but fundamentally unrepresentable. The phenomenologists spoke of an infinite duree (Bergson, 1889/1960; Merleau-Ponty, 1962; Schutz, 1973), undifferentiated immediate experience that our reflection edits into. For Kant and the phenomenologists, there is something beyond the reach of our writing and reflection toward which our inquiries must nonetheless reach. The inexpressible reality of the ding an sich or the infinite duree thus serves as a regulative ideal for human inquiry while remaining untouched by the representations.

Dewey's (1981c) conception of experience differs from this. It does not refer to some precognitive, precultural ground on which our conceptions of the world rest. Instead, it is a changing stream that is characterized by continuous interaction of human thought with our personal, social, and material environment:

> Because every experience is constituted by interaction between "subject" and "object," between a self and its world, it is not itself either merely physical nor merely mental, no matter how much one factor or the other predominates. . . . [experiences] are the products of discrimination, and hence can be understood only as we take into account the total normal experience in which both inner and outer factors are so incorporated that each has lost its special character. In an experience, things and events belonging to the world, physical and social,

> are transformed through the human context they enter, while the live creature is changed and developed through its intercourse with things previously external to it.
>
> *(p. 251)*

In other words, Dewey's ontology is not transcendental, it is transactional. The epistemological implications of this view are nothing short of revolutionary.[3] It implies that the regulative ideal for inquiry is not to generate an exclusively faithful representation of a reality independent of the knower. The regulative ideal for inquiry is to generate a new relation between a human being and her environment – her life, community, world – one that "makes possible a new way of dealing with them, and thus eventually creates a new kind of experienced objects, not more real than those which preceded but more significant, and less overwhelming and oppressive" (Dewey, 1981b, p. 175) In this pragmatic view of knowledge, our representations arise from experience and must return to that experience for their validation.

There are several features of this ontology of experience that make it particularly well suited for framing narrative inquiry as we are discussing it here. First, the temporality of knowledge generation is emphasized. Experience, for the pragmatist, is always more than we can know and represent in a single statement, paragraph, or book. Every representation, therefore, no matter how faithful to that which it tries to depict, involves selective emphasis of our experience. Dewey (1958) warns against obscuring the selection process, thus naturalizing the objects of our inquiry and treating them as if they are given:

> Honest empirical method will state when and where and why the act of selection took place, and thus enable others to repeat it and test its worth. . . . Under all the captions that are called immediate knowledge, or self-sufficient certitude of belief, whether logical, esthetic, or epistemological, there is something selected for a purpose, and hence not simple, not self-evident, and not intrinsically eulogizable. State the purpose so that it may be re-experienced, and its value and the pertinency of selection undertaken in its behalf may be tested.
>
> *(p. 271)*

Another way of saying this is that an honest empirical method will present inquiry as a series of choices, inspired by purposes that are shaped by past experience, undertaken through time, and will trace the consequences of these choices in the whole of an individual or community's lived experience.

In our view, narratives are the form of representation that describes human experience as it unfolds through time. Therefore, narratives are, arguably, the most appropriate form to use when thinking about inquiry undertaken within a pragmatic framework. Although narrative forms of representation are often used in inquiries framed by other philosophical frameworks, they are, in those cases, almost always regarded as having a degraded epistemic status; if the reality we seek to describe is presumed to be independent of our representations of it, then there is no need to tell the story of how our representation of the world emerged within a stream of experience nor how it returned to that experience.[4]

Second, a pragmatic ontology of experience emphasizes continuity, that is,

> the idea that experiences grow out of other experiences, and experiences lead to further experiences. Wherever one positions oneself in that continuum – the

> imagined now, some imagined past, or some imagined future – each point has a past experiential base and leads to an experiential future.
>
> *(Clandinin & Connelly, 2000, p. 2)*

It is important to note that this continuity is not merely perceptual; it is ontological. Experiences do not simply appear to be connected through time; they are continuous.

This conception of continuity is required by the pragmatic promotion of a transactional ontology. Rejecting centuries of speculation about what transcendent reality (God, eternal forms, pure substance) is needed to hold the amazing variety of human experiences together, William James (1909) states the basic principle of ontology of experience:

> The generalized conclusion is that therefore the parts of experience hold together from next to next by relations that are themselves parts of experience. The directly apprehended universe needs, in short, no extraneous transempirical connective support, but possesses in its own right a concatenated or continuous structure.
>
> *(p. 195)*

In other words, what you see (and hear, feel, think, love, taste, despise, fear, etc.) is what you get. That is all we ultimately have in which to ground our understanding. And that is all we need.

This continuity has important implications for the way we think about inquiry, narrative or otherwise. It reinforces the idea that inquiry is not a search "behind the veil" of appearances that ends in the identification of an unchanging transcendent reality. Instead, inquiry is an act within a stream of experience that generates new relations that then become a part of future experience. It also problematizes the boundaries of inquiry. If experience is continuous, then the initial parameters we set up for our inquiries are themselves a form of relation that can and should be questioned in the course of ongoing research. Dewey (1976) explains it as follows:

> It intimates that while the results of reflection, because of the continuity of experience, may be of wider scope than the situation which calls out a particular inquiry and invention, reflection itself is always specific in origin and aim; it always has something special to cope with. For troubles are concretely specific. It intimates also that thinking and reflective knowledge are never an end-all, never their own purpose nor justification, but that they pass naturally into a more direct and vital type of experience, whether technological or appreciative or social.
>
> *(pp. 332–333)*

Referring to inevitable inferential spillover of our inquiries, Dewey describes experience as having something that "stretches." This stretch is almost "indefinitely elastic" and extends into realms of personal, aesthetic, and social meaning.

This brings us a third feature of a pragmatic ontology of experience that makes it particularly well suited for framing narrative inquiries – its emphasis on the social dimension of our inquiries and understanding. Narrative inquiries explore the stories people live and tell. These stories are the result of a confluence of social influences on a person's inner life, social influences on their environment, and their unique personal history. These stories are often treated as the epiphenomenal to social inquiry – reflections of important social realities but not realities themselves. Dewey (1981a) warns against this prejudice that condescends to impoverishing experience as a source of knowledge:

> The most serious indictment to be brought against non-empirical philosophies is that they have cast a cloud over the things of ordinary experience. They have not been content to rectify them. They have discredited them at large. In casting aspersions upon the things of everyday experience, the things of action and affection and social intercourse, they have done something far worse than fail to give these affairs intelligent direction. . . . To waste of time and energy, to disillusionment with life that attends every deviation from concrete experience must be added the tragic failure to realize the value that intelligent search could reveal among the things of ordinary experience. I cannot calculate how much of current cynicism, indifference, and pessimism is due to these causes and the deflection of intelligence they have brought about.
>
> *(pp. 40–41)*

It is stunning how well Dewey's warning here seems to describe the contemporary climate in many service professions – teaching, health professions, social work, urban planning, and so on. Narrow standards of effectiveness are imposed on an undertaking whose significance to those involved is both nuanced and manifold. And this imposition of procrustean standards of evidence threatens to drain the meaning of that service from both the service providers and those receiving services. In contrast, narrative inquiry is an approach to the study of human lives conceived as a way of honoring lived experience as a source of important knowledge and understanding:

> Narrative inquiry is a way of understanding experience. It is collaboration between researcher and participants, over time, in a place or series of places, and in social interaction with milieus. An inquirer enters this matrix in the midst and progresses in the same spirit, concluding the inquiry still in the midst of living and telling, reliving and retelling, the stories of the experiences that made up people's lives, both individual and social.
>
> *(Clandinin & Connelly, 2000, p. 20)*

Beginning with a respect for ordinary lived experience, the focus of narrative inquiry is not only a valorizing of individuals' experience but also an exploration of the social, cultural, and institutional narratives within which individuals' experiences were constituted, shaped, expressed, and enacted – but in a way that begins and ends that inquiry in the storied lives of the people involved. Narrative inquirers study an individual's experience in the world and, through the study, seek ways of enriching and transforming that experience for themselves and others.

Viewed in this way, we can see that not only is a pragmatic ontology of experience a well-suited theoretical framework for narrative inquiries, narrative inquiry is an approach to research that enacts many if not all of the principles of a Deweyan theory of inquiry. In fact, we offer that narrative inquiry as we describe it is a quintessentially pragmatic methodology. What genealogy is to post-structuralist Foucauldian sociology, what critical ethnography is to critical theory, what experiments are to positivism, narrative inquiry is to Deweyan pragmatism.

Holding a Deweyan theory of experience as a constant, as we construct our map of narrative inquiry, allows us to see borders and borderlands between narrative inquiry and other forms of inquiry. It also allows us to see borderlands within the work of those of us engaged in narrative inquiry. A Deweyan view of experience allows for the study of experience that acknowledges the embodiment of the person living in the world (Johnson, 1987). Framed within this view of experience, the focus of narrative inquiry is not only on individuals' experiences but also on the social, cultural, and institutional narratives within which individuals' experiences are constituted, shaped, expressed, and enacted. Narrative inquirers study the individual's experience in the world, an experience that is storied both in the living and telling and that can be studied by listening, observing, living alongside another, and writing and interpreting texts.

This constant view of experience understood from a Deweyan perspective and of narrative inquiry as the study of experience understood in this way makes possible an understanding of borders and possible borderlands with other forms of research methodologies.

Border conditions

It is often helpful in describing phenomena to explain both what it is and what it is not. Having located the conceptual roots of narrative inquiry in a Deweyan ontology of experience, we can now contrast this with the philosophical assumptions that underlie other forms of scholarship. This, in turn, will permit us to make sense of the kinds of questions asked and methods employed in narrative inquiry. In what follows, we explore the conceptual border between narrative inquiry and social science grounded in three other philosophical traditions: post-positivism, Marxism, and post-structuralism.

Post-positivism

The contrast with post-positivism is perhaps the most frequently discussed in the literature on narrative inquiry. For example, Clandinin and Connelly (2000) described this conceptual border as the boundary between narrative inquiry and reductionist thinking. We realize that the literature on positivist and post-positivist epistemology and its implications for the social sciences is vast and beyond the scope of this chapter to summarize. Our modest goal here is to identify the most general features of this approach to social science inquiry and clarify its relation to narrative inquiry.

At the most general level, positivist philosophies begin with epistemological commitments and treat ontological commitments as secondary considerations. In other words, it begins with a theory of knowledge and, from there, ventures into claims about the nature of reality This approach to philosophy was developed in the 19th century as a reaction to the proliferation of baroque and confusing metaphysical claims about natural and social phenomena. Whether it is notions of corpuscular ether that moves objects, the influence of God on human souls, or evidence that someone was practicing witchcraft, positivism rejected any claims about reality that could not be grounded in empirical observations of the facts of experience.

Over the last century, positivist philosophers moderated their ambitions. Whereas early positivists sought to produce verifiable descriptions of reality, later post-positivists concluded that descriptions cannot be verified in any final way; they can only be falsified. Thus, they are willing to admit into the category of knowledge only those statements that can be demonstrably falsified by procedures that can be made public but that – when tried – have not proven false. The conception of reality that underlies this theory of knowledge is called critical realism and is the subject of considerable debate. Adherents minimally maintain (1) that reality is independent of our minds and (2) that something is real if it can bring about observable consequences that permit for public testing of a claim about the world (Bhaskar, 1997; Phillips & Burbules, 2000).

It is important to note, here, that this is not a naive realism, the idea that we have direct knowledge of the world without any mediation by our senses, social influence, or the like.[5] The critical realist can in fact claim that "there is no conflict between seeing our scientific views as being about objectively given real worlds, and understanding our beliefs about them as subject to all kinds of historical and other determinations" (Norris, 1999, p. 39).

Rather than deny the various social and cultural influences on social science inquiry, the post-positivist seeks to identify methodological procedures that can help communities deal critically with the many mediations of our experience of the world in a way that permits an identification of a reality that we all share. The virtue of this epistemologically conservative stance is that it provides a very stable consensus about a knowledge base for social science inquiry. The drawback is that the price of this stability is that large regions of human experience that influence human affairs – personal meaning, love, hate, aesthetic considerations, religious experience, narrative coherence of individual lives – are often placed outside the bounds of that inquiry.

Narrative inquiry, by way of contrast, begins with an ontology of experience. From this conception of reality as relational, temporal, and continuous, it arrives at a conception of how that reality can be known. This ontology is fundamentally different from that of a critical realist. The critical realist can admit the existence of an infinite variety of private impressions, personal significances, and personal meanings. However, she reserves the term *reality* for something beyond our immediate experience that structures everyone's experience similarly. Following Dewey, the narrative inquirer takes the sphere of immediate human experience as the first and most fundamental reality we have. Building on Dewey, the narrative inquirer focuses on the way the relational, temporal, and continuous features of a pragmatic ontology of experience can manifest in narrative form, not just in retrospective representations of human experience but also in the lived immediacy of that experience.

Following from this ontology, the narrative inquirer arrives at a very different conception of knowledge than the post-positivist. Whereas post-positivists seek a description of a reality that stands outside human experience, the narrative inquirer seeks a knowledge of human experience that remains within the stream of human lives. In other words, narrative inquiry does not merely describe this or that feature of someone's experience. It is simultaneously a description of, and intervention into, human experience; it acknowledges that descriptions add meaning to experience, thus changing the content and quality of the experience. Dewey (1981a) describes this irreducible interplay of description and intervention as follows:

> Knowledge or science, as a work of art, like any other work of art, confers upon things traits and potentialities which did not previously belong to them. [It] . . . is an act which confers upon non-cognitive material traits which did not belong to it. It marks a change by which physical events exhibiting properties of mechanical energy, connected by relations of push and pull, hitting,

> rebounding, splitting and consolidating, realize characters, meanings and relations of meaning hitherto not possessed by them.
>
> *(p. 126)*

Such recursive knowledge effects might be regarded as a design flaw in a post-positivist inquiry on human meaning, one that creates feedback loops that distort the data and undermine the researchers' ability to identify falsifiable claims. For the narrative inquirer, the fact that the inquiry is altering the phenomena under study is not regarded as a methodological problem to be overcome. It is the purpose of the research.

These differences in a general conception of inquiry call for different styles and approaches to scholarship on human experience. Clandinin and Connelly (2000) described how a focus on the temporal nature of human experience requires a particular kind of thinking. To think as a narrative inquirer is to think of events as happening over time; each event or thing has a past, present as it appears to us, and implied future. This temporality has semiotic implications. In narrative inquiry, an action is

> seen as a narrative sign . . . it is necessary to give a narrative interpretation of that sign before meaning can be attached to it. Without understanding the narrative history of the child [individual], the significance or meaning of the performance [action], the sign, remains unknown.
>
> *(pp. 30–31)*

This view of action can be contrasted to post-positivist research in which

> an action is taken as directly evidential. There is an equation connecting action and meaning, connecting performance and cognitive level. In narrative thinking [inquiry], however, there is an interpretive pathway between action and meaning mapped out in terms of narrative histories.
>
> *(p. 31)*

Clandinin and Connelly (2000) also describe a difference between narrative inquiry and post-positivist research based on the treatment of the context of human meaning. In post-positivist research, while the influence of context is acknowledged, the purpose of research design is to limit attention to that context. The ideal is often considered an experiment in which all contextual influences can be controlled or at least accounted for. In narrative inquiry, multiple contexts beyond the researcher's control – such as spatial contexts, cultural contexts, social contexts, institutional contexts, place contexts, and people contexts – are always present. Narrative inquiry is, following this, a relational form of inquiry. Describing the way people go about making sense of their experience within these contexts, and contributing to that ongoing sense making, is the purpose of narrative inquiry.

There is a trade-off involved in embracing a robust engagement with the temporal and contextual nature of human experience. What narrative inquirers gain in the proximity to ordinary lived experience and the scope of their considerations, they, at times, sacrifice in certainty. Narrative inquirers work with an attitude of knowing that other possibilities, interpretations, and ways of explaining things are possible. This sense of uncertainty or tentativeness is one of the most visible and remarked on the differences between narrative and post-positivist inquirers. It often inspires exchanges in which both forms of research are grossly misrepresented. Post-positivists can accuse narrative inquirers of being confused about the object they are describing, self-indulgent, and substituting opinion for knowledge. Narrative inquirers accuse post-positivists of being naive about the nature of human experience, inhumanly procrustean in their conception of knowledge, and politically complicit with government powers that want to silence whole regions of human experience.

Such hyperbolic exchanges are, in the opinion of these authors, unhelpful. It is better to look more closely at the practice of each type of research and critique specific commitments. For narrative inquirers, a sense of tentativeness in representing their own experiences or the experiences of others is the necessary condition for conceiving of a form of inquiry whose object is the transformation of lived human experience. In other words, narrative inquirers must think of any description of human meaning as tentative, if they are to keep alive the possibility that the description can change the quality of the experience being described.

The challenge for the narrative inquirer, therefore, is less one of achieving the highest possible grade of epistemic clarity and is instead how to integrate ethical and epistemic concerns – how to put knowledge in the service of enhancing human experience. The post-positivist conception of knowledge has a role to play in refining narrative inquiry. False or delusional representations of human experience are unlikely to enhance that experience in any sustainable way. But falsehoods are not the only risk about which narrative inquirers are concerned. They are also concerned with missing heretofore unrealized possibilities in human experience. As William James (1897) exclaimed in "The Will to Believe and Other Essays in Popular Philosophy,"

> Believe truth! Shun error! – these, we see, are two materially different laws; and by choosing between them we may end by coloring differently our whole intellectual life. . . . We must remember that these feelings of our duty to either truth or error are in any case only expressions of our passional life. Biologically considered, our minds are as ready to grind out falsehood as veracity, and he who says, "Better go without belief forever than believe a lie!" merely shows his own preponderant private horror of becoming a dupe. He may be critical of many of his desires and fears, but this fear he slavishly obeys. He cannot imagine anyone questioning its binding force. For my own part, I have also a horror of being duped; but I can believe that worse things than being duped may happen to a man in this world. . . . Our errors are surely not such awfully solemn things. In a world where we are so certain to incur them in spite of all our caution, a certain lightness of heart seems healthier than this excessive nervousness on their behalf. At any rate, it seems the fittest thing for the empiricist philosopher.
>
> *(p. 721)*

Marxism and critical theory

Post-positivism is not the only philosophical neighbor with which narrative inquirers negotiate border conditions. Less frequently explored, but often more morally and politically charged, is the border between narrative inquiry and approaches to social analysis grounded in some form of Marxism, including but not limited to the work of Marxist sociologists, critical theorists, critical ethnographers, and post-Marxists.

Narrative inquirers and Marxist-influenced scholars working in the applied social sciences often share an interest in analyzing the way large institutions dehumanize, anesthetize, and alienate the people living and working within them. They also share an interest in resisting those effects by producing a scholarship that intervenes in this process by helping people develop a more robust sense of the reality around them and their agency within that reality. What is different between their approaches is their underlying conception of that reality.

As with post-positivism, the literature on Marxist, critical theory, and post-Marxist social theory is vast and beyond the scope of this chapter to summarize. Our modest goal here is to identify the most general features of these conceptions of social science inquiry and clarify its relation to narrative inquiry. If narrative inquiry traces its philosophical roots to Dewey's philosophy, then contemporary critical theory can be said to trace its philosophical roots to Marxist philosophy. Like Dewey and the pragmatists, Marxist philosophies begin with ontological commitments and treat epistemological commitments as important subsequent considerations. The differences between the two lie in the details of their ontological commitments.

For the Marxist, the fundamental motivation for their analysis is the observation that large-scale social arrangements conspire not only to physically disempower individuals and groups but also to epistemically disempower people. In other words, systems of oppression in modern capitalistic societies include the means by which the sources of that oppression are obscured. This process of deflecting attention from the real causes of oppression is no mere momentary distraction. It involves, according to Marxist theorists, sustained deflections of thought perpetrated by the most cherished and respected traditions of our cultures: religion, nationalism, and liberal humanism.

Marx's term for this deflection of attention from the real cause of oppression was *ideology*. Ideology has been such a generative idea in western social inquiry that it has acquired many definitions (Hawkes, 2003). For our purposes we will let ideology refer here to a system of thought and practice that gives rise to false consciousness in individuals and communities. False consciousness is a condition in which a person acquires a habit of thinking and feeling that prevents him or her from noticing and analyzing the real causes of his or her oppression.

It is the Marxist critique of humanism that is germane to our discussion. Humanism, according to this view, is an ideological system. The false consciousness it produces is an exclusive attention to individuals and individual human experience as a source of knowledge. The humanist idea that all knowledge must begin in the observations and content of individual consciousness leaves people trapped in their inherited ideologies. This is the charge that Marxist-influenced scholars most often bring to bear on the work of narrative inquirers. By focusing on individual experience as a source of insight, the larger social conditions that shape the narratives in which people live go unexamined. Marx and Engles warned that humanist ideologies simultaneously shape institutions that distort human experience and then point to that distortion as the fundamental condition of truth. The result is an inversion of reality and falsehood.

> Consciousness can never be anything else than conscious existence, and the existence of men is their actual life-process. If in all ideology men and their circumstances appear upside-down as in a camera obscura,[6] this phenomenon arises just as much from their historical life-process as the inversion of objects on the retina does from their physical life-process. . . . We set out from real, active men, and on the basis of their real life-process we demonstrate the development of the ideological reflexes and echoes of this life-process. The phantoms formed in the human brain are also, necessarily, sublimates of their

> material life-process, which is empirically verifiable and bound to material premises.
>
> *(Marx, 1846/1972, p. 118)*

Over the last century, this early formulation of "false consciousness" has been critiqued, refined, and elaborated by many social theorists (Adorno, 2000; Augoustinos, 1999; Horkheimer, 2005; Lukacs, 1972; Wetherell, 1999). These critiques have focused on the class-identity essentialism that underlies the juxtaposition of false consciousness and a proletariat consciousness that is free from the distortions of ideology (Laclau & Mouffe, 1987). They have also examined the limits of processes of representation to actually describe ideology (Jameson, 1992; Marcuse, 1964; Zizek, 1999). In most cases, however, some version of Marxist anti-humanism – the idea that ordinary individual experience is distorted by ideology and is, therefore, not a trustworthy source of insight about the social challenges we face – has remained a central analytical commitment of critical theory and post-Marxist scholarship.

This rejection of individual experience as a valid source of knowledge stands in clear contrast to the commitments of narrative inquiry as we have presented it. Precisely understanding that difference, however, requires a careful examination of the philosophical assumptions underlying each tradition. A casual read of the idea of "false" consciousness may give the impression that the first commitment of Marxist-influenced theorists is epistemological – an idea of how to discern truth from falsehood. It is, instead, an ontological principle that ultimately anchors their analysis – the assertion that the material conditions of society precipitate ideologies that shape and distort our ability to understand our world. These material conditions precede and influence epistemological fashions in ways that function to protect and reproduce a grotesquely unequal distribution of human wealth and social power. It is, therefore, in the fundamental reality of these material conditions that Marxist-influenced scholars seek explanation for social and psychological phenomena.

> In the social production which men carry on they enter into definite relations that are indispensable and independent of their will; these relations of production correspond to a definite stage of development of their material powers of production. The sum total of these relations of production constitutes the economic structure of society – the real foundation, on which rise legal and political superstructures and to which correspond definite forms of social consciousness. The mode of production in material life determines the general character of the social, political and spiritual processes of life. It is not the consciousness of men that determines their existence, but on the contrary, their social existence determines their consciousness.
>
> *(Marx, 1964, p. 51)*

Although it may seem extremely abstract, understanding the ontological as opposed to epistemological starting point of Marxist-influenced social theory is necessary for understanding the style and content of this scholarship as well as its relationship with narrative inquiry. A mode of inquiry founded in epistemological commitments – such as positivism – takes accurate description of the world as its primary objective. Epistemic principles, in this case, determine the way the accuracy of research conclusions will be assessed. A mode of inquiry founded in ontological commitments – such as Marxism or critical theory – takes transformation of those ontological conditions as its primary objective.[7] For the Marxist-influenced scholar, research and analysis is an intervention that seeks to change the material conditions that underlie oppressive social conditions.

As remarked on earlier, narrative inquiry shares with Marxism an explicit grounding in ontological commitments as well as the goal of generating scholarship that transforms the ontological conditions of living. The differences between these two traditions of inquiry are located in the specifics of those commitments and their conception of intervention. Scholarship grounded in Marxism privileges the macrosocial material conditions of life as the primary influence on human life and thinking. The relational texture of everyday life, including the personal, religious, historical, and cultural narratives that provide meaning to that life, are treated as derivative of the macrosocial conditions of life. Furthermore, these narratives are frequently considered obstacles to be overcome on the way to a more realistic understanding of the causes of human experience.

The narrative inquirer, by way of contrast, privileges individual lived experience as a source of insights useful not only to the person himself or herself but also to the wider field of social science scholarship generally.[8] As described in the comparison to post-positivism, this approach to analyzing human experience is grounded in a pragmatic relational ontology. It takes the immediacy of lived experiences, specifically its narrative qualities, as a fundamental reality to be examined and acted on. According to this view, all representations of experience – including representations of the macrosocial influences on that experience – ultimately arise from first-person lived experience and need to find their warrant in their influence on that experience. Dewey (1981a) is unequivocal on the latter point:

> Thus here is supplied, I think, a first rate test of the value of any philosophy which is offered us: Does it end in conclusions which, when they are referred back to ordinary life-experiences and their predicaments, render them more significant, more luminous to us, and make our dealings with them more fruitful? Or does it terminate in rendering the things of ordinary experience more opaque than they were before, and in depriving them of in "reality" even the significance they had previously seemed to have?
>
> *(p. 18)*

In privileging lived experience as the ultimate source of, and site of, validation for knowledge, the narrative inquirer does not exclude the possibility of analyzing the oppressive effects of macrosocial conditions. Many social theorists who ground their work in a pragmatic ontology examine the macrosocial conditions of oppression (de Lauretis, 1986; Hook, 1987; Sullivan, 2001, 2006; West, 1989), as do many narrative inquirers (Chang & Rosiek, 2003; Hadden, 2000; Henry & Tator, 2005; Laubscher & Powell, 2003; Maher & Ward, 2002; Sconiers & Rosiek, 2000). However, ultimately, narrative inquirers demur at the Marxist contention that individual lived experience needs to be approached first as the product of ideologies, meaning that the first step in social inquiry is the critique of ideologies. For the narrative inquirer, a person's experience must be listened to on its own terms first, without the presumption of deficit or flaw, and critique needs to be motivated by the problematic elements within that experience. Consequently, the intervention envisioned by the narrative inquirer focuses first on the qualities of lived experience; it is in collaboratively transforming the narratives within which people live that narrative inquiry seeks to lay the foundations for social change. Without such foundations rooted in the storied experiences of ordinary people, it is believed that efforts at social change are condemned to either be ineffective or hollow exercises of externally imposed authority.

Herein lies the most important difference in the practice of inquiry of these two traditions of scholarship. For the Marxist-influenced scholar, the insistence on beginning inquiry in the lived experience of individuals can at best seem overly burdensome. For problems with a clearly macrosocial provenance, this would be like requiring an injured patient to describe their wounds at the cellular level before providing medical care – an unreasonable and dangerous delay of action. At worst, in the Marxist view, the narrative inquirer appears to be the willing dupe of humanist ideologies that function to deflect any attempt to analyze the real causes of oppression. They would say that narrative inquiry stays within the comfortable zone of private experience and provides no leverage for insisting that the mostly middle- and upper-class professionals who conduct and read the research examine their complicity with institutionalized oppression.

Narrative inquirers, on the other hand, often find scholarship grounded in Marxism at best condescending. It approaches people's experience with the presumption of deficits that only the Marxist academic can remedy. At its worst, the narrative inquirer can find scholarship grounded in Marxist theory to be imperialist and self-defeating. By preemptively dismissing the lived experience of persons as a possible source of insight, it simply replaces one totalizing source of external authority – be it church, state, or post-positivist social science – with another. The result is the continued disempowerment of exactly those persons the Marxist-influenced scholars seeks to emancipate.

This dismissal of lived experience is particularly egregious when applied to communities who have been historically silenced by processes of colonialism, patriarchy, homophobia, and other forms of oppression. Stone-Mediatore (2003) describes this excess as follows:

> Worse still, when we treat experience-based narratives as mere ideological artifacts, we reinforce the disempowerment of people who have been excluded from official knowledge production, for we deny epistemic value from a central means by which such people can take control over their own representation.
>
> *(p. 2)*

When reciprocal criticisms between different research paradigms reach the level of mutual recrimination and inspire an unwillingness to listen across disciplinary differences, they are not constructive. This need not be the outcome in this case. There is, in our opinion, much that narrative inquirers can gain from a continued dialogue with Marxist-influenced social theorists. Scholarship grounded in Marxist philosophy serves as a much-needed tonic for Pollyannaish liberal social policy that seeks a solution to all social problems through programs of individual self-improvement. It has also provided some of the most cogent challenges to liberal social science that cravenly ignores the possibility that large-scale socioeconomic conditions can explain both individual behavior and the way researchers choose the unit of analysis for their scholarship. There is nothing that makes such myopias a necessary feature of narrative inquiry. However, by taking the experience of the individual as the starting point and the site of validation for narrative inquiries, the risk of slipping into self-insulating habits of attention and analysis is high.

The question of whether narrative inquiry as a field can avoid this risk is ultimately an empirical question. The development of a narrative inquiry research community that can avoid simply reproducing narratives that support macrosocial systems of oppression, and can instead contribute to the amelioration of oppressive conditions, will depend on (1) educating narrative inquirers for whom the promotion of social justice is a central commitment, (2) the increased inclusion of voices examining experiences of oppression in the narrative inquiry literature, and (3) regular dialogue with scholars in other disciplines who can provide constructive political critique of narrative inquiry practices and texts.

Post-structuralism

A third scholarly community with which narrative inquirers negotiate border conditions are post-structural social and cultural theorists. Post-structuralism and the more diffuse post-modern cultural developments to which it contributed are often considered the natural home to narrative inquiry. Post-structuralism focuses attention on the linguistic and narrative structure of knowledge. It raises fundamental and highly technical questions about the ways we represent the world and makes compelling arguments for encouraging epistemic and methodological diversity in the social sciences. Lyotard (1984), in his watershed work *The Postmodern Condition: A Report on Knowledge*, explained the narrative connection as follows:

> In the first place, scientific knowledge does not represent the totality of knowledge; it has always existed in addition to, and in competition and conflict with, another kind of knowledge, which I will call narrative in the interests of simplicity (its characteristics will be described later). I do not mean to say that narrative knowledge can prevail over science, but its model is related to ideas of internal equilibrium and conviviality next to which contemporary scientific knowledge cuts a poor figure.
>
> (p. 7)

There can be little question that narrative inquirers have benefited from the widespread influence of post-structuralist critiques of a narrowly and naively conceived scientism. These critiques have made audiences more receptive to the idea that there may be other ways of knowing that merit scholarly attention. However, narrative inquiry as we present it here cannot ultimately be grounded in post-structuralist theories about knowledge. To understand the reasons for this epistemic immiscibility, a brief review of the conceptual history of post-structuralism will be necessary.

Post-structuralism traces its roots to the linguistic structuralism of Ferdinand de Saussure (1959). Saussure challenged Aristotelian notions of an ideal one-to-one correspondence between a word and its object. Using the term *signifier* to denote a linguistic sign and *signified* to denote the object to which the sign referred, Saussure argued that, despite a few notable exceptions, the relation between words and their objects was essentially arbitrary. A signifier maintained a stable relationship to its signified, according to Saussure, through its embedded relationship with a whole system of signs, la langue, the language (See graphic below).

The full story of the development of contemporary post-structuralism from Saussurean linguistics is beyond the scope of this chapter. It would suffice to say here that 20th-century anthropologists (e.g., Levi-Straus), psychoanalysts (e.g., Lacan), sociologists (e.g., Foucault, Buarillard), literary critics (e.g., Barthes, Spivak), philosophers (e.g., Derrida), and feminists (e.g., Kristeva, Butler) picked up Saussure's theories, elaborated on them, and extended their application to almost every area of study in the humanities and social sciences. For our purposes, the most important of these elaborations was the application of structuralism to the study of the academic disciplines themselves.

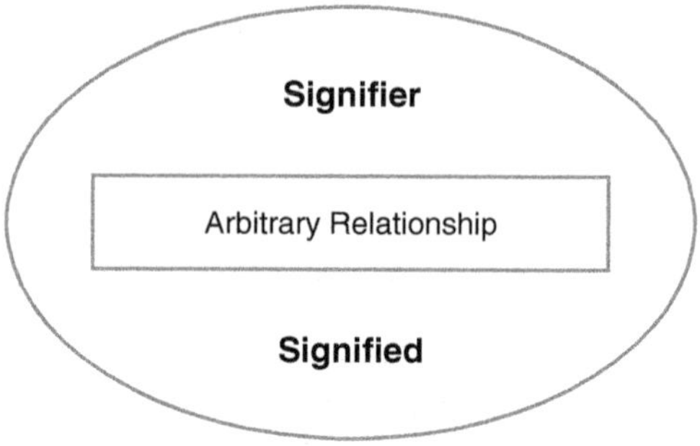

Academic disciplines are often thought to be defined by an object of study. The existence of the object and normative views about its ideal state are assumed to precede research on it. A scholar's method of study is chosen because it uniquely suits the object. For example, "mental illness" is assumed to have preexisted and inspired the development of the field of psychiatry. "Intelligence" is often assumed to exist in individuals and this fact is thought to justify the development of methods of measuring the characteristic. "Race" was long presumed to exist and the science of eugenics was presumed to be the study of the differences between human races. In each case, the object of study had clear normative binaries built in before inquiry began: illness/health, intelligent/unintelligent, white/non-white, and so on.

Post-structuralists used Saussure's theories to invert these assumptions. They took Saussure's argument about the arbitrary relationship between signifiers and signified and extended it to the relationship between an academic discipline and its object of study (See graphic below).

They argued that a close examination of the history and rhetoric of the human sciences revealed that objects of scholarly attention within disciplines often shift in ways that are unrelated to the accumulation of empirical evidence. What keeps a disciplinary community stable instead is its relationship to wider social and historical discourses, discourses that are shaped by and express a variety of competing interests that have little to do with the reality of the object of study. Just as words retain a somewhat stable meaning because they are embedded in a larger system of language, disciplinary discourses remain stable because they are embedded in a larger system of social discourses.

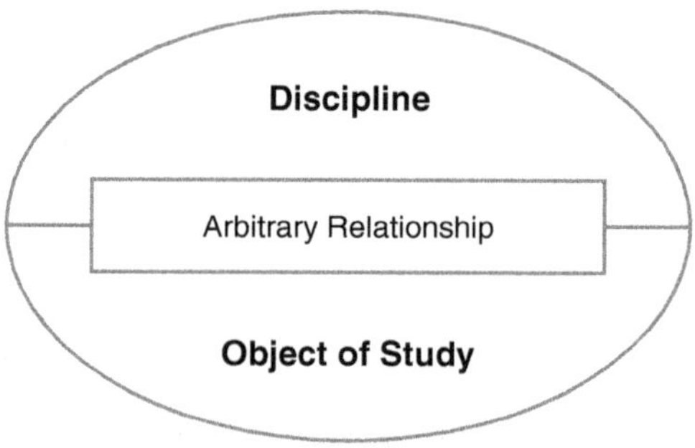

The result is an inversion of the traditional conception of an academic discipline. Instead of the object of study defining the process of inquiry, the process of inquiry creates the object that it examines. This social production of the object of inquiry serves to legitimate the norms associated with that object. Foucault (1982) explains,

> I would like to show with precise examples that in analyzing discourses themselves, one sees the loosening of the embrace, apparently so tight, of words and things, and the emergence of a group of rules proper to discursive practice. These rules define not the dumb existence of a reality, nor the canonical use of a vocabulary, but the ordering of objects. . . . [This presents us with] a task that consists of not – of no longer treating discourses as groups of signs (signifying elements referring to contents or representations) but as practices that systematically form the objects of which they speak.
>
> *(p. 176)*

If it is not the objects, but instead various human interests expressed through social discourses, that ultimately shape academic disciplines, then the enlightenment project of establishing a knowledge base beyond politics becomes impossible. The norms that guide our inquiry become an effect of, not a refuge from, the operation of power:

> Power and knowledge directly imply one another. . . . There is no power relation without the correlative constitution of a field of knowledge that does not presuppose and constitute at the same time power relations.
>
> *(Foucault, 1977, pp. 27–28)*

What emerges from this analysis is a powerful argument for encouraging epistemic and methodological diversity in the social sciences. The interdependent relationship between knowledge and power implies that oppression operates, in part, by artificially narrowing the range of what counts as legitimate knowledge. Remarking on the relation between power and narrative forms of knowledge, Lyotard (1984) elaborates,

> In the West, narrative knowledge has been subjugated by scientific knowledge. The latter is "governed by the demand for legitimation" and, as a long history of imperialism from the dawn of Western civilization demonstrates, cannot accept anything that fails to conform to the rules (the requirement for proof or argumentation) of its own language game.
>
> *(p. 27)*

What also emerges from this analysis is a deep ambivalence about social science that seeks to intervene in the lives of those it studies. Post-structuralism provides analytic tools that help surface the way allegedly objective social science inquiry has served the function of legitimating arbitrary and hurtful social practices. Post-structuralism does not, however, make the development of alternative normative commitments part of its project. Just because our way of knowing the world is mediated by power and human interests it does not mean that there is an alternative way of knowing that escapes this condition. The gap between our descriptions of the world and the actual world is, for the post-structuralist, ultimately unbreachable.[9] What we are left with is an infinite series of supplemental descriptions of the world, and descriptions of those descriptions, of which we need to remain suspicious. Post-structuralist social analysis self-consciously locates itself as one more of these redescriptions.[10]

Here, then, we can see both the similarities and the differences between post-structuralist social analysis and narrative inquiry. Narrative inquiry seeks to examine experience with an eye to identifying new possibilities within that experience. It maintains that knowledge gained from that experience has a linguistic structure; specifically, it maintains, with Lyotard, White, Jameson, and others, that some knowledge is narrative in form.

For the post-structuralist, however, our narrative knowledge has an entirely discursive provenance. Signs can only rely on other signs for their meaning, and thus inquiry does not deal with lived experience itself. Such experience may exist. But as soon as we speak or write about it, we have moved into the process of re-presentation. Representations depend on other representations and discursive systems for their meaning. Consequently, the post-structuralist researcher may listen to stories that individual persons tell her or him. But in so doing she or he will not be interpreting those experiences as immediate sources of knowledge and insight; instead, she or he will be listening through the person's story to hear the operation of broader social discourses shaping that person's story of their experience.

Narrative inquiry, by way of contrast, begins with a pragmatic ontology that treats lived experience as both the beginning and ending points of inquiry. Various social and cultural influences may come into play during the inquiry. As Clandinin and Connelly (2000) note,

> In narrative inquiry, people are looked at as embodiments of lived stories. Even when narrative inquirers study institutional narratives, such as stories of school, people are seen as composing lives that shape and are shaped by social and cultural narratives.
>
> *(p. 43)*

In a narrative inquiry, these social and cultural influences are not treated only as the occasions for critical exposure. They are treated as resources to be used in the pursuit of always tentative and partial ameliorations of experience. This is, of course, a normative project. The norms, for better or worse, must come from within the lived experience being studied. This translates into a collaborative ethic for inquiries, one in which researchers trained in the academy do not presume a transcendent perspective that explains away the stories they and their participants live as mere effects of preexisting social discourses. Clandinin and Connelly (2000) express a narrative inquirer's ambivalence about post-structuralism and post-modernism as follows:

> Because nothing is, as it seems, the only things worth noticing are the terms, the formal structures, by which things are perceived. One does not teach, one mindlessly reproduces a social structure; one does not have emotionally credited intentions, one has preset expectations; one does not have experiences that are one's own, one merely moves forward by contextual design. . . . Persons, they argue, can never see themselves as they are because they are always something else; specifically, they are whatever social structure, ideology, theory or framework is at work in the inquiry. Because narrative inquiry entails a reconstruction of a person's experience in relation to others and to a social milieu, it is

> under suspicion as not representing the true context and the proper "postera" by formalists.
>
> *(p. 39)*

The use of the term *formalist* here may be confusing to some, because in the field of literary criticism, post-structuralism emerged as a critical alternative to a school of thought known as formalism.[11] In the above passage, Clandinin and Connelly use the term more generally. The point they make is that once our representations of experience are assumed to be unmoored from any genuine relation with that experience, then all that is left to analyze is the formal relationship between different discursive systems.

So why not accept the post-structural emphasis on formal symbolic relations, besides the fact that some might find it distasteful? A precise philosophical answer requires returning to the way post-structuralism is grounded in the application of Saussurean ideas about the operation of language to the whole of human experience. Rosiek and Atkinson (2005) explain the limitation of this view as follows:

> At a logical level, the presumption that all signifiers have an arbitrary relationship with the things they signify is questionable at best. This view of semiotics, taken as an article of faith by most post-structuralists (Derrida, 1974; Sherriff, 1989), is based on an extrapolation of the characteristics of linguistic signs to all other signifying activity. . . . Without a sound defense of a general arbitrariness in the sign relation, the complete collapse of individual experience into social dynamics is not possible.
>
> *(p. 12)*

There are alternative semiotic theories that pay more attention to individual embodied experience as a source of meaning. For example, Charles Sanders Peirce (1991), arguably the founder of the pragmatic philosophical tradition, argued that meaning required a signifier, a signified, and an embodied interpreter of the sign. Peirce recognized that some meaning existed primarily at a linguistic level in the formal relations between signifiers. Other meaning, however, arises from more immediate less socialized experiences. Physical pain, visual stimulation, viscerally experienced affections, abrupt disconfirmations of one's expectations, and so forth are also sources of meaning. Additionally, according to Peirce, the encounter with any sign – linguistic or not – is mediated by embodied habits of interpretation, habits that have a history in the individual and in their community. Thus, when a person loves, his or her love is not a floating signifier that simply acquires meaning because the object of affection fits the category of loveable. It is also a habit of relating to an individual with a unique history and for whom there is no substitute.

The existence of such alternative semiotic theories does not foreclose debates between post-structuralists and narrative inquirers. The post-structuralist scholar, like the Marxist-influenced scholar, can still accuse the narrative inquirer of being at best naive about the way social forces shape personal experience and the social construction of knowledge. At worst, they can accuse narrative inquirers of creating a program of research that, through its commitment to an ontology of experience, functions to silence forms of analysis that cannot be readily reconciled with those commitments. The narrative inquirer can respond that the post-structuralist's privileging of macrosocial discursive formations as an exclusive unit of analysis is excessive. Yet such macrosocial influences exist and must be considered. However, the claim that they are all that exists, and that therefore nothing is to be learned from a study of experience as lived, is at best condescending and unjustified. At worst, in its exclusive preoccupation with critique, post-structuralism can be accused of sacrificing real possibilities for amelioration and political engagement.

As we have stated before, divisiveness in interdisciplinary exchanges is not helpful. In our view, the differences between narrative inquiry and post-structuralist analysis are more a matter of emphasis. Each form of emphasis comes with its attendant risks. Narrative inquirers choose to take their risks with people and the stories they live and tell. Sometimes this means working within problematic social discourses longer than the post-structuralist would. In the following, Cornel West (1993) describes the kind of decision that ultimately must be made at this philosophical boundary:

> It takes us right to the center of a dialogue between various postmodern theorists, who would put forth a social constructivist thesis, and pragmatists, who themselves claim to endorse a social constructivist thesis, but do not render in their own writings a consciousness of the degree to which they are deploying terms which themselves are constructs.
>
> Now see, I would opt for the latter. . . . I would opt for the pragmatist who does in fact affirm social constructs from culture to culture, civilization to civilization. Why? Because it is so unavoidable, given the kind of socialization and acculturation human beings undergo in a given culture . . . we can accent the constructive character of the individual deed and what have you. Once we have done that, I am not sure we have done as much as the post-modern theorists think we have.
>
> *(pp. 51–52)*

Having identified some of the border conditions of what we are calling the field of narrative inquiry, we now turn to an exploration of the way those borders blur and run together – in other words, to an exploration of the borderlands of narrative inquiry.

Borderlands of narrative inquiry

Borders are abstractions. They exist as clear demarcations of territory only on maps but do not show up so clearly in the real world (Clandinin & Connelly, 1995). The preceding review of the philosophical territory in which narrative inquiry takes place highlighted the differences between four traditions of inquiry. In our effort to make these distinctions clear, we spoke in terms of epistemological and ontological differences. In the practice of research, however, such philosophical exactness is often a luxury. The actual business of interpreting human experience is messier. As researchers we find ourselves drifting, often profitably, from one paradigm of inquiry into another. We do not cross borders as much as we traverse borderlands.

Although we believe attention to the philosophical assumptions that distinguish narrative inquiry from other forms of research can be very useful to a narrative inquirer, experience has also taught us that some caution is in order. The temptation to reify borders, to think of them as real and necessary features of experience, is often strong, especially for academics. As some feminist philosophers warn,

> This tendency to dichotomize human experiences is persistent, powerful, and pernicious. Dualistic categories are such an organizing force because they

> provide a simple classification system that allows even the most complex and elusive qualities to be compared and contrasted in bold, clear terms.
>
> *(Belenky, Bond, & Weinstock, 1997, p. 119)*

To avoid this pitfall, it is important to respectfully examine, rather than conveniently ignore, the cases that don't fit our categorizations and dichotomies.

Fortunately, much work has already been done in this regard. Clandinin and Connelly (2000) have described the places where narrative inquiry intersects with other ways of thinking as "bumping places," conceptual spaces where different traditions of inquiry come together and where tensions become apparent. Clandinin and Connelly note that all inquirers come to their inquiries with their own views, attitudes, and ways of thinking. Our personal narratives of inquiry may

> coincide with or cross a boundary to varying degrees with the actual inquiries that we undertake. Almost all of us – it is almost unimaginable that we could not – come to narrative inquiries with various versions of formalistic and reductionistic histories of inquiry . . . we are forever struggling with personal tensions as we pursue narrative inquiry . . . narrative inquirers need to reconstruct their own narrative of inquiry histories and to be alert to possible tensions between those narrative histories and the narrative research they undertake.
>
> *(p. 46)*

Huber and Keats Whelan (in press) employ the language of "borders." Citing Gloria Anzaldúa's writing on Mestisa consciousness, they write about "a struggle of borders, both interior and exterior." They draw our attention to the close connection between the struggles within each of us and our struggle with external forces as we locate ourselves in the landscape of narrative inquiry. These interior and exterior struggles, according to these authors, do not take the form of clear and distinct borders. Instead, they are better thought of as borderlands in which scholars situate themselves.

In what follows, we play with the idea of borderlands, those spaces that exist around borders where one lives within the possibility of multiple plotlines. This way of understanding the spaces around the philosophical borders we have described fits with a view of a landscape that does not have sharp divides that mark where one leaves one way of making sense for another. Anzaldúa (1987) writes of a borderland as a

> vague and undetermined place created by the emotional residue of an unnatural boundary . . . a constant state of transition. Los atravesados live here . . . those who cross over, pass over, or go through the confines of the "normal."
>
> *(p. 3)*

Although Anzaldúa is writing of individuals' experiences as they compose themselves in crossing cultural and national boundaries, the idea of a borderland is helpful for understanding the tensions that exist for those of us who work within the broad plotlines of narrative inquiry. Narrative inquirers frequently find themselves crossing cultural discourses, ideologies, and institutional boundaries. In this work they often encounter both deep similarities and profound differences between their own experience and those with whom they work, neither of which can be reduced to the other.

The result is less a harmonious single explanation of their world than it is an expanded understanding of the tensions and conflicted possibilities in the stories people live. Maria Lugones (1992) notes that Anzaldúa affirms this dissonance. She writes of a "mestiza consciousness [which] is characterized by the development of a tolerance for contradiction and ambiguity, by the transgression of rigid conceptual boundaries, and by the creative breaking of the new unitary aspect of new and old paradigms" (p. 34).

We need to be careful in appropriating Anzaldúa's words, so as not to engage in an imperialist whitewashing of her work. Narrative inquiry does not take as its primary focus the intersection of processes of colonization, patriarchal oppression, and racist exclusion that Anzaldúa made it her life's work to engage. All of these systemic injustices and their intersections, however, do find their way into narrative inquiries because they are a part of people's lives and lived stories. Furthermore, the institutional terrain in which narrative inquirers often struggle to locate themselves are similarly fraught with power struggles over whose voices are worth listening to. Therefore, as narrative inquirers locate themselves within the broad ideas of what it means to engage in narrative inquiry, they too seem to enter into a liminal space, where conceptual boundaries are still in the making and the possibilities for what we might do are diverse. Thus, although Anzaldúa was not originally writing about narrative inquiry, we think her ideas apply here.

What Anzaldúa teaches us is that borders are never clean and clear but are blurred as regions overlap and come together. A view of borderlands understood as Anzaldúa explicated them is a view that fits well with the borderland spaces inhabited by narrative inquiry as it bumps up against post-positivism, Marxism, and post-structuralism but it also fits with the borderland spaces that exist within the broad field of narrative inquiry.

Borderland spaces with post-positivism

As we considered these borderland spaces, we began to see that there is no sharp divide; there are blurred borders and researchers are more or less clear about how they can engage their research questions and practices depending on their place on the landscape in relation to narrative inquiry and post-positivist forms of inquiry. Adopting a view of borderlands between narrative inquiry and post-positivism, we began to see that researchers, working from a post-positivist view and searching for ways to understand phenomena, sometimes design their research in ways that allow them to draw on practices similar to those narrative inquirers might use.

For example, post-positivist research that attempts to understand how contexts, understood temporally, influence, shape, and are shaped by people's actions shift researchers toward examining the context-dependent and temporal nature of human thinking generally. As they search for ways to study the shaping influence of context over time they begin to engage in practices that might be seen as having an affinity with the practices of narrative inquirers who are also interested in studying how context shifts individuals' storied experiences over time. Narrative inquirers, in turn, often find this kind of post-positivist research affirming and illuminating of their own inquiry projects.

These affirmations and illuminations can lead narrative inquirers deeper into the borderlands, where the priorities of post-positivist research begin to replace the priorities of narrative inquiry. For example, some narrative inquirers search for ways to speak to a sense of "the universal case" (Clandinin & Connelly, 2000, p. 32). Some narrative inquirers, unable to live with the tension produced by constantly proliferating counter narratives, search for ways to ameliorate this tension by seeking universal themes in which the narrative tensions can be contained. In that search, they move into the borderlands with post-positivist research, which takes the identification of generalizable patterns in human experience as its primary goal (Clandinin & Connelly, 2000). This desire to speak to the universal comes, we think, from being immersed in an academic world that encourages us to speak to the universal. Thomas King (2003) describes this impulse as an attraction to

> dichotomy, the elemental structure of Western society. And cranky old Jacques Derrida notwithstanding, we do love our dichotomies. Rich/poor, white/black, strong/weak, right/wrong, culture/nature, male/female, written/oral, civilized/ barbaric, success/failure, individual/communal. We trust easy oppositions. We are suspicious of complexities, distrustful of contradictions, fearful of enigmas.
>
> *(p. 25)*

As narrative inquirers move further into this borderland, the desire to speak of general trends, of the context free, and to provide a stable knowledge base for social science inquiry stands in tension with a narrative inquiry view that knowledge of human experience begins and must return to the stream of particular human lives. This tension can be a source of new ideas and rich interdisciplinary dialogue. It can also become the cover for forms of academic violence.

Take, for example, the researcher who listens to people's stories, not as a prelude to collaboratively enhancing those persons' continuing experience but instead as a prelude to identifying common themes and universal narrative structures. On the one hand, important insights about narrative aspects of human experience might be revealed in such a study. On the other hand, from our Deweyan view, such a study severs the narratives from the relational, temporal, and continuous features of experience that give it meaning. The story is thus ripped from the personal history of the one living it and is treated as fixed data, much as one might treat numerical data. We use the word *ripped* deliberately, to highlight not only the decontextualization of the story but also the power and status differentials that are often involved when social scientists conduct research on, as opposed to with, people. (See a discussion of this point in Tsai's chapter in this volume.)

Tracking the lines of epistemic and ethical responsibility in this kind of research becomes more difficult in the borderlands, where paradigmatic standards become blurred. As a result, these borderland disputes within the broad field of narrative inquiry are frequently glossed over. We, however, see the importance of naming the struggle of living in the borderlands and acknowledging both the possibilities and the violence that accompany the emergence of subtly different but nonetheless conflicting ontological and epistemological stances.

Borderland spaces with Marxism

As in the borderlands between narrative inquiry and post-positivism, we see researchers working from a Marxist-influenced view sometimes asking research questions and raising concerns that resemble narrative inquiry in many respects. Most frequently, this movement is inspired by a felt need to bring a Marxist-influenced critique of the macrosocial sources of oppression into practical relation with immediate experience. Critical ethnographer Barry Kanpol (1997) describes the questions he encountered in his travels along this borderland as follows:

> I have over the last few years or so begun to ask these problematic questions: To what end do critical educators theorize? Why is theory so devoid of personal narrative? What relationship has critical theory to the everyday life-world of those who work in the trenches, such as teachers, administrators, students and researchers? Why doesn't critical analysis and practice seriously find its way into public schools?

Once the importance of personal narratives to critical theoretic analysis is acknowledged, many political purposes are ascribed to narrative inquiry. Critical race theorist Richard Delgado (1989) made exactly this point in his widely cited article "Legal Storytelling: Storytelling for Oppositionists and Others: A Plea For Narrative," which highlights three ways that attention to people's stories can be an important way of responding to macrosocial forms of oppression. First, he argues, it serves a healing function:

> So, stories – stories about oppression, about victimization, about one's own brutalization – far from deepening the despair of the oppressed, lead to healing, liberation, mental health. . . . Storytelling emboldens the hearer, who may have had the same thoughts and experiences the storyteller describes, but hesitated to give them voice. Having heard another express them, he or she realizes, I am not alone.
>
> *(p. 2437)*

Second, it can contribute to the transformation of oppressors. Silence is an essential part of processes of macrosocial oppression. Inequality and injustice are sustained, in part, by the ways in which privileged members of society insulate themselves from the suffering of others. Attending to the narratives of marginalized groups can disrupt this insularity.

> Yet, stories help oppressed groups in a second way – through their effect on the oppressor. Most oppression, as was mentioned earlier, does not seem like oppression to those perpetrating it. It is rationalized causing few pangs of conscience. The dominant group justifies its privileged position by means of stories, stock explanations that construct reality in ways favorable to it.
>
> *(Delgado, 1989, p. 2437)*

Finally, Delgado (1989) argues that paying attention to people's stories opens up possibilities for generating new stories in which we can all live:

> Listening to stories makes the adjustment to further stories easier; one acquires the ability to see the world through others' eyes. It can lead the way to new environments. . . . Listening to the stories of outgroups can avoid intellectual apartheid. Shared words can banish sameness, stiffness, and monochromaticity and reduce the felt terror of otherness when hearing new voices for the first time. . . . If we would deepen and humanize ourselves, we must seek out storytellers different from ourselves and afford them the audience they deserve. The benefit will be reciprocal.
>
> *(p. 2439)*

As we noted above, for the narrative inquirer, a person's experience needs to be listened to on its own terms first, without the presumption of deficit or flaw. Critique of that experience needs to be motivated by the problematic elements within that experience. For the critical scholar drawn into the borderland with narrative inquiry, such commitments do not come easily. It requires that they simultaneously acknowledge that an individual's experience is shaped by macrosocial processes of which she or he is often unaware and that the same individual's experience is more than the living out of a socially determined script. We see some of this struggle in Shari Stone-Mediatore's (2003) book *Reading Across Borders: Storytelling and Postcolonial Struggles*, in which she writes,

> Feminist epistemologists, for instance, have warned that we cannot rely on experience to counter ideology because experience itself is formed through ideological processes. Furthermore, as feminists in the Marxist tradition emphasize, the "reality" that we encounter is a product of human history, but everyday experience tends to confront such historical reality as if it were mere fact. As Sandra Harding puts it, "our experience lies to us."
>
> (p. 99)

As she enters a borderland space between Marxist-influenced views and narrative inquiry, Stone-Mediatore does not want to lose track of the large-scale material conditions that shape human life, but she also wants to credit the force of the experiences of individuals who live in marginal positions in dominant narratives. As she searches for ways to study experience, she begins to engage in practices that might be seen as having an affinity with the practices of narrative inquirers who are also interested in studying individual's storied experiences as shaped by cultural, institutional, and social narratives. Citing the work of other transnational feminists in this methodological borderland, she observes that

> these critics explore concrete ways that the most disempowered people can use resources in their daily lives to challenge the discourses and institutions that keep them in subservient positions . . . they . . . investigate how we might transform lived experiences of discontent into critical knowledge and political consciousness. They recognize narration to be key in the transformation of experience into useful knowledge.
>
> (p. 126)

We see this struggle to reconcile respect for the experience of individuals with a concern about the way ideologies distort experience in critical ethnography informed by feminist scholarship, such as that done by Michelle Fine and Lois Weis (Fine, 1987; Fine & Weis, 2003). As early as her landmark work in New York schools in the 1980s, Fine wanted to hear the stories of experience of the high-school students even as she wanted to engage in a macrosocial analysis. Focusing on the silencing of voices that she defines as "the process by which contradictory evidence, ideologies, and experiences find themselves buried, camouflaged, and discredited" (Fine, 1987, p. 157), she attends to the voices of Deidre, Alicia, Monique, and Patrice. An example of the borderland struggle is evident when Fine writes that students' voices helped her see that, for her, "participation was encouraged, delighted in, and a measure of the 'good student.' For these adolescents, given their contexts of schooling, 'participation' signified poor discipline and rude classroom behavior" (Fine, 1987, p. 167). It was, it seems, as she listened first to the stories of the students' experiences that she began to attend differently to what she was hearing. In her later work with Weis, we continue to see her working in the borderland of contradictions between narrative inquiry and Marxist-influenced scholarship. It is in this borderland space between acknowledging the macrosocial dimensions of oppression and attending to the voices of youth, teachers, and others that Fine and Weis see the possibility for "facilitating individual and collective movements toward social change and social justice" (Fine & Weis, 2003, pp. 4–5).

Approaching from the other side of the border, the narrative inquirer drawn to the borderland with Marxist-influenced scholarship also faces struggle. These narrative inquirers often experience conflict as they recognize their own and others' complicity with institutionalized oppression and find it difficult to continue listening to the storied experience of participants. The more attention a researcher pays to macrosocial structural processes of oppression – be it patriarchy, white supremacist ideologies, institutionalized homophobia, or market economies commodifying every aspect of our lives – the less it may seem that individuals and their experiences make a difference. Focusing on the details of personal experience can feel like escapism.

The need to respond to the structural conditions of oppression is often most acutely felt by narrative inquirers who have previously done service in urban communities or remote rural communities where poverty rates are high and the maldistribution of wealth and resources is most felt. However, scholars who begin their analysis from a position of service to those among us who suffer most, often do so because they feel respect for members of these communities. Frequently, the researchers are members of the communities themselves. Consequently, they want to listen to the stories of the people they seek to serve. They prefer to conduct research with, not on, the people with whom they work.

It is this commitment to listening and collaboration, on the one hand, and an awareness that large-scale social systems set people up to perpetuate their own oppression, on the other hand, that can lead a researcher to the borderlands between narrative inquiry and critical-theoretic scholarship. We offer no easy resolution to this tension. Instead, we offer a caution. Ultimately, the narrative inquirer traveling in this borderland will find it necessary to steer between the Scylla of political naïveté and the Charybdis of collecting stories from participants only to treat them as examples of an oppressive social structure. The former can render narrative inquiries irrelevant to the most pressing social justice concerns. The latter can end up dismissing the lived experience of persons as a possible source of insight and thus simply replace one habit of silencing voices from the margins with another similar habit.

Borderland spaces with post-structuralism

Perhaps the most highly trafficked theoretical and methodological borderland of the three we discuss here is the one between narrative inquiry and post-structuralism. As described in the preceding sections, narrative inquirers share a use of linguistic terms for describing human knowledge and experience with post-structuralists. Consequently, many scholars draw liberally from both traditions when conducting their research. Differences in the underlying ontological assumptions of these two theoretical frameworks, however, occasionally surface in this borderland, producing tensions, confusions, as well as new possibilities for analysis.

The tensions are similar to those found in the previous theoretical borderlands we have described. For example, post-structuralists share with post-positivists a primary focus on description of broad patterns in human activity as distinct from narrative inquirers' focus on individuals' experience. Despite the profound differences between these two theories, each has its way of minimizing what people learn struggling to live in the interstices of these broad patterns of human activity, be they behavioral or discursive, cognitive or cultural. Stone-Mediatore (2003) speaks to the borderland spaces created between post-positivism, post-structuralism, and narrative inquiry. Referring to post-positivist research paradigms broadly as "empiricist," she explains,

> Neither empiricist nor poststructuralist theories of experience can account for the subversive force of many marginal experience narratives . . . both schools presume that stories of experience are mere unreflective reports of spontaneous awareness. As a result, both obscure the capacity of writers to grapple with muted, contradictory, or even traumatized experience. Moreover, both overlook the capacity of readers to attend to phenomena that are only intimated by metaphors or tension within texts, phenomena that are not directly articulated because they defy our categories for representing experience.
>
> *(p. 2)*

Post-structuralists also share with critical theory scholars a concern that large-scale social processes can condition individual experience so thoroughly that individuals cannot recognize the operation of those processes. This only reinforces their skepticism about truth claims based on personal experience. The difference between post-structuralists and critical theory scholars, as described earlier, is that the post-structuralist sees no escape from discursive processes, no way to finally anchor even scholarly representations in an extradiscursive reality.

Consequently, post-structuralists who find themselves in the borderlands with narrative inquiry often arrive there less because they consider the people's stories sources of new knowledge about social reality and more because they are attracted to the productive power of stories. They are looking for a way to move beyond description of the formal qualities of social discourses to transformative intervention but need a mode of intervention that is not totalizing:

> What is sought is a reflexive process that focuses on our too easy use of taken-for-granted forms and that might lead us towards a science capable of continually demystifying the realities it serves to create. [I envisage] an altogether different approach to doing empirical inquiry which advocates the creation of a more hesitant and partial scholarship capable of helping us to tell a better story in a world marked by the elusiveness with which it greets our efforts to know it.
>
> *(Lather, 1991, p. 15)*

Scholars influenced by post-structuralist theory and attracted to the productive power of stories frequently focus on exploring the use of narrative representations in educational research. They frame the purpose of crafting narrative representations in different ways, sometimes emphasizing political and rhetorical value, at other times their aesthetic value, and at other times their ability to foster emotional and moral responses to a topic. Across these purposes, however, lies a sense that narratives can make things happen in ways that other forms of representation cannot. Sconiers and Rosiek (2000) explain this as follows:

> When used in the postmodern sense, narrative research treats all representations of educational events – informant's as well as researcher's – as partially fictionalized (re)presentations whose meaning exists in a contested space between

> authors and their audiences (Hall, 1992; Kincheloe, 1997; Stake & Kerr, 1995). In this case, the researcher's project is not to escape the textual play of meaning by establishing privileged access to "one true account" of a classroom event, but to participate constructively in an intertextual dialogue about the meaning of these events (Denzin, 1997). When used in the arts-based, performative sense, narrative research can employ fictionalized accounts of events as a way of pointing to as yet unrealized possibilities within that experience (Eisner, 1995; Noddings, 1995; Stake & Kerr, 1995) or as a means of producing the conditions that make certain meanings possible (Butler, 1997; Conquergood, 1991; Lather, 1997).
>
> *(p. 400)*

The promise of this focus on using narrative modes of representation in social science research is that it may "open up an imaginative space for us to recognize alternative identities and ways of life" (Stone-Mediatore, 2003, p. 99) or "lift the veil of conventionality from my eyes as they subtly raise disturbing questions about the necessity and desirability of comfortable, familiar . . . discourses and practices" (Barone, in press). The danger is that the ambition to generate new and better versions of our world will presumptively erase or displace the stories people are already living. The goal of transformation inevitably involves hubris and raises the question "Whose transformation?" Where the motivation is more aesthetic than political, we see narrative inquirers occasionally becoming entranced by a particularly striking metaphor through which they choose to read their participants' stories. They become so caught up in the metaphor that they no longer attend to the stories of experience but, rather, attend to how the stories of experience fit within the entailments of the metaphor. The threat of colonialism and dehumanization looms large.

For those approaching this borderland from the other side, starting closer to narrative inquiry as we have described it, the attraction to post-structuralist theory is often similar to the attraction to critical theory. Concern about the way broad systems of social oppression obscure people's ability to see their own participation in those systems inspires a search for language that can express ambivalence about insights that arise from within stories as lived, without completely discounting first-person experience as a source of important knowledge.

For example, in a study of the experiences of four white teachers who taught in aboriginal schools, Kennedy (2001) struggled to attend to her participants' stories of experience while simultaneously attending to how theoretical constructions of race shaped the teachers' stories. The tension of the borderland was evident as she struggled to listen to the reconstruction of the teachers' experiences in relation to others and to a social milieu without being caught into attending only to the social structure of race. She wrote of trying to snag the race thread in individuals' experiences as it emerged rather than beginning with it preemptively. Within this borderland space, Kennedy frequently finds her work being read for the post-structuralist terms that apply:

> A person is a member of a race, a class, a gender, and may be said to have varying degrees of power in any situation. Part of the tension for a narrative inquirer is to acknowledge these truths while holding to a different research agenda.
>
> *(Clandinin and Connelly, 2000, p. 45)*

This borderland tension and struggle is also evident in the work of Soreide (in press). In her paper titled "Narrative Construction of Teacher Identity: Positioning and Negotiation," Soreide explores how the discourse communities of five Norwegian elementary school teachers shape their teacher knowledge landscapes. She shows how the teachers draw from the available discourses to compose and to construct their teacher identities. Her struggle emerges when she wants to treat each individual's experience as a unique case, deserving respect and attention tailored to their situation and personal history, even as she wants to use their words to illustrate and illuminate how broader social discourses condition their experience. Soreide uses post-structuralist theory to analyze the stories teachers tell of themselves – that is, what Soreide calls their ontological narratives. Instead of presenting these narratives as derivative of the discourses, she attempts to show how the teachers' subject positions were used as a resource by the teachers in constructing their personal narratives of teacher identity. Soreide writes in the borderland between narrative inquiry and its attention to individual experience and the post-structuralist's privileging of macrosocial discursive formations as a unit of analysis. She turns uneasily in both directions, that is, to the individual's narratives of experience as source of identity and the macrosocial discursive formations to show how teacher identity is context dependent, negotiable and negotiated, shifting, multiple, and contradictory.

Another striking example of the struggles inherent in the borderland between narrative inquiry and post-structuralist research is found in Borland's (1991) description of her feminist oral history research with her grandmother. She described how her grandmother, Beatrice, recounted her life "in a highly structured and thoroughly entertaining narrative . . . to her folklorist-granddaughter, who recorded her words on a tape for later transcription and analysis" (p. 63). Beatrice and her granddaughter, however, did not interpret this narrative in the same way, and this later led to conflicts between the two. The grandmother wanted her stories of experience to be both the starting and ending points of the inquiry. Borland writes that her analysis of those stories was informed by "contemporary feminist conceptions of patriarchal structures, which my grandmother does not share" (p. 69). Borland found herself in the borderland between narrative inquiry and post-structuralism as she wants to attend to her grandmother's experience but does not want to abandon her feminist theories. Borland speculates that some form of polyphonic representation may be needed to honor both these interpretations:

> I am suggesting that we might open up the exchange of ideas so that we do not simply gather data on others to fit into our own paradigms once we are safely ensconced in our university libraries ready to do interpretation. By extending the conversation we initiate while collecting oral narratives to the later state of interpretation, we might more sensitively negotiate issues of interpretive authority in our research. . . . At the very least, it would allow us to discern more clearly when we speak in unison and when we disagree. Finally, it would restructure the traditionally unidirectional flow of information out from source to scholar to academic audience by identifying our field collaborators as an important first audience for our work. Lest we, as feminist scholars, unreflectively appropriate the words of our mothers for our own uses, we must attend to the multiple and sometimes conflicting meanings generated by our framing or contextualizing of their oral narratives in new ways.
>
> *(p. 73)*

As these examples illustrate, the narrative inquirer who lives in the borderland spaces with post-structuralist researchers lives in spaces that do not allow for easy oppositions. As narrative inquirers live in such spaces, we need to find ways to stay open to complexities, contradictions, and enigmas. As we do this, we acknowledge the richness and complexity as well as the possibility for tension, violence, and strong disagreement that make these borderland spaces.

Looking back across the borderlands

We began this section by acknowledging that borders, philosophical or geographic, become less clear the closer you get to them. We offered, therefore, that it was better to speak of borderlands, regions of shared influence between different research traditions. Before we close, we should also acknowledge that these influences themselves lack clear edges. Even when a researcher's primary philosophical commitments are clear, other scholarly paradigms can shape their work with important findings, by posing pressing questions or by offering critique from outside. In other words, the influence of, say, positivism on narrative inquiry does not abruptly end as much as it tapers off depending on who you are talking to and what you are talking about.

Consequently, the influence of our philosophical neighbors can be seen even far from what we have described as borderlands. We can see what we might call borderlands *within* the community of narrative inquirers. Some narrative inquirers are more interested in the structure of professional identity narratives. Others are more interested in the difficulty some individuals have in addressing the big picture social justice issues in our world. Others are more interested in working with people to aesthetically craft new narrative representations of experience. Some find themselves working to combine these interests and others. Such differences of emphasis and interest, we offer, are not simply idiosyncratic. They can often be traced to the scholarly literature being read by a given narrative inquirer.

These borderlands within, just like the borderlands with other traditions, can create tensions and provoke strong disagreements. Ultimately, however, we see these multiple influences that overlap and shade into one another as contributing to the richness and complexity of narrative inquiry.

Shared commitments: commonplaces on the narrative inquiry landscape

In this chapter, we laid out an understanding of narrative inquiry that emerges from Dewey's theory of experience. As we did this, we created a map that positioned narrative inquiry alongside, but distinct from, post-positivist, Marxist, and post-structuralist forms of inquiry. In doing so we suggested there were borderland spaces between these various forms of inquiry, borderlands in which these distinctions become blurred and difficult to identify. We attempted to show how these borderlands were spaces of tension and struggle and how these struggles and tensions become apparent within differing research practices and texts. We ended by saying these borderland struggles are echoed to some extent in the differences we see within and among narrative inquirers.

In this section, we want to affirm that amid the influence of our philosophical neighbors, there is something distinctive about narrative inquiry that marks it as narrative inquiry. There are affinities and commonplaces among those of us who engage in narrative inquiry. These multiple influences and tensions enhance the field of narrative inquiry rather than overwhelm it.

The most defining feature of narrative inquiry, as we have presented it, is the study of experience as it is lived. As noted throughout this chapter, experience is what is studied in narrative inquiry and we argued for a Deweyan view of experience. This shared commitment to the study of experience is central to narrative inquiry. Within this focus, there are additional shared commitments in narrative inquiry. Connelly and Clandinin (2006), based on their own work with narrative inquiry and based on a review of others' writing about narrative inquiry (Josselson, 1993; Lieblich, 1995; McAdams, 1996; Mishler, 2000; Polkinghorne, 1988), identified three further commonplaces of narrative inquiry – attention to temporality, sociality, and place – which specify dimensions of narrative inquiry spaces and mark out the landscape space of narrative inquiry.

The first commonplace, temporality, attends to Dewey's notion of continuity in experience – that is, that every experience both takes up something from the present moment and carries it into future experiences. Events, people, and objects under study are in temporal transition and narrative inquirers describe them with a past, a present, and a future.

The second commonplace, sociality, points toward the simultaneous concern with both personal and social conditions. This commonplace connects with Dewey's notion of interaction – that is, that people are always in interaction with their situations in any experience. By personal conditions Clandinin and Connelly (2000) mean the feelings, hopes, desires, aesthetic reactions, and moral dispositions of the person, whether inquirer or participant. By social conditions they mean the existential conditions, the environment, surrounding factors and forces, people and otherwise, that form the individual's context.

Another important dimension of the sociality commonplace is the relationship between participant and inquirer. Narrative inquirers are always in an inquiry relationship with participants' lives. They cannot subtract themselves from relationship. Narrative inquirers, throughout each inquiry, are in relationship, negotiating purposes, next steps, outcomes, texts, and the other concerns that go into an inquiry relationship. Nor can they pretend to be free of contextual influences themselves. As Rosiek (2005) points out, practitioners and their academic collaborators both "face similar conflicts between the discourses of their professional training and the discourses of the non-academic communities in which they live and work" (p. 269). In narrative inquiry, research questions and texts are ones where inquirers give an account of who they are in the inquiry and who they are in relation to participants.

The third commonplace, place or sequences of places, draws attention to the centrality of place, that is, to the specific concrete, physical, and topological boundaries of place where the inquiry and events take place. This commonplace recognizes that all events occur in some place. It draws attention to borderland tensions because those who work from post-positivist, post-structuralist, or Marxist positions may wish to escape the limitations of place in the interests of generalizability. For narrative inquirers, the specificity of location is important. The qualities of place and the impact of places on lived and told experiences are crucial. As Basso (1996) writes,

> As places animate the ideas and feelings of persons who attend to these same ideas and feelings animate the places on which attention has been bestowed, and the movements of this process – inward toward facets of the self, outward toward aspects of the external world, alternately both together – cannot be

> known in advance. When places are actively sensed, the physical landscape becomes wedded to the landscape of the mind, to the roving imagination, and where the latter may lead is anybody's guess.
>
> *(p. 107)*

As an inquiry proceeds temporally, place may also change and narrative inquirers need to stay awake to how place shifts the unfolding stories of lives.

These commonplaces are ideas that hold us together. They are commonplaces or touchstones that allow narrative inquirers to understand their research as occupying a distinct place on the methodological landscape.

Concluding thoughts

Not everyone who engages in narrative inquiry will be inclined to dwell on its underlying philosophy at length. However, given the explosion of research under the broad heading of narrative inquiry, we feel opening up the debate about the philosophical roots of narrative inquiry as a research methodology brings a helpful clarity to the field. More important, in our view, it helps us not to waste energy on conflicts born of confusion and serves as an important starting point for helping narrative inquirers to be good neighbors in the broader community of scholars. As we continue to develop the ideas of narrative inquiry, we hope it enables us to recognize the good neighbors in others, even if they speak different theoretical languages.

As we reflect on our conceptual cartography of narrative inquiry, we are struck by the energy generated by those interested in studying people's lives. This rush to narrative inquiry and the willingness to move into the borderlands with narrative inquiry suggests an eagerness to understand in more complex and nuanced ways the storied experiences of individuals as they compose storied lives on storied landscapes.

We are also struck by the enthusiasm for narrative ways of thinking, for narrative ways of understanding knowledge and identity that cuts across disciplines and professions. As Rita Charon (2006), a leader in bringing narrative practices to medicine, writes,

> We search the horizon – astronomers, oceanographers, artists, musicians, doctors, novelists, geneticists – seeking ways to recognize ourselves and those who surround us, yearning to place ourselves within space and time (and infinity), dramatizing our stubborn beliefs that life means something and that we ourselves matter.
>
> *(p. 69)*

What Charon draws our attention to is that stories matter and that, increasingly, we are interested in knowing the stories that all people live and tell. As we, and other narrative inquirers now know, inquiry, narrative inquiry, into those stories that people live and tell, also matters.

Notes

1 For example, a Mercator map of the globe preserves relative shapes and permits a viewing of the entire globe but makes objects appear larger the farther they are from the equator. A globe preserves both shape and size, but all areas cannot be viewed simultaneously. However, what area is selected as a center for the map shifts what is seen as marginal. For example, a map with North America in the center makes other areas marginal. A map

that moves Asia from the margin to the center shifts how North America and Asia are seen. Something similar happens when the North Pole is in the center of the map. Each projection serves a purpose but also involves limitations in usefulness and accuracy.

2 Quotes from *The Collected Works of John Dewey* are copyright © 1986 by the Board of Trustees, Southern Illinois University, reproduced by permission of the publisher.

3 In the opinion of the authors, while Dewey's views are revolutionary, the revolution in the human sciences that his philosophy points to is yet to occur.

4 More will be said about this comparison in later sections.

5 Many who are attracted to narrative inquiry can be tempted to oversimplify the positivist position as a prelude to rejecting it. This does not advance the cause of narrative inquiry nor does it make for sound foundations of scholarship. For an economical summary of positivist and post-positivist epistemologies, see Phillips and Burbules (2000) and Archer, Bhaskar, Collier, Lawson, and Norrie (1998).

6 A *camera obscura* was an instrument used by artists during the Middle Ages to cast an image onto paper by means of mirrors. Because the image was inverted, a lens was needed to correct it.

7 Epistemic questions about the accuracy of an analysis will inevitably arise in the course of such inquiry; however, epistemic standards would be adopted as a means to ontological intervention.

8 This utility, it perhaps should be pointed out, would not simply be in the form of a case illustration of ideologically distorted false consciousness – although narrative inquiry could, in fact, provide such illustrations.

9 Derrida (1972/1982) called this gap *différance,* of which he said:

> In fact "Older" than Being itself, such a *différance* has no name in our language. But we "already know" that if it is unnamable, it is not provisionally so, not because our language has not yet found or received this name, or because we would have to seek it in another language, outside the finite system of our own. It is rather because there is no name for it at all, not even the name of essence or of Being, not even that of "differance," which is not a name, which is not a pure nominal unity, and unceasingly dislocates itself in a chain of differing and deferring substitutions.
> (p. 26)

10 This emphasis on description may seem to move post-structuralism closer to positivism. Such proximity, if it exists, would be limited at best. The premise underlying post structuralism is that our representations of the world (signifiers) cannot, by their very nature, achieve some kind of uniquely faithful relationship to the things that describe (signifieds). Given this assumption, the post-positivist ideal of assembling knowledge only from discrete falsifiable statements is both naive and nonsensical. Post-structuralists interpret post-positivism, like all epistemologies, as a discursive formation that functions primarily as a mode of social control masquerading as an ideal rationality.

11 These latter formalists approached the interpretation of literature with an eye to the formal qualities of the text alone, whereas the post-structuralists insisted on historicizing the meaning of the text and interpreting it in relation to the broader context of the entire social and cultural moment in which it was produced and read.

References

Adorno, T. (2000). *The Adorno reader* (B. O'Connor, Ed.). Boston, MA: Blackwell.

Anzaldúa, G. (1987). *Borderlands/La Frontera: The new mestiza*. San Francisco, CA: Aunt Lute Books.

Archer, M., Bhaskar, R., Collier, A., Lawson, T., & Norrie, A. (Eds.). (1998). *Critical realism: Essential readings*. New York: Routledge.

Augoustinos, M. (1999). Ideology, false consciousness and psychology. *Theory & Psychology*, *9*(3), 295–312.

Barone, T. (in press). A return to the gold standard? Questioning the future of narrative construction as educational research. *Qualitative Inquiry.*

Basso, K. (1996). *Wisdom sits in places: Landscape and language among the Western Apache.* Albuquerque, NM: University of New Mexico Press.

Belenky, M. F., Bond, L. A., & Weinstock, J. S. (1997). *A tradition that has no name.* New York: Basic Books.

Bergson, H. (1960). *Time and free will: An essay on the immediate data of consciousness* (F. L. Pogson, Trans.). New York: Harper & Brothers. (Original work published 1889)

Bhaskar, R. (1997). *A realist theory of science* (2nd ed.). New York: Verso.

Borland, K. (1991). "That's not what I said": Interpretive conflict in oral narrative research. In S. Gluck & D. Patai (Eds.), *Women's words: The feminist practice of oral history* (pp. 63–75). New York: Routledge.

Chang, P., & Rosiek, J. (2003). Anti-colonial antinomies: A case of cultural conflict in the high school biology curriculum. *Curriculum Inquiry, 33*(3), 251–290.

Charon, R. (2002). Meaning and anticipation: The practice of narrative ethics. In R. Charon & M. Montello (Eds.), *Stories matter: The role of narrative in medical ethics.* London: Routledge.

Charon, R. (2006). *Narrative medicine. Honoring the stories of illness.* Oxford: Oxford University Press.

Clandinin, D. J., & Connelly, F. M. (1995). *Teachers' professional knowledge landscapes.* New York: Teachers College Press.

Clandinin, D. J., & Connelly, F. M. (2000). *Narrative inquiry: Experience and story in qualitative research.* San Francisco, CA: Jossey-Bass.

Connelly, F. M., & Clandinin, D. J. (1990). Stories of experience and narrative inquiry. *Educational Researcher, 19*(5), 2–14.

Connelly, F. M., & Clandinin, D. J. (2006). Narrative inquiry. In J. Green, G. Camilli, & P. Elmore (Eds.), *Handbook of complementary methods in education research* (pp. 375–385). Mahwah, NJ: Lawrence Erlbaum.

de Lauretis, T. (1986). Through the looking glass. In P. Rosen (Ed.), *Narrative, apparatus, ideology: A film theory reader* (pp. 360–372). New York: Columbia University Press.

Delgado, R. (1989). Storytelling for oppositionists and others: A plea for narrative. *Michigan Law Review, 87*(8), 2411–2441.

Derrida, J. (1982). *Margins of philosophy* (A. Bass, Trans.). Chicago, IL: University of Chicago Press. (Original work published 1972).

de Saussure, F. (1959). *Course in general linguistics.* New York: McGraw-Hill.

Dewey, J. (1938). *Experience and education.* New York: Collier Books.

Dewey, J. (1958). *Experience and nature.* New York: Dover.

Dewey, J. (1976). *The middle works, 1899–1924: Vol. 10. Journal articles, essays, and miscellany published in the 1916–1917 period* (J. A. Boydston, Ed.). Carbondale, IL: Southern Illinois University Press.

Dewey, J. (1981a). *The later works, 1925–1953: Vol. 1. Experience and nature* (J. A. Boydston, Ed.). Carbondale, IL: Southern Illinois University Press.

Dewey, J. (1981b). *The later works, 1925–1953: Vol. 4. The quest for certainty: A study of the relation of knowledge and action* (J. A. Boydston, Ed.). Carbondale, IL: Southern Illinois University Press.

Dewey, J. (1981c). *The later works, 1925–1953: Vol. 10. Art as experience* (J. A. Boydston, Ed.). Carbondale, IL: Southern Illinois University Press.

Fine, M. (1987). Silencing in public schools. *Language Arts, 64*(2), 157–174.

Fine, M., & Weis, L. (2003). *Silenced voices and extraordinary conversations: Reimagining schools.* New York: Teachers College Press.

Foucault, M. (1977). *Discipline and punishment: The birth of the prison* (A. Sheridan, Trans.). New York: Pantheon.
Foucault, M. (1982). *The archaeology of knowledge*. London: Routledge.
Hadden, J. (2000). A charter to educate or a mandate to train: Conflicts in theory and practice. *Harvard Educational Review, 70*(4), 524–536.
Hawkes, D. (2003). *Ideology (the new critical idiom)*. New York: Routledge.
Henry, F., & Tator, C. (2005). *The colour of democracy: Racism in Canadian society*. Toronto, Ontario, Canada: Nelson Thomson.
Hook, S. (1987). *Paradoxes of freedom*. Amherst, NY: Prometheus Books.
Horkheimer, M. (2005). *Eclipse of reason*. New York: Continuum International.
Huber, J., & Keats Whelan, K. (in press). Entangled lives: Enacting transient social identities. In S. Kouritzin, N. Piquemal, & R. Norman (Eds.), *Qualitative research: Challenging the orthodoxies*. Mahwah, NJ: Lawrence Erlbaum.
Hurwitz, B., Greenhalgh, T., & Skultans, V. (2004). *Narrative research in health and illness*. Oxford: Blackwell.
James, W. (1897). *The will to believe: And other essays in popular philosophy*. New York: Longmans, Green.
James, W. (1909). *The meaning of truth*. New York: Longmans, Green.
Jameson, F. (1992). *Postmodernism, or, the cultural logic of late capitalism*. Durham, NC: Duke University Press.
Johnson, M. (1987). *The body in the mind: The bodily basis of meaning, imagination and reason*. Chicago, IL: University of Chicago Press.
Josselson, R. (1993). A narrative introduction. In R. Josselson & A. Lieblich (Eds.), *The narrative study of lives* (pp. ix–xv). Newbury Park, CA: Sage.
Kanpol, B. (1997). Reflective critical inquiry on critical inquiry: A critical ethnographic dilemma continued. *Qualitative Report, 3*(4). Retrieved July 27, 2006, from www.nova.edu/ssss/QR/QR3–4/kanpol.html
Kennedy, M. (2001). *Race matters in the life/work of four, white female teachers*. Unpublished doctoral dissertation. University of Alberta, Edmonton, Canada.
King, T. (2003). *The truth about stories*. Toronto, Ontario, Canada: House of Anansi Press.
Laclau, E., & Mouffe, C. (1987). Post-Marxism without apologies. *New Left Review, 66*, 77–106.
Lather, Patti. (1991). *Getting smart: Feminist research and pedagogy with/in the postmodern*. New York: Routledge.
Laubscher, L., & Powell, S. (2003). Skinning the drum: Teaching about diversity as "other." *Harvard Educational Review, 73*(2), 203–222.
Lieblich, A. (1995). *Seasons of captivity: The inner world of POWS*. New York: State University of New York Press.
Lieblich, A., Tuval-Mashiach, R., & Zilber, T. (1998). *Narrative research: Reading, analysis and interpretation*. Thousand Oaks, CA: Sage.
Lugones, M. (1992). On borderlands/La Frontera: An interpretive essay. *Hypatia*, 7(4), 31–37.
Lukacs, G. (1972). *History and class consciousness*. Boston, MA: MIT Press.
Lyotard, F. (1984). *The postmodern condition: A report on knowledge* (G. Bennington & B. Massumi, Trans.). Minneapolis, MN: University of Minnesota Press.
Maher, F., & Ward, J. (2002). Sexism in the classroom. In F. Maher & J. Ward (Eds.), *Gender and teaching* (pp. 1–18). Mahwah, NJ: Lawrence Erlbaum.
Marcuse, H. (1964). *One-dimensional man*. Boston, MA: Beacon.
Marmon Silko, L. (1997). *Yellow woman and a beauty of the spirit*. New York: Touchstone.
Marx, K. (1964). *Selected writings in sociology and social philosophy* (T. B. Bottomore, Trans.). London: McGraw-Hill.

Marx, K. (1972). *The German ideology*. In R. C. Tucker (Ed.), *The Marx-Engels reader* (pp. 110–166). New York: W. W. Norton. (Original work published 1846)

McAdams, D. P. (1996). *The stories we live by*. New York: Guilford Press.

Merleau-Ponty, M. (1962). *Phenomenology of perception* (C. Smith, Trans.). London: Routledge & Kegan Paul.

Mishler, E. (2000). *Storylines: Craft artists' narratives of identity*. Harvard, MA: Harvard University Press.

Norris, C. (1999, Autumn). Bhaskar interview. *Philosophers' Magazine*, p. 34.

Peirce, C. S. (1991). *Peirce on signs: Writings on semiotic* (J. Hooper, Ed.). Chapel Hill, NC: University of North Carolina Press.

Phillips, D., & Burbules, N. (2000). *Postpositivism and educational research*. Lanham, MD: Rowman & Littlefield.

Piles, S., & Thrift, N. J. (1995). *Mapping the subject: Geographies of cultural transformation*. London: Routledge.

Polkinghorne, D. E. (1988). *Narrative knowing and the human sciences*. Albany, NY: State University of New York Press.

Rosiek, J. (2005). Toward teacher education that takes the study of culture as foundational: Building bridges between teacher knowledge research and educational ethnography. In G. Spindler (Ed.), *New horizons in the ethnography of education*. Mahwah, NJ: Lawrence Erlbaum.

Rosiek J., & Atkinson, B. (2005). Bridging the divides: The need for a pragmatic semiotics of teacher knowledge research. *Educational Theory*, *55*(4), 231–266.

Schutz, A. (with Luckman, T.). (1973). *The structures of the life-world* (R. Zaner & H. T. Engelhardt Jr., Trans.). Evanston, IL: Northwestern University.

Sconiers, Z. D., & Rosiek, J. L. (2000). Historical perspective as an important element of teachers' knowledge: A sonata-form case study of equity issues in a chemistry classroom. *Harvard Educational Review*, *70*(3), 370–404.

Soreide, G. (in press). Narrative construction of teacher identity: Positioning and negotiation. *Teachers and Teaching: Theory and Practice*, *12*(5).

Sorrell, K. (2004). *Representative practices: Peirce, pragmatism and feminist epistemology*. New York: Fordham University Press.

Spanbauer, T. (1992). *The man who fell in love with the moon*. New York: Grove Press.

Stone-Mediatore, S. (2003). *Reading across borders: Storytelling and knowledges of resistance*. New York: Palgrave Macmillan.

Sullivan, S. (2001). *Living across and through skins: Transactional bodies, pragmatism, and feminism*. Bloomington: Indiana University Press.

Sullivan, S. (2006). *Revealing whiteness: The unconscious habits of racial privilege*. Bloomington, IN: Indiana University Press.

Vaz, K. (Ed.). (1997). *Oral narrative research with black women*. Thousand Oaks, CA: Sage.

West, C. (1989). *The American evasion of philosophy: A genealogy of pragmatism*. Madison, WI: University of Wisconsin Press.

West, C. (1993). *Beyond eurocentrism and multiculturalism. Vol. I: Prophetic thought in postmodern times*. Monroe, ME: Common Courage Press.

Wetherell, M. (1999). Beyond binaries. *Theory & Psychology*, *9*(3), 399–406.

Zizek, S. (1999). *The ticklish subject: The absent centre of political ontology*. New York: Verso.

15

A RETURN TO METHODOLOGICAL COMMITMENT

Reflections on narrative inquiry

Vera Caine, Andrew Estefan and D. Jean Clandinin

Introduction

Since the late 1980s/early 1990s, social science researchers have taken a narrative turn in understanding experience (Pinnegar & Daynes, 2007). It was during this time that researchers began to specifically develop a research methodology called narrative inquiry (Connelly & Clandinin, 1990). During the early years of narrative inquiry's development as a research methodology, many important and subtle distinctions were highlighted that shaped differences between narrative research and narrative inquiry. However, in the years since then, narrative inquiry and narrative research have become terms that are frequently used almost interchangeably in the research literature, without a distinction of the different ontological and epistemological traditions underlying narrative research approaches. Riessman and Speedy (2007) point out that "narrative inquiry in the human sciences is a 20th century development; the field has 'realist', 'postmodern', and constructionist strands, and scholars and practitioners disagree on origin and precise definition" (p. 429). It is thus not always clear, when the term narrative inquiry is used, what ontological and epistemological stances are at play. This diversity in the ways in which what is called narrative inquiry is taken up both enriches and concerns those of us engaged in narrative inquiry Without a clear sense of the epistemological and ontological commitments for those of us working in the field, much is blurred and much becomes tension-filled.

What is apparent in the development of narrative inquiry, however, is how interwoven narrative ways of thinking about phenomena are with narrative inquiry as research methodology. It is "the interweaving of narrative views of phenomena and narrative inquiry that marks the emerging field and that draws attention to the need for careful uses and distinctions of terms" (Clandinin & Rosiek, 2007, p. 36). As we argue for greater clarity regarding what counts as narrative inquiry, it is important to see that we are also arguing for an understanding of narrative inquiry beyond a research methodology. It is also an argument for a narrative view of experience.

Reprinted with permission. Acknowledgement; Caine, V., Estefan, A., & Clandinin, D. J. (2013). A return to methodological commitment: Reflections on narrative inquiry. *Scandinavian Journal of Educational Research*, *57*(6), 574–586. doi:10.1080/00313831.2013.798833

This broader argument allows us to understand experience beyond the lens of the researcher; we see experience as lived in the midst, as always unfolding over time, in diverse social contexts and in place, and as co-composed in relation. We also see the pedagogical possibilities and long-term commitment to those we work alongside that come from this interweaving of a narrative view of experience with narrative inquiry as methodology.

As the three authors of this paper engaged in our various research projects, we listened to and read studies that described the use of stories and narratives as part of what is named narrative inquiry. We heard people talk about telling good stories, representing research findings as stories, or using stories to tell – in more compelling ways – of problems, encounters, or observations. These uses of story and narrative appear to have been co-opted under the label "narrative inquiry," and we are troubled by this co-optation. In these moments, we return to our understandings of narrative inquiry and see the importance of making our ontological and epistemological commitments visible. We understand narrative inquiry as both phenomenon and methodology (Clandinin & Connelly, 2000) and this forms the basis for ways we know how to be, and live, as researchers and as people in relations.

In what follows, we consider the methodological commitments of narrative inquiry in an attempt to highlight distinctions and to more clearly frame the ontological commitments we hold as narrative inquirers. As we do this, we distinguish our commitments from research practices that use stories as data; view narrative and story as representational form, as content analysis, and as structure; or treat stories as the phenomena under study. We try to make evident how and why narrative inquiry is different from forms of narrative analysis used within other qualitative research methodologies, such as thematic analysis, linguistic analysis, structural analysis and, more recently, visual analysis. Stories or narratives are also used as data in other qualitative methodologies, such as phenomenology, ethnography and case study. Narrative or story forms of representation are also used as ways of representing results or findings in various qualitative and quantitative methodologies and are increasingly seen as an effective approach to knowledge translation and knowledge mobilization. By showing our methodological commitments, which shape and are shaped by ontological commitments, we hope the differences between narrative inquiry and these other uses of narrative in research will become evident.

First and foremost, narrative inquirers begin with an interest in experience (Clandinin & Connelly, 2000). A narrative inquiry, therefore, proceeds from an ontological position, a curiosity about how people are living and the constituents of their experience. Narrative inquiry does not proceed from a realist, constructionist, or postmodern position; instead, how we seek to understand and evoke experience arises from within the inquiry (Clandinin & Rosiek, 2007). We understand the inquiry as a negotiated research practice. As much as narrative inquiry arises from puzzles around people's experience, thinking or inquiring narratively involves an ontological commitment. A narrative ontology precedes the emergence of research puzzles and calls forth obligations and commitments. A narrative ontology implies that experiences are continuously interactive, resulting in changes in both people and the contexts in which they interact (Dewey, 1938, 1981). It is through this experience that people's lives are composed and re-composed in relation with others who are also living storied lives. It is through story that people are able to understand, make meaning of, and relate experiences, because story is how people make sense of their existence (Clandinin, Huber, & Murphy, 2011). A narrative ontology thus calls upon researchers to enter into what Dewey (1934) termed "ordinary experience," both theirs and their participants' – that is, to enter the practice and artistry of lives lived.

It is in how we live out our research puzzles alongside our participants that our ontological commitment becomes evident in the complexities of entering the field of experiences as they are being lived; as we attend to lived, relived, told, and retold stories of experience; and as we begin to craft our always negotiated research texts. We see this commitment as extending beyond the immediacy of the research puzzle and have come to understand that narrative inquirers hold responsibilities and obligations for, and toward, the people whose stories are lived and told.

The ontological commitment of a narrative inquirer shapes each stage of a narrative inquiry. As we consider our research puzzles we draw upon our own experiences, which orient us to the inquiry. As we negotiate entry into the field our ontological commitment makes possible a relational means of researching, of being able to "work out" what to do in the field, how to work with participants, and decide together what we want to achieve as our inquiry unfolds. This ontological stance underpins a central epistemological commitment of narrative inquirers, that experience is knowledge for living (Dewey, 1938; Clandinin & Connelly, 2000). To engage deeply with experience, an ontological commitment is, then, a relational commitment. It is a commitment to a form of togetherness in research that seeks to explore how we are living in the midst of our stories.

Telling a story: beginning a narrative inquiry in the midst of an inquirer's life

Imagine we told you a story about a young girl leaving her parents' home without money, a map, or a passport and traveling across borders to find herself sleeping underneath bridges alongside the river in the midst of Paris. The young girl finds herself among a gentle crowd. Being chased each night by the police at various and unpredictable hours, sleep becomes impossible, and in these sleepless hours, the young girl befriends Jose. They spend each night sitting on a bench beside the bridge, their bodies leaning into each other, their hands and lips touching on occasions only to reaffirm their presence within a place and space of kindness, unsettledness, ambiguity and brutality.

Beginning to retell the story: from telling to retelling in narrative inquiry

We could depart from the story at the end of the last sentence to discuss substantive issues of at-risk youth, of first experiences of homelessness, of troublesome stories of police, of state authority, and of marginalization; or we could tell stories of friendship. We could tell a story that seems to start with leaving and, perhaps, foreshadows leaving as well. Yet as narrative inquirers, we cannot so easily depart at the last sentence. It is hard to see the definitive beginning or end of the experiences about the young girl and Jose, their social contexts, their lives across time, and the places in which they live and eventually meet. We cannot so easily depart if we want to understand experiences in the past, present, and future. Wonders continue to emerge and we attend to them as narrative inquirers, as people.

Narrative inquiry, defined as both research methodology and a view of phenomena, is the intimate study of an individual's experience over time and in context(s) (Clandinin & Connelly, 1994, 2000). John Dewey's (1938, 1958) view of experience is cited most often as the philosophical underpinning of narrative inquiry (Clandinin & Rosiek, 2007). Dewey's criteria of experience, interaction, and continuity enacted in situations provide the grounding for the attention paid in the three-dimensional narrative inquiry space to temporality, place, and sociality (Clandinin & Connelly, 2000).

From a narrative view of experience, we attend to place, temporality, and sociality within our own life stories and within the experiences of participants. Within this space, each story told and lived is situated and understood within larger cultural, social, familial, and institutional narratives. Narrative inquiry is marked by its emphasis on relational engagement, whereby the understanding and social significance of experience grows out of a relational commitment to a research puzzle. For these reasons it is important that narrative inquirers carefully consider who they are, and who they are becoming, in the research puzzle. The researcher's presence and investment is an important feature of narrative inquiry research. In studying and understanding experience narratively, researchers recognize the centrality of relationships. Amidst these relationships, participants relate and live through stories that speak of their experience (Crites, 1971).

The young girl in the story is Vera. Alongside colleagues and friends, Vera returns to her early childhood experiences often. Sliding backward in time and over places, she attends to the sociality dimensions of narrative inquiry. Her felt experiences, her emotions, her aesthetic responses to the social events in which she found herself so long ago and again now become evident. In this way she begins to retell, to inquire into her experiences of those long-ago times that are called forward.

Embedded in the retellings of these early experiences is a notion that each story is always partial and contextual and offers new possibilities as the stories are retold. For Vera these early landscapes shape her research puzzles and how she thinks and lives as a narrative inquirer, as she wonders about home, belonging, bodies, contradictions, and uncertainties. Richardson (1997) deepens our understanding as she describes how a

> story of a life is less than the actual life, because the story told is selective, partial, contextually constructed and because the life is not yet over. But the story of a life is also more than the life, the contours and meanings allegorically extending others, others seeing themselves, knowing themselves through another's life story, re-visioning their own, arriving where they started and knowing "the place for the first time."
>
> *(p. 6)*

Richardson also reminds us of Clandinin and Connelly's (2000) understanding of the difference between the telling and living out of stories. In the living out of her stories Vera sees that her earlier story fragment alludes to the deeper conditions of human life, but that the story told is not a fixed text; it is composed in, and out of, the living. As narrative inquirers, we stay as close to people's experiences as we can.

In retelling her early experiences, Vera also recognizes that her and Jose's experiences allowed for silent and unspeakable stories, stories that can possibly be traced on people's skin, and stories that are visible but also hidden (Prosser, 2007). As Vera recalls the shape of Jose's body, the colour of his skin and eyes, she notices how fragmented her memory has become and how much has been left unsaid. It is through the questions Jean asks, and the places which Vera returns to alongside Jose, that new retellings become possible. Jean's commitment to understanding her experiences over time allows new puzzles to emerge, while also honoring that some of the experiences will never be told. As narrative inquirers we understand that people also live their stories in "what they do not say. They live them in attending to the words of others rather than their own words" (Neumann, 1997, p. 107). Reflecting on Neumann's words, we also attend to ethical obligations in our relationships, and stay mindful that our words might call forth or shift attention in new and unsettling ways.

In the retelling, we contemplate our vulnerabilities and uncertainties and are reminded again that narrative inquiry is first and foremost a relational research methodology, and, while it is research, it is also a transaction between people, which makes ethical issues and concerns about living well with others central to the inquiry (Clandinin & Connelly, 2000). We are reminded of Clandinin and Rosiek's (2007) discussion of Dewey's notion of ontology as transactional. Within this pragmatic view, "our representations arise from experience and must return to that experience for their validation" (p. 39). This is a reminder that while we contemplate experience, we attend to participants and those we come to know in the telling and living of experience.

Telling another story: beginning again in the midst

I was born into the story of the adopted child, unwanted and given away to somebody else. I grew into stories of the boy who grew up knowing he was different: the fat kid, the kid who knew he liked the other boys and not the girls, and who walked home from school with either my own blood or other people's spit on my face and school shirt. There are still times, even recently, when I am forced to return to these stories, because they are still being lived by others in contexts and times that I left behind long ago. But even though I am not there, fragments of this story have traveled with me across continents, through time, serving as a constant reminder that we are our stories, and our stories are what we need to learn, to live, and to live well. Today, I live and see the world and my work through a lens that compels questions about how our stories shape us, and our relationship with the world in which we live. It is in these moments that I *cannot not* be a narrative inquirer. I talk back and forth with many lived and told stories; this back-and-forth talk allows me to begin to retell and relive my experience.

Beginning to retell the story

In a narrative inquiry, stories are not just a medium of learning, development, or transformation, but also a life. As Andrew tells and writes the above story, we begin to see how strongly our early childhood experiences shape us and how important it is to see them in the context of Andrew's life now. They are not fixed stories. They open up new wonders about composing a life in the midst – in the midst of Andrew's life, his parents' lives, and his life yet to be lived. In narrative inquiry it is inquiry into the experiences that compose a life, a dwelling within the three-dimensional narrative inquiry space composed of place, temporality, and sociality, (Clandinin & Connelly, 2000) that are foregrounded. Gunn Allen (1998) speaks of a journey of life:

> my life, like my work, is a journey-in-between, a road. [. . .] We live on the road that the dead walk down. We ride it out of town and back. By its meanders we discover what is there, what is not. By its power we are drawn into a confluence of minds, of beings, of perceptions, of styles.
>
> (*p. 191*)

The notions of journey, movement, and continuity speak to Carr's (1986) term of narrative coherence – we seek narrative coherence in the "telling and retelling, to ourselves and to others, the story about what we are about and what we are" (p. 97). We do not see narrative coherence as the orderly linking together of experiences into a neat chronological frame. Instead, it arises from sitting with stories, with each other, as we seek to compose ourselves in relation. Perhaps Andrew's and Vera's told story fragments speak to their search for narrative coherence on what seems like a road they have walked back and forth, a journey they now take as colleagues.

Narrative coherence is one of the ways to open up how we think about methodological commitment. As researchers we become part of participants' lives and are often drawn in to participants' ways of seeking narrative coherence. This way of researching is different to the practice of interrogating a research text such as a transcript – reaching into it as if it were life – and extracting "the story" that foregrounds experience and voice. Riessman (2008) reminds us that "stories do not fall from the sky" (p. 105). Nor can they simply be plucked from a research transcript. Narrative inquirers understand data as field texts that are to be experienced as they are lived and told as narrative compositions. Living *is* field text, and field texts are co-compositions of lives (Clandinin, Huber, & Murphy, 2011) lived in rich narrative contexts. Insofar as being able to describe, evoke, and represent experience, then, for narrative inquirers a transcript alone simply will not do. As Andrews (2007) reminds us:

> Stories are not only the way in which we come to ascribe significance to experiences . . . but they are one of the primary means through which we constitute our very selves . . . we become who we are through telling stories about our lives and living the stories we tell.
>
> *(pp. 77–78)*

As Andrew begins to retell his story he attends to the unfolding and enfolding of time, of moving from and to places, and to his inner responses to the events he experienced in different places. In the inquiry, the intergenerational as well as social, cultural, familial, and institutional narratives begin to emerge and draw forth our ontological commitment. Andrew's story reminds us that we are always in the midst.

The relational and ethical as shaping the ontological commitments of narrative inquirers

The first responsibility of narrative inquirers is always to participants. The negotiations of entry and exit, as well as the representation of experience, are central ethical concerns. These responsibilities are not simply considerations of method or what to do when researching with participants. Embedded within the practices of entry, exit, and representation is a relational knowing (Hollingsworth, Dybdahl, & Minarik, 1993) – a recognition that an embodied response is drawn forth within each relationship and within our memory and imagination (Bruner, 2002; Sarbin, 1998, 2004). In this way, we have come to understand that our thinking as narrative inquirers grows out of being-in-relation. This thinking, our sensitivity to a relational orientation, is a methodological consideration that organizes what it is that counts as knowledge, as inquiry, and as knowledge of the practice for narrative inquirers.

Through attending to the relational in-between spaces in narrative inquiry, possibilities arise to discover new ways of knowing and understanding, and also for profound change. We are reminded that "in-between" spaces are spaces where we ask one another "who" and not "what" we are (Arendt, 1958). These in-between spaces are filled with uncertainty and indeterminacy. They are places of liminality; the betwixts and betweens, which, we argue, require attention to context(s), relationship(s), and time to explore narratively. As Lorde (1981) points out, it is in these in-between spaces that we recognize that our necessity for interdependence is not threatening, but rather is the spark for creativity. From experience that arises in the betwixt places, Andrew thinks about his more recent experiences and research interests, and he locates passion, energy, and a commitment to those with whom he engages in research. The intersections of who he was, who he is now, where he wants to go, and with whom, transform the betwixt into the becoming, a narrative coherence that is laden, and that becomes an ontological and ethical commitment to a relational mode of research. This composition of a self in the midst of lives and relationships necessitates a shift in attention from methodological considerations about prescribing how to construct research correctly, to sensitivity to the conditions around which we *become with* each other.

To enter into these relationships often requires the imaginative leap of the skeptical or cautious "as-if" (Greene, 1995) towards imaginary stories. Entering into relationships also requires a "believing-in." Narrative inquiry is about exploring and understanding lived experience and, as we live as narrative inquirers, we also know that our relational responsibilities are first to participants, but also to our relationships with participants and to what is called forth in us. As Vera returns to her experiences alongside Jose she wonders if Jose is still alive, if he too remembers their time together.

Imagination and memory interwoven in ontological and methodological commitments

While imagination can never "take leave of the other" (Kearney, 1988, p. 218), it must continuously search for the spirit of play. Lugones (1987) offers that playfulness "is marked by openness to surprise and self-construction as a way to understand oneself in a relational way, by traveling to each other's worlds, as a place of imagination" (p. 180). Imagination, Kearney (1988) argues, "needs to be able to laugh with the other as well as to suffer" (p. 367). In this laughter and suffering, this play with the other, this narrative inquiry, our imagined relationship is central. It allows us to attend in new ways. As we engage with our own stories and with the stories of participants, we are invited to enter into relationships alongside them. These relationships invite us into more playful ways of being as we world-travel; a relational journey in which we come alongside others and ourselves, in different times, places, and relationships.

It is perhaps the notion of play as a feature of imagination and relationship that helps us arrive at new meanings and understandings of the stories of ourselves, of others, and of the relational spaces where we come together with participants. Our understanding of imagination is shaped by Sarbin's (1998, 2004) definition of imagination as a perceptual and embodied knowing. Imagination influences not only our own life stories and stories to live by (Connelly & Clandinin, 1999), but also how we understand and construct the narrative accounts (Clandinin & Connelly, 2000) of others and of ourselves in relation with others. Our life writing, our stories over time and places and relationships, focus on memory and on the present moment of our experience, on being, as well as our future. Stories to live by are fluid, always shaped by the embodied, temporal notion of becoming, and link knowledge, context, and identity (Connelly & Clandinin, 1999). They are also, as Andrew's story reminds us, shaped by our ability to live with stories – to live with difficult stories that cannot be forgotten. Maybe these are unfitting stories, stories that resist the easy telling, that are awkward and jagged (Raoul, 2007), but unfitting stories are also stories to live by and a relational ontology requires that we do not turn first to the inquiry as a way to make these stories fit. Representation, as the act that arises from our relational ontology, necessitates our living with the unfitting story rather than with attempts to tame, sanitize, or analyze. As narrative inquirers we attend to difficult stories and experiences, we stay with them; we dwell alongside participants in possible ways of retelling them. As Bruner (2002) points out, it is the interplay between memory and imagination that informs and shapes our experiences, our memories of our life stories, and our imagining of stories to live by. Understanding life stories and stories to live by requires an attentiveness and wakefulness within the relationships we enter as narrative inquirers.

Moving from retelling to reliving

Some of the early writing for this paper was done in preparation for a conference presentation in Paris. Vera knew her return to Paris would open up new retellings of her story alongside Jose, and would lead her to other stories of meeting with Jose in different times and places. While she first met Jose in Paris, she last saw him in Amsterdam with his girlfriend Veronica. Veronica was dying of AIDS and the complications of long-term substance use at the time – her own body and Jose's silent stories of his relationship with Veronica remind Vera of her own fragility and nested stories. It is in this last physical encounter with Jose that Vera begins to feel her body's gait shifting to a new rhythm, one shaped by these early stories and by stories that seek ways of understanding experience from a place of relationships. The experiences wrote a new story into her body, one that Vera recognized only many years later. It is the experience of her shifting pattern of walking that we now see as a methodological happening. Often our understanding as narrative inquirers does not come instantaneously, or quickly, or by engaging in clever analysis. Instead our understanding deepens as we retell and relive our lived stories over time, place, and social contexts.

As we inquire into Vera's stories, we enlarge our meaning of place as carrying an "emotional sense of belonging, discursive spaces, imaginative and virtual landscapes, as well as political divisions and cultural distributions" (Fenwick, 2005, n.p.). Expanding on the concept of belonging, May (2001) explores being at home, belonging, as "an in-between state of being within and without our selves. [. . .]. 'Being at home' in this sense is a state of forgetting ourselves in living our relationality" (p. 228). Honoring this living of our relationality is key to narrative inquiry. In these moments we know that not only does our life matter, but so also do the lives of others, and that the stories we each tell, once told to each other, are important moments through which we interconnect. These stories speak of and about our experiences, and of and about our relationships with others. These retellings allow us as narrative inquirers to move forward and backward, inward and outward, and keep our knowing always located in place(s).

Beginning and ending narrative inquiries in the relational midst

Attending to the whole of human life and to life in relational spaces is marked by ambiguity, messiness, and beauty (Freeman, 2007). Connecting our life as researchers and our everyday experiences to those of others, and to new places on the landscapes, can challenge our understandings and perceptions. "In the hearing of others' stories [. . .] we can metaphorically lay our stories alongside another's, seeking resonances and reverberations that help us imagine who we might become" (Clandinin & Raymond, 2006, p. 103). While Jose, like research participants, was only temporarily physically present in our lives, it is Sarris (1997) who helps us see that there is never a way to tell a final story:

> [S]tories are inner things: you're interacting with a living story. The way western man is taught to read is to find meaning, the symbols. Instead I say no, a story is not something you figure out the meaning of but something you carry with you the rest of your life to talk back and forth with.
>
> *(Sarris, p. 229)*

Although Dewey is most often invoked in narrative inquiry to provide a philosophical underpinning for conceptualizing experience, he also offered other ideas that speak to the artistry or craft of a narrative inquiry that does not attempt to offer a final story. Dewey suggested that our senses are complicit in the uptake and interpretation of meaning. Although senses are physical and physiological mechanisms, they are activated and used in relation with place, time, and people. We listen casually, with purpose, and with pre-understandings that arise from earlier experiences. Ears are not simply passive recipients of a story, but rather tools that filter, add to, and refract stories in different ways (Dewey, 1934). Although we illustrate this idea with reference to one sense, hearing, it does not require a large leap of imagination to think about how engagement of the senses in a relational research context grounds inquiry in an embodied, connected process that works to develop an understanding of experience. Put differently, in the context of a narrative inquiry, the production of research texts follows the art of engagement in a storied research relationship that is never final, and could always be otherwise. It is the artistry of relationship that allows for understanding and acts of representation to follow, the purpose of which is not, as Dewey (1934) reminded us, to emphasize forms of high art or the exemplar of experience, but rather to experience and show the wonder of a life lived on a richly storied landscape.

By being narrative inquirers we have come to see understanding from an intimate place of experiences. Experience in our world is grounded in a relational in-between space where we attend to the multiple dimensions of looking backward and forward, inward and outward, and pay attention to places simultaneously as spaces of being, becoming, and possibility. This sense of the possibility of becoming otherwise (Greene, 1995) can be seen in the way described by Basso (1996, p. 59): "That story is working on you now. You keep thinking about it. That story is changing you now, making you want to live right."

Stories are ubiquitous and ancient (Clandinin, 2006). Stories as they are lived, told, retold, and relived circulate in and fill spaces between people. They offer us insights into experiences and resonate in ways that help us to learn and form connections with others. A relational and transactional ontology precedes narrative inquiry research, because stories are about what happens to and between people. That we are living stories means that the connection between researcher and participant begins long before formal research contact. One might say that Andrew has been in a relationship of sorts with research participants since he was about ten years old. This context, while not yet a "relationship," holds, incubates, and clarifies or even extends the puzzles and research interests of the narrative inquirer. The construction of a relational space is not an accidental result of mulling over the plans for a research proposal or an ethics submission. These relational considerations are, by contrast, the fundament of a narrative inquiry. Creating spaces that allow us to tell stories of self are one of the ways that we foster development of identity for researcher and participants (Clandinin & Cave, 2008). This cannot be achieved by treating stories as reductionist artifacts of a research process.

Vera last saw Jose 25 years ago. Those early childhood experiences have stayed with her in so many ways and shaped who she is today; a reminder that the story is always still working on us. As we look backwards, forwards, and sideways, in this paper we see that as narrative inquirers we resist telling the good story, the story with beginnings and endings, with resolutions, and with illustrative powers (Downey & Clandinin, 2010). Life as it is lived is not neat, tidy, or formulaic. Nor does it easily fit within the confines and conventions of the good story. As such, we resist the good story because it does not reflect our ontological and epistemological positions as narrative inquirers. Instead, being-in-relation guides our work and the stories of experiences that arise from it.

Coming to what our ontological commitments mean for us as narrative inquirers

Those of us who are engaged in understanding our commitments in, and to, narrative inquiry need to stand back and carefully consider our commitments as we dance along in Geertz's (1995) metaphoric parade. We need to start a conversation among those of us who name narrative inquiry as our methodology and our phenomena, so that we do not continue to talk past each other. We must insist we name our ontological commitment from the outset.

At the outset of this article, we drew attention to the multiplicity of methods labeled narrative inquiry. In some of what is called narrative inquiry, narratives and stories are data collected by researchers. People tell their stories to researchers. The stories and narratives are the study data. There is usually an assumption that the stories are waiting to be told and, when asked, people will tell their stories usually according to the western tradition of a beginning, middle, and end, with a plot line, characters, and resolution. Sometimes these stories and narratives follow other cultural formats, but the underlying assumptions are the same. In other work named narrative inquiry, all oral texts are considered as stories or narratives. In other work named narrative inquiry, more careful attention is paid to the larger and smaller contexts in which stories are told. There is attention to the larger sociopolitical narratives in the context as well as to the trust and relationship between researcher and participant. In all of this, however, narratives or stories are the object of analysis.

When one moves from story or narrative (as data) to analysis, there are multiple forms of narrative analysis. Texts are created from the told stories and these texts can be analyzed using different analytic frames (Josselson, Lieblich, & McAdams, 2003; Riessman, 1990; Chase, 2005).

Sometimes research is named narrative inquiry when the research texts are composed as narratives. As so many people say in considerations of representation, they want to tell a story. Audiences listen to stories and learn from stories. We hear comments such as "the audience will remember the stories." Narrative is seen as one of a number of possible representational forms, but it seems to be becoming an increasingly popular one, particularly when researchers are speaking to the public or media.

We see our understanding of narrative inquiry differently. Narrative inquiry is both the phenomenon under study and the methodology for its study. Narrative inquiry is how we understand human experience. It carries with it a view of the phenomenon of experience. We live storied lives in storied landscapes (Connelly & Clandinin, 1999). As Marmon Silko (1996) reminds us, we are in landscapes, part of the landscapes, not objective viewers of the landscape. Narrative inquiry works from the understanding that who we are – our stories to live by – are fundamentally narrative in nature (Clandinin & Connelly, 2000). The narrative nature of experience, viewed from within narrative inquiry, necessitates considerations of relational being and knowing, attention to the artistry of and within experience, and sensitivity to the nested and overlapping stories that bring people together in research relationships. Within this view of narrative inquiry we need to attend closely and make explicit our ontological and epistemological assumptions. As we consider questions of methodological and ontological commitment, we need to continue conversations about what the field should attend to in narrative inquiry in order to deepen important methodological considerations.

References

Andrews, M. (2007). Exploring cross-cultural boundaries. In D. J. Clandinin (Ed.), *Handbook of narrative inquiry: Mapping a methodology* (pp. 489–511). Thousand Oaks, CA: Sage Publications.

Arendt, H. (1958). *The human condition*. Chicago, IL: University of Chicago Press.

Basso, K. (1996). *Wisdom sits in places: Landscape and language among the western Apache*. Albuquerque, NM: University of New Mexico Press.

Bruner, J. (2002). *Making stories: Law, literature, life*. Cambridge, MA: Harvard University Press.

Carr, D. (1986). *Time, narrative, and history*. Bloomington, IN: Indiana University Press.

Chase, S. E. (2005). Narrative inquiry: multiple lenses, approaches, voices. In N. K. Denzin & Y. S. Lincoln (Eds.), *The SAGE handbook of qualitative research* (3rd ed., pp. 651–680). Thousand Oaks, CA: Sage Publications.

Clandinin, D. J. (2006). Narrative inquiry: A methodology for studying lived experience. *Research Studies in Music Education, 27*, 44–54.

Clandinin, D. J., & Cave, M. (2008). Creating pedagogical spaces for developing doctor professional identity. *Medical Education, 42*(8), 765–770.

Clandinin, D. J., & Connelly, F. M. (1994). Personal experience methods. In N. K. Denzin & Y. S. Lincoln (Eds.), *The SAGE handbook of qualitative research* (pp. 413–427). Thousand Oaks, CA: Sage Publications.

Clandinin, D. J., & Connelly, F. M. (2000). *Narrative inquiry: Experience and story in qualitative research*. San Francisco, CA: Jossey-Bass Publishers.

Clandinin, D. J., Huber, J., & Murphy, M. S. (2011). Familial curriculum making: Re-shaping the curriculum making of teacher education. *International Journal of Early Childhood Education, 17*(1), 9–31.

Clandinin, D. J., & Raymond, H. (2006). Note on narrating disability. *Equity and Excellence in Education, 39*(2), 101–104.

Clandinin, D. J., & Rosiek, J. (2007). Mapping a landscape of narrative inquiry: Borderland spaces and tensions. In D. J. Clandinin (Ed.), *Handbook of narrative inquiry: Mapping a methodology* (pp. 35–75). Thousand Oaks, CA: Sage Publications.

Connelly, F. M., & Clandinin, D. J. (1990). Stories of experience and narrative inquiry. *Educational Researcher, 19*(5), 2–14.

Connelly, F. M., & Clandinin, D. J. (1999). *Shaping a professional identity: Stories of educational practice*. New York: Teachers College Press.

Crites, S. (1971). The narrative quality of experience. *Journal of the American Academy of Religion, 39*(3), 291–311.

Dewey, J. (1934). *Art as experience*. New York: Berkley Publishing Group.

Dewey, J. (1938). *Experience and education*. New York: Collier Books.

Dewey, J. (1958). *Experience and nature*. New York: Dover.

Dewey J. (1981). *The later works, 1925–1953: Volume 10. Art as experience* (J. A. Boyston Ed.). Carbondale, IL: Southern Illinois University Press.

Downey, C. A., & Clandinin, D. J. (2010). Narrative inquiry as reflective practice: Tensions and possibilities. In N. Lyons (Ed.), *Handbook of reflection and reflective inquiry: Mapping a way of knowing for professional reflective practice* (pp. 383–397). Dordrecht, Netherlands: Springer.

Fenwick, T. (2005). *Tidying the territory: Clarifying our terms and purposes of integrated learning and work*. Paper presented at the International Conference on Work and Lifelong Learning, Toronto, ON.

Freeman, M. (2007). Autobiographical understanding and narrative inquiry. In D. J. Clandinin (Ed.), *Handbook of narrative inquiry: Mapping a methodology* (pp. 120–145). Thousand Oaks, CA: Sage Publications.

Geertz, C. (1995). *After the fact: Two countries, four decades, one anthropologist*. Cambridge, MA: Harvard University Press.

Greene, M. (1995). *Releasing the imagination: Essays on education, the arts, and social change*. San Francisco, CA: Jossey-Bass Publishers.

Gunn Allen, P. (1998). *Off the reservations: Reflections on boundary-busting, border-crossing loose cannons*. Boston, MA: Beacon Press.

Hollingsworth, S., Dybdahl, M., & Minarik, L. (1993). By chart and chance and passion: Learning to teach through relational knowing. *Curriculum Inquiry, 23*(1), 5–36.

Josselson, R., Lieblich, A., & McAdams, D. P. (Eds.). (2003). *Up close and personal: The teaching and learning of narrative research*. Washington, DC: American Psychological Association.

Kearney, R. (1988). *The wake of imagination*. Minneapolis, MN: University of Minnesota Press.

Lorde, A. (1981). The master's tools will never dismantle the master's house. In C. Moraga & G. Anzaldua (Eds.), *This bridge called my back: Writings by radical women of color* (pp. 98–101). Watertown, MA: Persephone Press.

Lugones, M. (1987). Playfulness, "world"-travelling, and loving perception. *Hypatia, 2*(2), 3–19.

Marmon Silko, L. (1996). *Yellow woman and a beauty of spirit: Essays on Native American life today*. New York: Touchstone Books.

May, J. (Ed.). (2001). *Time space: Geographies of temporality*. London: Routledge.

Neumann, A. (1997). Ways without words: Learning from silence and story in post Holocaust lives. In A. Neumann & P. L. Peterson (Eds.), *Learning from our lives: Women, research, and autobiography in education* (pp. 91–120). New York: Teachers College.

Pinnegar, S., & Daynes, J. G. (2007). Locating narrative inquiry historically: Thematics in the turn to narrative. In D. J. Clandinin (Ed.), *Handbook of narrative inquiry: Mapping a methodology* (pp. 3–34). Thousand Oaks, CA: Sage Publications.

Prosser, J. (2007). Visual methods and the visual culture of schools. *Visual Studies, 22*(1), 13–30.

Raoul, C. (2007). Postscript: Unfitting stories, undisciplined research. In C. Raoul, A. Henderson, & C. Paterson (Eds.), *Unfitting stories: Narrative approaches to disease, disability and trauma* (pp. 297–305). Waterloo, ON: Wilfred Laurier University Press.

Riessman, C. K. (1990). *Divorce talk: Women and men make sense of personal relationships*. New Brunswick, NJ: Rutgers University Press.

Riessman, C. K. (2008). *Narrative methods for the human sciences*. Thousand Oaks, CA: Sage.

Riessman, C. K., & Speedy, J. (2007). Narrative inquiry in the psychotherapy professions. In D. J. Clandinin (Ed.), *Handbook of narrative inquiry: Mapping a methodology* (p. 426–456). London: Sage.

Richardson, L. (1997). *Fields of play: Constructing an academic life*. New Brunswick, NJ: Rutgers University Press.

Sarbin, T. R. (1998). Believed-in imaginings. In J. DeRivera & T. Sarbin (Eds.), *Believed-in imaginings: The narrative construction of reality* (pp. 15–30). Washington, DC: American Psychological Association.

Sarbin, T. R. (2004). The role of imagination in narrative construction. In C. Daiute & C. Lightfoot (Eds.), *Narrative analysis: Studying the development of individuals in society* (pp. 5–20). Thousand Oaks, CA: Sage Publications.

Sarris, G. (1997). The truth will rise. In L. Crozier-Hogle & B. Wilson (Eds.), *Surviving in two worlds: Contemporary Native American voices* (pp. 225–234). Austin, TX: University of Texas Press.

16

REVERBERATIONS OF NARRATIVE INQUIRY

How resonant echoes of an inquiry with early school leavers shaped further inquiries

D. Jean Clandinin, Sean Lessard and Vera Caine

Introduction

In this paper we draw on two studies, one study (Clandinin et al., 2010) that is finished and a second (Caine et al., 2010) that grew out of this first finished project. These two projects have been undertaken with two different, but overlapping, groups of researchers: the first included Pam Steeves, Yi Li, Joy Ruth Mickelson, George Buck, Marni Pearce, Vera Caine, Sean Lessard, Claire Desrochers, Marion Stewart, Marilyn Huber, and Jean Clandinin; the second included three members of the previous group, Sean Lessard, Vera Caine, and Jean Clandinin and added Simmee Chung, Trudy Cardinal, Shauna Bruno, Florence Glanfield, and Dwayne Donald. The researchers in both studies work within the Centre for Research for Teacher Education and Development, a research space in which collaborative research is valued. Our purpose in this paper is not to report the results of either study but to show how the work in one study shaped our work in the design and living out of a subsequent project.

Our scholarly and personal interests intertwine in both of these projects as we understand lives narratively, as unfolding, enfolding, nested compositions (Clandinin & Connelly, 2000; Clandinin et al., 2006). Following Dewey's (1938) ideas on education as experience, we work with others to attend to lives in the making, lives in motion. For the most part, Clandinin has come alongside teachers, student teachers, children, parents and others as their lives met in schools and, while she may have spent time with them in places such as homes and other social places, they began their inquiries together in schools. By this we draw attention to how schools were the common ground of meeting and to how they moved in and out of schools, telling, in their words, actions, and bodies, stories of their knowing and of their identities (Clandinin & Connelly, 1995; Clandinin & Connelly, 1996). Caine's studies have been alongside young women as they composed their lives outside of schools (Caine, 2010a), as well as alongside a teacher and students in a classroom (Caine, 2010b).

Reprinted with permission. Acknowledgement: This paper was first published in 2012 in the journal Educacao, Sociedade & Culturas [Education, Society & Cultures], the journal of the Centre for Research and Intervention in Education (CIIE-UP), of the Faculty of Psychology and Education Sciences of the University of Porto (FPCEUP), Portugal. Reverberations of narrative inquiries. Educacao, Sociedade & Culturas, 36,7–24. Available online: www.fpce.up.pt/ciie/revistaesc/ESC36/ESC36 D.Jean Sean&Vera.pdf

In the completed study, *A narrative inquiry into the experiences of youth who left school early* (Clandinin et al., 2010), we became intrigued by the life-composing of youth who left school prior to high school completion so we might learn more about their storied experiences, recognizing that their lives in school were only part of their much larger life compositions. We were interested in learning of their lives and, perhaps through learning about their lives, we wanted to learn more about our lives as educators and more about schools. Our overall intentions were, in part, to learn about what we call stories of school and about how we might begin to shift those stories. The research was not an intervention study, but we hoped that what we learned might shift policies and practices around youth who left school prior to graduating.

Our research puzzles were to explore how the experiences of youth shaped their leaving school early and to explore how their experiences of leaving school early shaped their lives. Our puzzle was situated in a concern for understanding youths' life-making in all of the layered complexities of their lives in and out of schools. In this narrative inquiry, we, a group of 11 researchers, came alongside, that is, engaged in a series of conversations with, 19 youth. The criteria for inclusion of participants were that the youth had to be between the ages of 18 to 21, have left school before graduating, and had been out of school for more than a year. We invited youth whose life experiences were diverse, that is, they lived in rural, urban, and suburban places, included males and females, youth of diverse heritages, youth of different family groupings, youth of different socio-economic groupings and so on. We did not engage with the youths' previous teachers or meet these youth in schools. We met the youth in the midst of their complex, ongoing lives, lives that had not yet included high school graduation. We engaged with each youth in a series of conversations shaped by our overall research puzzles around how their lives shaped their leaving of school and how leaving school shaped their lives. We met in coffee shops, offices, cafes, diners, libraries – two of the youth also took us back to the junior high schools they had attended. As we thought about our work we played with the term story constellations (Craig, 2007) to think about the diverse set of story constellations that the youth lived within as they engaged with us in the study. While Craig used the idea of story constellations to illustrate the web of stories from which, and within which, we are each composing lives, the term, for us, also directed our attention to the constellation of places within which the youth lived as well as to the places within which they shared their lives with us.

The field texts (or data) (Clandinin & Connelly, 2000; Connelly & Clandinin, 2006) were, for the most part, transcripts of one-on-one conversations with each youth. We also wrote field notes on our conversations with the youth and on other contacts we had with the youth. Some of the youth engaged in drawing about their experiences and some youth also shared memory box artifacts.

We engaged in two levels of what might be called analysis or interpretation. In the first level of analysis, as we moved from field texts to research texts, each inquirer composed a narrative account of his/her unique experiences with the young person with whom s/he had engaged in conversations. Some inquirers worked with only one youth, others worked with more than one. Following Clandinin and Connelly (2000), we were attentive to the three dimensional narrative inquiry space of sociality, temporality and place. We drafted narrative accounts and negotiated them with each participant until each youth felt we had an account that represented something of who they were and were becoming. The term narrative account, or perhaps narrative accounting, allows us to give an account, an accounting, a representation, of the unfolding of lives, both participants and researchers, at least as they became visible in those times and places where our stories intersected and were shared. Narrative accounts are a way, then, to show the layered relationships between researcher and participant as we make visible how we co-compose. In using the term narrative account, we strive for a sense of being responsible to each other and to our negotiated relationships as well as to our negotiated texts. We work toward a sense of mutuality and co-composition in what we write.

In the second level of analysis, all 11 members of the research team looked across the 19 individual narrative accounts to inquire into resonant threads or patterns that we could discern. We engaged in this process as a collaborative research team. We did so in order to offer a deeper and broader awareness of the experiences of early school leavers with an overall intention to open up new wonders and questions about early school leaving and, in part, to help us learn more about schools and how to shape them in ways that might be more responsive to the life-composing of all youth. We identified six resonant threads.

Narrative accounts in the first study

In the overall study, the team of 11 researchers composed 19 narrative accounts. We share only fragments from three of the accounts here because of space limitations. These fragments are drawn from much longer narrative accounts. All of the accounts were negotiated with participants. The participants all have pseudonyms. We share from the accounts of two youth with whom Clandinin worked and from one of the accounts of a youth with whom Lessard worked.

1. Andrew (Jean Clandinin)

As I listened to Andrew tell of the place of sports in his life, he said "it has always been about basketball, in junior high too, but, like the teachers in junior high, they seemed more caring and understanding so I kinda like got along with them, like really well". Sports were the central thread in his life and it was being able to play sports, particularly basketball, that kept him involved.

> I'd just go to school and play basketball and I had good times in doing, like, school stuff, so, and in high school, it was a big change from how the teachers were in junior high to high school so then that's like when I was, I just, like, really focused on just wanting to play basketball.

Andrew continued to play sports, mainly basketball, both in and out of school, during his junior high school years. He spoke of the support of his junior high school physical education teacher whose daughter he met while playing "club basketball". By the end of junior high school he had to choose one sport and concentrate on it and he chose basketball. He did, however, mention that when he was in Grade 11 he played some volleyball on the school team "for fun".

When it came time to choose a high school, Andrew selected a high school because of their interest in having him play basketball. As he said, "'cause I just liked the, I had been talking to the coach since I was in, like Grade 6, so, kinda like had a bond there so I decided to go there". He agreed when I said, "So it's been about basketball for a long time". Andrew's story of himself was composed around being a basketball player.

By the time he was in high school, Andrew was not particularly interested in any subject area. As he said,

> I was interested just 'cause I know I needed that to go somewhere else with basketball, but it wasn't really something, like, I'd just make sure I'd get, like, a high percentage, I'd just make sure I'd get, like, the passing grade just so I could keep playing. So I wasn't really putting all my hard work into it [school work].

Andrew left high school in his final term of Grade 12.

2. *Skye songmaker (Sean Lessard)*

"I didn't always understand my work and I am too shy to ask for help, I felt dumb." She told me often during our conversations that she struggled with the schoolwork and it was different than what she had learned on the reserve; the pace was too fast. She told me: "Do you know that I am actually smart, Lessard? I was the class valedictorian in my grade nine class at the reserve". I replied by simply saying, "I know you are".

She told me about her feelings coming to a new place and how she often felt low as a student. She told of one of her first days in class. The class went to a driving range to play golf. She was excited because golf was her favourite sport. However, she missed the school bus because she was not familiar with public transportation in this new city. She arrived late to the driving range having walked there alone. The teacher stopped class and told everybody to "look at who is late". He asked where she was. She replied, "I am not a city person, I got lost". He laughed and said, "Are you sure about that? Are you sure you didn't get lost at the mall?". With everyone looking at her, they laughed. Skye did not remember many stories from high school but this story stayed with her long after. She said, "I felt like quitting right there and going home. But then he would have been right about me". That day at the driving range, "I felt like he thought I was just another dumb Indian".

The girls (Skye and her sisters who had unexpectedly joined Sean and Skye in the conversation) recalled times in the past when their mom and dad taught them sports, dancing, and culture. (In this work with Skye, Sean used the term culture to draw attention to cultural teachings and traditions.) They laughed when they told stories and corrected each other along the way. As they told stories, they moved backwards in time to intergenerational connections they shared with their cultural roots. They told me they had been practicing and learning about culture and traditional dancing since they were babies. I know by walking alongside them that their cultural roots come from a place. The passing down of knowledge through participation is a thread that weaves throughout their lives. The cultural stories and knowledge started before them, before their parents, as they told stories about their grandfather, a gifted man, a song maker and singer. He was a very spiritual person with special gifts. The girls spoke proudly of their grandmothers and grandfathers and how culture had always existed in their family.

Skye left high school before graduating.

3. *Truong (Jean Clandinin)*

Truong became a father to a daughter two and a half years ago. His daughter lives with her mother, but Truong and his mother have access to the child on the weekends. He describes his daughter as putting "joy in my life".

> When I see her laughing and playing around it's just like the greatest thing. So when she, like, you know, she gives me like kisses and hugs and stuff, it's like

> it's a good thing to me right because I'm not used to it, like, I've never kissed my mom in my life that I can remember. I've never, I've maybe hugged her once my whole life so I mean this kind of stuff is different to me. But she is my daughter and I do love her. And she is, she is the joy in my life.

I wonder if his daughter has, in some ways, interrupted the stories he was living and telling. Did her arrival and his knowing he was a father shift the trajectory of his forward looking story?

As we talked, Truong spoke of his experiences of leaving school. He had played on the volleyball team in Grades 10 and 11 and had experienced a great deal of success. But Grade 12 was different.

> And then Grade 12 came around and there was no more volleyball (. . .) and so I was, like, whatever, I don't really feel like going to school anymore. I got kicked out second semester of Grade 12. Like, I did go to my classes and stuff but I was more of, oh I'm late, forget it, I don't want to go anymore or you know, stuff like that and I just didn't have motivation to go anywhere.

In Grades 10 and 11, he said

> If I was late I'd still go to school, if I didn't have a ride to school I would bus to school but in Grade 12 if I didn't have a ride I was, ah, I'm staying home today. If it's cold or, like, I bussed to school in Grade 10 a couple of times during the winter and stuff, right, and like, you know, but that's 'cause I had a game or practice or something after school so I wanted to be there.

As he looked back over this time in high school, he said, "the only things I really cared about in high school were basically my friends and volleyball".

He had a "distinctive hair style" and was described as "the Asian guy with the bangs 'cause I had, like, spiky hair with two long strands coming down the sides". He spoke of his teachers in high school in the following way:

> Like a lot of teachers, I don't know if they liked me (. . .) but a lot of coaches and teachers and stuff knew who I was. They knew me for, like, the person that I was and stuff but the principal or the student counsellor or whatever didn't really care, didn't, like, I've known a lot of kids that got so many chances, like they, they fought or whatever, they got kicked out of school and then they would come back and everything's good and stuff, right, but with me it was like OK, come to the office, you're expelled because you skipped too much. And I'm like OK well, what am I going to do, I'm not going to cry about it right?

As Truong told me these stories about not being given second chances as others had been, I sensed he had learned to accept such treatment and to not fight back. He described that he "was like my own person with my own friends". Truong has tried to complete high school. He tried to register "when I was about 18 or 19" in order to "finish up". He attributes his desire to complete high school to the birth of his daughter. He became a father at 19. "That's why I kind of wanted to go back to school and finish up too 'cause she was my motivation for it."

Truong has spent his life taking care of others with whom he has relationships. He worked from when he was about 15, at first with "under the table pay" when he "washed dishes and stuff for the restaurant" where his mom was the cook. The money he earned then was to "just kind of take care of myself and my mom didn't have to worry about me too much right, like, I'd have lunch money or whatever". He learned early to help out with the finances at home, to take care of himself to save his mother from even more financial worry.

Truong has been a watchful big brother to his two younger siblings. "I built the rep of people being scared of me and stuff like that so my little brother and my little sister can go through school peacefully." He learned to live and tell stories of himself as a tough guy, someone to be scared of, in order to provide his siblings with protection from harm. As he said, "I kinda lived the life that I lived basically for them to go through school and I've tried, I did everything that I can for them to graduate and stuff right, to go through school peacefully".

Truong left high school before graduating.

These fragments of three narrative accounts offer some sense of the lives of the youth, particularly something of how their lives shaped their leaving of school and how leaving school early shaped their lives.

Resonances across the narrative accounts

In the second level analysis as a collaborative group, we looked across the narrative accounts and identified what we called resonant threads, threads that echoed and reverberated across the accounts. In what follows we provide brief explanations of each thread.

Thread 1: conversational spaces

The importance of conversational spaces for telling and retelling life stories (Clandinin & Connelly, 2000) became evident in the research conversations. We wondered if such conversation spaces along the way might have helped some of the youth feel less alone in composing their lives within complex institutional, social, cultural, linguistic and familial narratives (Clandinin et al., 2006).

Thread 2: relationships

The importance of relationships to the youths was multidimensional and became visible throughout our research. The participants' relationships with family, peers, programs of study, and teachers, as well as the interruption of relationships through disruptions and transitions, exemplified the significance of relationship – connection and association – when we thought about early school leaving.

Thread 3: identities

The youths were composing their identities on elementary, junior high, and senior high school landscapes as well as on complex home and community landscapes. While they saw themselves composing who they were and were becoming, they did not tell their stories as dropouts. A number of them actively resisted the label of dropout, telling their stories around plotlines of "not in school, for now". Their forward looking stories included school.

Thread 4: complexities across time

Looking across multiple narrative accounts, we were struck by the complexity of stories lived when whole lives were considered. When early school leaving was seen as a complex set of storied events composed over time, the notion of a discrete decisions or factors in dropping out of school became problematic. Complexity in composing lives over time became evident in the lives of the youths who left school early.

Thread 5: responsibilities

Relational responsibility threads were evident in many of the narrative accounts. Many of the youths were composing lives in which they struggled to balance conflicting responsibilities on home, school, and community landscapes. At times it seemed as though they were trying to compose lives that allowed them to shift between, and across, multiple responsibilities. The institutional, familial, and cultural narratives (Clandinin et al., 2006) in which they were embedded shaped their experiences.

Thread 6: cultural, social, and institutional narratives

All stories are embedded within social, cultural, institutional, and familial narratives that shape, and are shaped by, individual's stories to live by (Connelly & Clandinin, 1999). As we attended to the cultural, social, familial, linguistic, and institutional narratives within which the youth composed their lives, we noted competing plotlines that shaped their stories to live by. The youths' stories spoke of, and to, contradictions between cultural narratives, familial narratives, and stories of school. Caught sometimes in these contradictions, youth were humiliated or embarrassed in front of other students and teachers. Within the institutional landscape, composing an identity seemed to be more challenging than passively accepting one. We understood in deeper ways that there were stories that lived in schools about individuals who were seen only within those institutional, cultural, and social narratives. We understood how difficult it was for the youth to negotiate stories to live by outside the plotlines of those institutional, cultural, and social narratives. Institutional stories such as the "Aboriginal story", the "athlete story", and the "gender" story shaped institutional narratives, that is, stories of school, and sometimes became, in Carr's (1986) terms, a story to live out or to live up to. Being shaped by those institutional plotlines shaped many tensions for youth.

These six resonant threads spoke to the complexities of the lives the youth were composing. Their lives awakened us to what might be possible if we engaged with their stories as a way to open up or disrupt current stories of schools to allow for the reimagining of schools.

Lingering wonders shape another study

As we ended the first study, we wrote our report (Clandinin et al., 2010) for the funding agency and had further conversations with those youth who indicated they wanted to be in touch. What we learned lingered with the three authors of this paper. The ways that these particular youths' lives had been shaped by their leaving of school youth influenced us a great deal and the reverberations in our stories were intense. School seemed different for each of us now that we saw the ways that these particular youths' lives had been shaped by their leaving of school and by their lives as lived both in and out of schools. Some wonders stayed with us in quite profound ways.

We realized that the early school-leaving rate was particularly high for youth of Aboriginal heritage as well as for some immigrant and refugee youth. We also knew that the move from junior high school to senior high school was a difficult time for many youth and, for some, the transition was just too difficult. They could not negotiate the liminal space of the transition from junior high school to high school (Clandinin, 2011). We only met youth who attended high school in our first study. However, we learned from the participants about the difficulties they had experienced as they moved from junior high schools to high schools.

Current study: coming alongside Aboriginal youth and families

We began to imagine a second study (Caine et al., 2010), one that grew out of those lingering wonders. We proposed a new narrative inquiry into the educational experiences, both in and out of school, of youth and families of Aboriginal heritage. The research puzzles that shaped our second study were around the educational experiences of youth and their families. Our research puzzles were framed around collaboratively inquiring into the "educational (home/community/school) experiences of Aboriginal youth and families and the ways that these experiences are shaped by cultural, social, historical, linguistic, and institutional narratives" and to "explore, through narrative inquiry, the possibilities for Aboriginal youth and families to restory their school experiences in a way that will enable educators and educational policy makers to create more educative spaces in school".

This time we wanted to come alongside youth who were between 12 and 15 years old, that is, while they were still attending junior high school. We had come to realize from the first study and from our experiences with youth that junior high was a significant time and place in youths' lives. We wanted to come to know them and to hear their stories of education and schooling and we wanted them to metaphorically and literally "take us home" so we might hear their families' stories of education and schooling. We knew there were intergenerational reverberations from the stories of residential schools that shaped many Aboriginal people's stories of school (Young, 2005).

We spent a long time in the design of the narrative inquiry considering how we would come to meet the youth and to spend time with them. In part, our care with the design of the second study was a reverberation from our experiences with the youth in the first study. We realized we needed a space, that is, a physical place and time, to connect with the youth. We wanted to be outside of the hours of the regular school day so we would neither be in a teacher's classroom nor need to be accountable to the mandated curriculum. We gained permission to work in a junior high school with a fairly high population of urban Aboriginal youth (40% of youth self-identified as First Nations, Inuit, or Métis), but was also a school where Aboriginal youth from a nearby reserve attended school. In our original proposal to the Social Sciences and Humanities Research Council of Canada, one of our funding agencies, we appeared to have conveyed an almost utilitarian sense of the space, that is, it would be a space where we could meet junior high students and form relationships with them.

We negotiated, with the permission of the school principal, to meet in a mostly unused classroom in an after school time, a time when school clubs happen, that is, during the time between the 2:37 p.m. afternoon dismissal and 4:00 p.m. We knew the space needed to be invitational and we also wanted it to be purposeful. As we talked about what would happen in that afterschool, in-school, space, we linked it back to our wonders about a resonant thread from our earlier study, the one about conversational spaces.

Creating conversational spaces?

We spent a great deal of time wondering and talking about what conversational spaces might look like. We did not see them as the kinds of spaces that are sometimes created in schools around what is seen as a deficit or problem that one youth or a group of youth are experiencing. Too often those kinds of spaces create a kind of deficit lens from which to view youth. Through such a lens, the youth are seen as less than, rather than in their life complexities. In part, our attentiveness to the kind of space we were designing was another reverberation from the first study. We wondered how to create spaces where we might learn to attend more to the voices of youth in attempts to change the stories of school. In the first study, as we listened to the youths' stories, we saw schools as narrowly defined places for students to gain prescribed knowledge, skills, and attitudes. In their stories, we heard them speak of leaving their multiplicity, the wholeness of who they are and the stories they are in the midst of living, at the door of the school.

Now with the opportunity for this new study, could the space we created in the school for a small group of youth working together with us over two years and while they were still attending school be a conversation space where we could hear youths' stories of their whole lives, a space in which they could tell of their multiplicity, the wholeness of who they are, and the stories they are in the midst of living? We knew that conversational spaces are not spaces to exchange and confirm already familiar understandings, but, rather, are characterized by emergent occasions for exploring other possible stories. They are relational spaces characterized by mutuality and possibility, where embodied, lived tensions become resources or triggers for telling and retelling stories. Because we also wanted the youth to take us to their families in order that we might learn more of their outside of school, familial curriculum making worlds (Huber, Murphy, & Clandinin, 2011), we also wanted to create a space where families would want their children to become engaged, knowing that it was a space in the school but outside the mandated school hours. This was a complex undertaking that required a great deal of imagination as we had not yet met the youth and we did not know much about the families. Lessard, as someone familiar with the particular school district in which we planned to work, had some insight into the school but we were, in many ways, trying to imagine up a space (Greene, 1995) that might work for the youth and their families, as well as for us, without knowing the youth and their families.

We decided to fill it with arts activities such as painting, drawing, beading, mask making, drum and rattle making, photography, collage making and so on. We saw art-making as one way to come alongside, to begin to build relationships with the youth. We also considered sports and other physical activities but decided on art-making so the youth could develop arts skills to represent their storied experiences. The invitations to join the space were open to all youth in the school, although we described it as a space for Aboriginal youth. Both Aboriginal and non-Aboriginal youth came to the afterschool space if they chose to. Their families signed consent forms for them to participate.

As we worked with the youth in the first year of the project, they also helped us shape the space with activities about which they wanted to learn more. In this paper we do not represent the results of our analysis of what was a shifting space as we moved from a focus on relationship building with the youth and engaging in arts activities in order to learn new art skills to a space where inquiring into the youths' and our lived and told stories began to dominate the space. That shift happened both because some of us (Cardinal, 2011; Chung, 2010) had begun one-on-one inquiries with individual youth and their families but, more importantly, we intentionally shifted what we were doing to an inquiry focus. In our second year, we engaged in conversations with the participating youth about how to begin to use art-making as a way to tell their stories, to inquire into their stories, and to represent the telling and retelling of their stories. As in our first study, the field texts (data) included transcripts of one-on-one conversations with youth, field notes on the activities in the club space, and artifacts that the youth created. The youth have taken up this work in thoughtful and engaged ways. In this paper, we focus our theorizing of this shifting conversational space as a space at the intersection of what we are now calling familial and school curriculum making (Huber et al., 2011).

Worlds of curriculum making and conversational spaces: interweaving concepts

Huber et al. (2011) developed an understanding of two worlds of curriculum making: familial curriculum making, and school curriculum making worlds. For many years now, Clandinin (Clandinin & Connelly, 1992; Connelly & Clandinin, 1988) has understood curriculum as a life-making process working from the idea of curriculum as a course of life. As Clandinin and her colleagues continued to focus on identities as stories to live by (Connelly & Clandinin, 1999), and on curriculum as a life-making process (Clandinin et al., 2006), they imagined "how curriculum could be seen as a curriculum of lives" (Huber & Clandinin, 2005, p. 318). Their understanding of the negotiation of a curriculum of lives as children's and teachers' lives met in classrooms was grounded in the idea that "the composition of life identities, "stories to live by" . . . [are] central in the process of curriculum making" (2005, p. 318).

As we used these ideas to reflect on the study with the youth who left school early, we heard many instances where the composing of stories to live by, like Andrew's stories to live by as a basketball player, and Skye's stories to live by as a strong student and a golf player, were integrally interwoven with their curriculum making in schools. When their stories to live by bumped against the mandated curriculum making, their stories to live by were interrupted and disrupted (Clandinin et al., 2006).

In the early work on curriculum making (Clandinin & Connelly, 1992; Clandinin et al., 2006; Connelly & Clandinin, 1988), curriculum making was seen as only occurring in schools. As we began the work with the early school leavers, we worked from this assumption and understood that, while youth came to school embodying and living out their experiences from out of school, curriculum making occurred in in-school places. However, Huber et al. (2011) argued there was another place of curriculum making. In their research they showed that families co-compose with their children and youth a kind of curriculum outside of school. They described various features of these places of familial curriculum making: features that attended to the multiplicity and diversity of people who engage in each child's familial curriculum making, the intergenerational features of the curriculum making, the place of response in familial curriculum making, and a view of life in the making. They found children and youth experienced many tensions as they moved between their familial and school curriculum-making places. Children embodied these tensions as they lived in these two curriculum-making places. In their work they showed ways in which attention to children's embodied tensions makes visible the gaps and silences children experienced as they lived in, and between, these two curriculum-making places.

The conceptualization of two curriculum-making places was useful as we revisited our first study with the youth who left school early. Many gaps and silences became visible as we attended to their lives in these two curriculum making places. We saw, for example, that Truong's responsibilities to care for others in his family did not fit in his school curriculum making. Thinking about Truong's two places of curriculum making, we became more attentive to the conflicting plotlines that Truong lived within.

Huber et al. (2011) also argued that these two places of curriculum making comprised two worlds in Lugones' (1987) understandings of "worlds" and ""world"-travelling". Lugones wrote that a "world" need not be a construction of a whole society. Lugones wrote from her experience as an "outsider to the mainstream", as a woman "of color in the US" (1987: 3) to develop her concept of world travelling. Drawing on her work, Huber et al. (2011) wrote that Lugones "saw herself as needing to "travel" to different worlds, worlds in which she constructs herself and her worlds in which she is "stereotypically" or "arrogantly" perceived or constructed by others" (2011, p. 108). Further they wrote that

> we see that not only are children's and youths' worlds of familial and school curriculum making shaped by differing physical places but also by differing ways of being and interacting and, therefore, of knowing and knowledge. In our exploration of the tensions children experienced in school curriculum making entered onto familial landscapes, we saw the emergence of conflicting stories.
> *(p. 108)*

As we revisited the work with the early school leavers using these ideas, we again saw many instances of the emergence of conflicting stories (Connelly & Clandinin, 1999), stories where the youth experienced stories where the plotlines in their stories to live by conflicted one with another. For example, in Skye's stories we heard her stories in which she was a top student, a strong golf player and a dancer. Her stories to live by were carefully nurtured in her familial curriculum making world. When she arrived in the urban school world, the world of school curriculum making, she learned she was constructed as an "Indian" who did not attend school regularly but spent her time at the mall. She carried this tension in her body as she moved between her familial world of curriculum making and the school world of curriculum making.

In Lugones' (1987) description of "worlds" and ""world"-travelling", she described that "those of us who are "world"-travellers have the distinct experience of being different in different "worlds" and of having the capacity to remember other "worlds" and ourselves in them" (p. 11).

As Huber et al. (2011) showed, children engage in this "world"-travelling over days, weeks, months and years as they move back and forth between home and school and, in this movement, experience multiple tensions in both worlds. Lugones described this "shift from being one person to being a different person" as "travel" (1987, p. 11). Travel is being constructed, and constructing oneself differently, in different worlds. For example, Skye, in composing and living out two different stories of who she is and who she is becoming in her school curriculum making world and familial curriculum making world, seemed to understand that she needed to animate both constructions of herself depending upon which curriculum making world she was inhabiting in any particular moment.

> In a "world" some of the inhabitants may not understand or hold the particular construction of them that constructs them in that "world". So, there may be "worlds" that construct me in ways that I do not even understand. Or it may be that I understand the construction, but do not hold it of myself. I may not accept it as an account of myself, a construction of myself. And yet, I may be *animating* such a construction.
>
> *(Lugones, 1987, p. 10, italics in original)*

Skye gave us a sense that she knew this as she stayed on the golf course rather than leave in the face of her teacher's racist remark. She knew that she was Aboriginal and her physical appearance, the skin she wore, animated the teacher's construction of her. She stayed but recognized her resistance to the stereotypical story of her that was called up by the teacher's remark.

We now are hearing similar stories from the youth in our current study, stories that construct them as Indian, Native, and often as less than. We also are hearing stories of their lives as dancers, grandchildren, siblings, and those who attend to, or are cared for by, others. In the art club, we struggled to create a space located in the physical place of school but within an afterschool time, a space we were attempting to construct as a space between multiple curriculum making worlds. In our struggle to shift the space by working alongside the youth and each other, we learned to travel to other worlds, both their other worlds and our other worlds, to be and interact in different ways. As we moved into the second year of the current study, we, too, noticed that the youth, and we, intentionally travelled with attentiveness to the living, telling, and retelling of their lives, our lives and our shared experiences. As we did this, conversational spaces began to open. In these moments of travel, we were reminded of our study with the youth who left school early. As we attended to who we were alongside the youth in school, memories of the older youth who had left school early were often in our minds.

We learned that as children and youth animate multiple constructions of themselves, that is, as they live by some stories in school and other stories at home, they seem to feel that when they are at school they need to hold silent the stories they live in their familial curriculum making worlds and their embodied tensions. As Skye stands on the golf course, she holds silent the stories of her familial curriculum making world, noting that if she left or spoke out, she could not be certain of the consequences. We came to know there were stories the youth tell of themselves but also stories they leave behind because there is no safe place to tell them, share them or celebrate them. As we work with them and with each other in the art club we see ourselves as composing a space for narrative inquiry through living, telling and retelling stories as well as a safe space to explore, improvise, and try out other possible tellings of who they might be and become.

What Huber et al. (2011) illustrated was two worlds of curriculum making, worlds in Lugones' (1987) sense that are filled with multiple and often conflicting constructions of children and youth. These ideas of worlds and world travelling borrowed from Lugones as a way to understand the worlds of curriculum making are helpful as we try to understand the conversational spaces we are co-creating with the youth and families of Aboriginal heritage. Being attentive to intentional conversational spaces makes visible the tensions between the worlds of curriculum making. Living within conversational spaces with youth such as in the art club space draws attention to the ways that attending to living in multiple worlds deeply shape the relationships, the stories to live by, and the responsibilities of youth, as well as of ourselves as researchers.

We wonder, as we work alongside each other and the youth, how the absence of conversational spaces leads us, sometimes, to turning inward and to silencing the stories that we live and tell. When youth awaken to stories of who they are, and are becoming, as Aboriginal youth in the institutional story of school, it shapes their lives. Once awakened to the plotline of who they are within the story of school, they begin to silence their lived and told stories. We saw that happening in Skye's stories and we see it happening with the youth in our art club. Sometimes this silencing makes it even more difficult to enter into conversational spaces, that is, to understanding the possibility of conversational spaces. The silence has become part of the youth's stories to live by. Disrupting or interrupting the silences is more difficult when it is a way of knowing who you are and are becoming.

Recursive reverberations

Now as we are in the midst of working with the youth and their families, we stand, look backward and inward, and see that each project recursively elaborates the ones that came before. The reverberations of previously lived stories alongside participants from earlier studies come into our current life living, telling and retelling. The stories of the youth who left school early shaped our stories at the time but also continue to shape our stories as we live our retold stories into the future. Our retold stories shape our reliving as we imagine and live out our current study. The stories of the youth who left school early mingle with ours and allow us to newly imagine this "becoming" conversational space in light of the echoes left behind by those who came before. The reverberations stretch across, and through, lives.

References

Caine, V. (2010a). Narrative beginnings: Travelling to and within unfamiliar landscapes. *Qualitative Health Research, 20*(9), 1304–1311. doi:10.1177/1049732310367500

Caine, V. (2010b). Visualizing community: Understanding narrative inquiry as action research. *Educational Action Research, 18*(4), 481–496. doi:10.1080/09650792.2010.524820

Caine, V., Clandinin, D. J., Glanfield, F., Dellaire, P., Whiskeyjack, C., Baydala, L., . . . Donald, D. (2010). *A narrative inquiry into the educational experiences of urban Aboriginal youth and families.* Funding proposal submitted to SSHRC, Ottawa, Ontario, Canada.

Cardinal, T. (2011). *Storied lives: A narrative inquiry into the experiences of Aboriginal youth and families.* Unpublished Doctoral Dissertation Proposal, University of Alberta, Canada.

Carr, D. (1986). *Time, narrative and history.* Bloomington, IN: Indiana University Press.

Chung, S. (2010). *A narrative inquiry into co-composing a curriculum of belonging as interwoven with identity making.* Unpublished Doctoral Dissertation Proposal, University of Alberta, Canada.

Clandinin, D. J., & Connelly, F. M. (1992). Teacher as curriculum maker. In P. W. Jackson (Ed.), *Handbook of research on curriculum* (pp. 363–401). New York: Macmillan.
Clandinin, D. J., & Connelly, F. M. (1995). *Teachers' professional knowledge landscapes.* New York: Teachers College Press.
Clandinin, D. J., & Connelly, F. M. (1996). Teachers' professional knowledge landscapes: Teacher stories, stories of teachers, school stories, stories of schools. *Educational Researcher, 25*(3), 24–30. doi:10.3102/0013189X025003024
Clandinin, D. J., & Connelly, F. M. (2000). *Narrative inquiry: Experience and story in qualitative research.* San Francisco, CA: Jossey-Bass.
Clandinin, D. J., Huber, J., Huber, M., Murphy, M. S., Murray-Orr, A., Pearce, M., & Steeves, P. (2006). *Composing diverse identities: Narrative inquiries into the interwoven lives of children and teachers.* London and New York: Routledge.
Clandinin, D. J., Steeves, P., Li, Y., Mickelson, J. R., Buck, G., Pearce, M., . . . Huber, M. (2010). *Composing lives: A narrative account into the experiences of youth who left school early.* Retrieved from www.elementaryed.ualberta.ca/~/media/elementaryed/Documents/Centres/CRTED/ComposingLives_FinalReport.pdf
Connelly, F. M., & Clandinin, D. J. (1988). *Teachers as curriculum planners: Narratives of experience.* New York: Teachers College Press.
Connelly, F. M., & Clandinin, D. J. (1999). *Shaping a professional identity: Stories of educational practice.* New York: Teachers College Press.
Connelly, F. M., & Clandinin, D. J. (2006). Narrative inquiry. In J. L. Green, G. Camilli, & P. B. Elmore (Eds.), *Handbook of complementary methods in education research* (pp. 477–488). Washington, DC: American Educational Research Association.
Craig, C. J. (2007). Story constellations: A narrative approach to contextualizing teachers' knowledge of school reform. *Teaching and Teacher Education, 23*(2), 173–188. doi:10.1016/j.tate.2006.04.014
Dewey, J. (1938). *Experience and education.* New York: Collier.
Greene, M. (1995). *Releasing the imagination: Essays on education, the arts, and social change.* San Francisco, CA: Jossey Bass.
Huber, J., & Clandinin, D. J. (2005). Living in tension: Negotiating a curriculum of lives on the professional knowledge landscape. In J. Brophy & S. Pinnegar (Eds.), *Learning from research on teaching: Perspective, methodology and representation* (pp. 313–336). Oxford, UK: Elsevier Ltd.
Huber, J., Murphy, M. S., & Clandinin, D. J. (2011). *Places of curriculum making.* London: Emerald Press.
Lugones, M. C. (1987). Playfulness, "world"-travelling, and loving perception. *Hypatia, 2*(2), 3–19.
Young, M. I. (2005) *Pimatisiwin: Walking in a good way: A narrative inquiry into language as identity.* Winnipeg: Pemmican Publications.

17

LIVING RELATIONAL ETHICS

D. Jean Clandinin, Vera Caine and Sean Lessard

As we wrote this book, we engaged in multiple conversations about the relational ethics which guided the living of narrative inquiries. We returned often to those narrative inquiries we had engaged in and those we read, published by other researchers whose work we had supervised. Through returning to multiple narrative inquiries we discerned what we identified at the outset as five dimensions of relational ethics at work in narrative inquiries. In order to do this, we revisited the theoretical resources that framed our nascent thoughts and returned to Clandinin's early writing with Connelly to trace the development of ethical matters in narrative inquiry. We also considered, and reconsidered, the writings and thoughts of numerous theorists and the teachings of indigenous Elders and scholars.

As we worked together in the narrative inquiry with Indigenous youth and families, the study we draw on most centrally throughout the book, we became wakeful to how we engaged in narrative inquiry with only tacit understandings of what a relational ethics for narrative inquiry might entail. In the late 1980s, Clandinin and Connelly began to explicitly conceptualize a research ethics for narrative inquiry. While they had not yet named narrative inquiry as a methodology, they already had a sense that other understandings of ethics would be needed in such close research relationships. Clandinin (1985) raised concerns about a different understanding of research ethics when she wrote that

> In terms of narrative it is appropriate to view this process as the negotiation of two people's narrative unities. The notion of narrative unity is borrowed from MacIntyre (1981) and is defined as a continuum within a person's experience which renders life experiences meaningful for the unity they achieve for the person. What we mean by unity is the union in a particular person in a particular place and time of all that he has been and undergone in the past and in the past of the tradition which helped to shape him. . . . The notion of narrative unity allows us the possibility of imagining the living out of a narrative as well as the revision of ongoing narrative unities and the creation of new ones.
> *(p. 365)*

Reprinted with permission. Acknowledgement; In Clandinin, D. J., V. Caine, & S. Lessard (2018) The relational ethics of narrative inquiry. London: Routledge. (Chapter 15, pp 186–203)

Connelly and Clandinin, having read and considered theorists such as Buber, Arendt, MacMurray and others, as theoretical resources, picked up on Clandinin's earlier writing and noted: "[b]ecause the study of personal practical knowledge requires intensive close working relationships with practitioners, fundamental ethical issues come close to the surface throughout the research, from negotiation of entry to the preparation of results" (Connelly and Clandinin, 1988b, p. 273). While they wrote of close working relationships with participants, they noted only the importance of "fundamental ethical issues." They continued to draw on MacIntyre's (1981) concept of narrative unity within and across lives as they outlined these fundamental ethical issues. In so doing, they attended much more closely to the negotiation of researcher and participant narrative unities. They began to conceptualize an underlying relational ethics in the following way:

> In everyday life, the idea of friendship implies a sharing, an interpenetration of two or more persons' spheres of experience. Mere contact is acquaintanceship, not friendship. The same may be said for collaborative research which requires a close relationship akin to friendship. Relationships are joined, as McIntyre implies, by the narrative unities of our lives.
>
> *(Connelly and Clandinin, 1988, p. 281)*

In what they wrote they signaled that something different than what was offered by university ethics boards was needed to think through these ethical issues. These ethical issues could not so easily be addressed, categorized, or resolved.

It was in 1990 that they named the methodology as narrative inquiry. At that time, Connelly and Clandinin attended more directly to ethics in narrative inquiry drawing most heavily on Noddings' (1984) work. In particular they pointed toward "the negotiation of entry" as highlighting "the way narrative inquiry occurs within relationships among researchers and practitioners, constructed as a caring community" (Connelly and Clandinin, 1990, p. 4). However, as we noted in Chapter 2, relational ethics as an appropriate and needed ethical stance in narrative inquiry was not explicitly named. By 2000, ten years later, Clandinin and Connelly (2000) wrote: "relationship lives at the heart of thinking narratively. Relationship is key to what it is that narrative inquirers do" (p. 189). By 2000, Clandinin and Connelly more clearly specified relational ethics in how narrative inquirers "attended to the maintenance of relationships with participants, now and in the future, as a first consideration. Ethical concerns needed to be reframed as concerns of 'relational responsibility'." In this way, ethics lives at the heart of narrative inquiry. Elsewhere, Clandinin, Caine, and Huber (2016) trace the development of ethics in more detail.

We continued to develop the idea of relational ethics in narrative inquiry but ethics was often drawn into the conversations as a way to think about how we were living with participants. After Clandinin and Rosiek wrote their chapter in the *Handbook of narrative inquiry: Mapping a methodology* (Clandinin, 2007), we began to write more about the relational ontology for narrative inquiry. The Clandinin and Rosiek (2007) chapter made increasingly visible the importance of relational ethics. As we searched for ways to understand the relational ontology of narrative inquiry, we more intentionally turned to concerns and questions of ethics. As Caine et al. (2013) note:

> a relational ontology requires that we do not turn first to the inquiry as a way to make these stories fit. Representation, as the act that arises from our relational ontology, necessitates our living with the unfitting story rather than

> with attempts to tame, sanitize, or analyze. As narrative inquirers we attend to difficult stories and experiences, we stay with them; we dwell alongside participants in possible ways to retell them.
>
> *(p. 581)*

However, it was not until we engaged in the work of writing this book that we turned our attention to directly discerning the dimensions of relational ethics.

While the most common meaning of dimension focuses on a measurable extent of some kind, our focus is on dimension as an aspect or feature of a thing. We do not intend to suggest that the dimensions of relational ethics are in any way measurable. We see these dimensions as particular aspects of relational ethics, as ways of living in relational ways. We were aware as we specified the dimensions of relational ethics that we were, in some ways, highlighting what could be seen as touchstones or markers of how to live a narrative inquiry in relationally ethical ways. When Clandinin and Caine (2013) laid out touchstones for judging the quality of narrative inquiries, they identified the first touchstone as relational responsibilities. They wrote that narrative inquiry spaces were "spaces of belonging for both researchers and participants; spaces that are marked always by ethics and attitudes of openness, mutual vulnerability, reciprocity, and care." Further, they noted that relational ethics in narrative inquiry are "an ethics of care" (Bergum, 1999; Noddings, 1984) and are "marked by responsiveness, as well as marked by short and long term responsibilities" (Huber et al., 2006). They draw attention to the ethical responsibilities which are

> [T]he ethics of everyday life (Charon and Montello, 2002); they guide all interactions with participants, including the negotiations of relationships with participants. Ethical understandings in narrative inquiry are marked by living in relational spaces that bring forth researchers' and participants' lived ethical understandings, complexities, and tensions. Living and being in a relational space, brings forth responsibilities where issues of attentiveness, presence, and response matter (Bateson, 1994; Lugones, 1987). It is marked by a process of self-reflection, contemplation, openness, and uncertainty (Bergum, 1999).
>
> *(Clandinin and Caine, 2013, p. 169)*

The way in which Clandinin and Caine framed the first touchstone foreshadows the five dimensions of relational ethics and what we have come to see through writing this book. However, in this book we have made more explicit the ways that relational ethics shape the design and living out of narrative inquiries from co-composing field texts and interim research texts to writing and making public final research texts. In this final chapter we return to the dimensions to gather our thoughts around each dimension but also to make visible the challenges around the living of these five dimensions in narrative inquiry. We return, at times, in the spirit of dialogue or conversation to some theoretical resources framed by wonders about what we have learned from attending closely to our experiences as narrative inquirers in particular studies. Drawing on concepts such as care, othering, mutuality, reciprocity, world-traveling, we return to the ethical dimensions.

In the midst: coming together on Pender Island

Part of our excitement as we began to plan the book and engage in writing to frame a book proposal had been the possibility of bringing other narrative inquirers together with us in order for them to also take a reflective turn on their own studies with an eye to relational ethics. We were excited by the idea of thinking alongside them and their work in terms of relational ethics.

Shaped by other experiences of writing retreats on book projects we invited a small group of narrative inquirers, Brenda Rossow-Kimball, Hiroko Kubota, Muna Saleh, Dustin Brass, and Jinny Menon, to join us at Jean's cottage on Pender Island for a two-day retreat in June, 2016. Prior to coming to join us we asked people to read our book prospectus that laid out the framework for the book, to write a draft chapter of how they thought of relational ethics in their own studies, and to read and be ready to respond to chapters authored by the others. We asked Elder Isabelle Kootenay, a key person in our narrative inquiry with the youth and their families, to join us. We also asked Jerry Rosiek, someone whose theoretical work in narrative inquiry had been a key source of insight, to join us.

Jean: encountering the uncertainty

Tasked with figuring out accommodations, helping people with travel schedules, and the challenges of finding ways to travel from airports to ferry terminals to the actual cottage, worrying about food for a group of ten kept me busy for many hours before the actual meeting. Organizing and arranging are things I know how to do. What I was less certain about was how we were going to create a kind of instant response group. While Sean, Vera, and I knew all of the people we invited, that was not the case for everyone else. We were mindful of the diversity within the group: some were faculty members, some were graduate students; some had teaching backgrounds, some had nursing backgrounds; some were indigenous, some were not; the list of ways of thinking about the diversity in the group seemed endless. While we intentionally asked these scholars to come together because of the diversity they reflect as a group, I now wondered how this would play out. We, too, had invited Elder Isabelle and I was worrying about protocol and how she would experience being in a group composed of researchers. I looked around the living room of the cottage and tried to imagine ten people gathered together. I counted plates, cups, glasses, cutlery. Vera and I arrived a day early and we planned meals and bought groceries. Jinny let us know at the last minute that her health would not allow her to travel. We readjusted plans just a bit. I worried about schedules and preferences. I worried about forgetting things. Mostly I just worried.

As I worried about the ordinary I knew that attending to these small matters was necessary. The stuff of everyday life is, I knew, what made it possible for people to feel at ease in a place. It mattered that there were some familiar and comfortable things. It mattered that we focused on ways to care for those whom we had invited. It mattered that we took care to make a conversational space. It mattered that we planned to prepare meals together and that we could enjoy working together. It mattered that we had a comfortable place where we could gather together as a group. These matters of everyday living were part of going slow, of coming alongside. Even finding ways to live in, and with uncertainty, were part of the everyday concerns that captured my attention.

I returned again and again to whether what we had imagined was possible. Was it possible to come together to continue what Sean, Vera, and I had already set in progress, that is, to deepen and make more explicit what we meant by relational ethics in narrative inquiry? The idea of writing such a book had lived in me for several years now. I wanted to think carefully about what it meant for me to live relational ethics in narrative inquiry. I had not moved much past my desire to write the book; until Sean, Vera, and I began to talk I had not imagined just what the book itself would look like. Now I doubted myself, sometimes thinking it would make more sense to study philosophical texts or to write with just Vera and Sean about our empirical studies. Why did we invite others? These moments of doubt were brief as I knew that we needed to think about relational ethics while we were in the midst of lives. That was the way we could best understand relational ethics.

As people spoke of who they were on that Friday evening, first at the dinner table and later sprawled comfortably around the living room, I felt the worries slip away. I still felt a bit worried about the shortness of the time we had together, and there were moments when I wanted to rush the dinner in order to get to the conversations. I knew that I could not do that. "Move slowly Jean," I admonished myself. "It will work, we will learn with each other. Listen carefully" were words I said as I breathed in and out.

Sean: coming to the writing weekend

Over a year later I so clearly recall my trip to Pender Island where we gathered as a writing group to think about the meanings of relational ethics in narrative inquiry. The trip stands out, in part, because I was traveling to a new place and, in part, because it was the first time that I traveled on a float plane. As I think closely with the experience I still remember the conversations with the pilot as well as with the passengers as I eagerly anticipated take off.

The trip was also the first time where I could spend a couple of days with Elder Isabelle Kootenay. Isabelle and I have been friends for many years now but this was the first time that I would be spending time with her outside the comforts of Alberta. I was looking forward to spending time with an Elder in this way. But my anticipation was also colored by my worries about how Elder Isabelle would get to the airport in Edmonton, about who would look out for her on the plane, about who would take care of her. We invited Elder Isabelle as she has been a guide and a fellow researcher alongside Jean, Vera, and myself. Her words mattered along the way in the research and her presence now at the writing retreat mattered deeply. It was not enough for us to say we had "consulted" an Elder in the process of writing and thinking about relational ethics. My worries, and those of Jean and Vera, led us to lay out careful plans: At the Edmonton airport Elder Isabelle would be met by Hiroko and Muna, two graduate students who were participating in the retreat. Isabelle and I messaged back and forth as her family member dropped her off at the airport in Edmonton. I also messaged Hiroko and Muna, ensuring they found her as they had not met her before. When I was assured they had found each other I was relieved, happy to know her travel would be easier.

I remember the rush of energy as people started to arrive at various times for the writing retreat. What stands out in my memory are the small conversations between friends and colleagues as we took moments throughout the weekend to take in the ocean air, breathing and admiring the peaceful beauty. The physical elements take me back to the details of the experiences alongside one another. Through the details of the geography, I found that I could more easily think with the conversations that took place. As I look back on these moments, I think about my initial ideas around ethics that were framed in an understanding that was closer to an institutional ethics board definition. I know how difficult I first found reframing my thinking to think more about particular understandings of relational ethics in narrative inquiry.

Living the conversational space within the weekend

Over the weekend we watched as Hiroko and Muna took care of Elder Isabelle in a thoughtful and attentive way with simple acts such as bringing her a cup of tea or accompanying her on the walk back to the cabin where they were sleeping. These small moments of care shifted the experience for Isabelle as she sat on the couch alongside new friends as we gathered for conversations about our work and about the book. The rhythm shifted as we moved from Friday greetings to Friday dinner and Friday conversations in the living room to Saturday morning breakfast and several hours of conversation in the living room and then small group writing, walking, and talking. Saturday evening involved pizza making followed by more conversations. Sunday morning, as we made and ate breakfast, we made forward-looking plans, always with a sense that we would see each other again. The conversations created spaces for sharing and ways forward so that we could better understand each other's work and thoughts.

We recall Isabelle's laughter alongside our own, as she helped prepare pizza dough as part of an experiment in baking pizzas in an outdoor oven. We all participated in the experiment in some way – some were making a fire in the oven, others prepared the pizza dough, while others chopped vegetables and other ingredients for pizza toppings. We can still hear the laughter as we pulled the first pizza from the fire, carefully scraping off the parchment paper from the charcoal crust. But with the joy woven into the cooking, even the burned pizza tasted delicious! Those hours of preparing food together further shifted the space as we talked again late in the evening about relational ethics. We attended to each other, the place, and the gift of shared conversations.

Isabelle's words, as well as her actions, were important during our time together. She reminded us to slow down in our thinking and in the process of coming together; she asked us to enjoy the opportunity to gather, to make and eat food together, and to share what we knew. She reminded us of the importance of conversation, of listening, and of response to each other. She also reminded us of the importance of walking, of silence, of sitting in contemplation with our surroundings, of honoring the place where we were and all of the animate and inanimate beings that were with us.

As we come to this last chapter, Sean writes:

> I believe Isabelle's presence and words mattered to all of us as she asked us to think about the food at each meal, as she engaged in playful laughter and conversation during the preparation of the food and each time before we ate. Although it was a new experience for many in the writing group, she said a few words in her Stoney Language, asking Whakan to guide us and to bless all of our relationships. She, too, asked Whakan to bless the food we were about to eat. In these small particular ways over the course of a writing weekend, openings and possibilities within ourselves and between relationships took root.

Five dimensions of relational ethics in narrative inquiry

We identified five interrelated dimensions in the relational ethics of narrative inquiry: the necessity of engaging with world-traveling with imagination, improvisation, and playfulness; the necessity of moving slowly in ways that allow for listening and living; the necessity of ethical understandings as always in process, in the making, with wakefulness to the ongoingness of experience; the necessity of always engaging with a sense of uncertainty and not knowing that acknowledges living ethically as living within liminal spaces that position us in places of dis/ease; and the necessity of understanding that ethical relations are always lived embodiments, that ask us to be still and to attend carefully to, and with, silence and contemplation. While we wrote chapters for each dimension and, in some ways attempted to pull them out as separate, we know that these dimensions are interwoven and cannot be pulled apart one from another. We have come to know that it is difficult to live some aspects of these dimensions, as they carry with them particular challenges.

A turn towards challenges of living relational ethics

By early Saturday afternoon, we had been talking for four or five hours. We took a break and a small group stayed behind to gather thoughts and do some writing. As we talked about our studies we began to consider questions around the challenges of living relational ethics in narrative inquiry. It was the beginning of a conversation that Sean, Jean, and Vera picked up each time they gathered.

Challenges embedded in playfulness and world-traveling

We described one dimension of relational ethics as engaging with imagination that calls forth the need to "world" travel (Lugones, 1987) and to do so with loving perception and playfulness. Engaging in this way calls us to be open to living in improvisational ways that are part of co-composing fields and field texts and composing research texts. We draw heavily on Lugones' concept of world-traveling. As Sean considered the challenges of living relational ethics with playfulness and world-traveling, he wrote:

> I am sitting today far removed from the moments within the U of A arts club, far away physically from the youth I was able to meet and connect with through the narrative inquiry. I did not imagine in those beginning moments of the research how the lives of some youth would intertwine so deeply with mine and how my experiences with them could flash back when I slow down and return to these places in my memory.
>
> But I need to also name the difficult spaces and challenges I enter into as a narrative inquirer. I am faced with challenges related to relational ethics, trying to negotiate what living relational ethics means and how it looks within a research study. The challenges stir up various feelings within me: some feelings tinged with regrets; some feelings of uncertainty if I did the right thing; some feelings about whether if I had lived differently what might have happened, what might the story have been.
>
> I write with reminders of Thomas King who reminds me about the ethics in relationships and with Richard Wagamese who nudges me with his words that "Actions, born of contemplation are wiser than those made in quiet desperation." I write this and feel these words throughout my body as I return to my experience with youth.
>
> Jean and Vera, my response group, admonish me to not engage in smoothing over stories, recalling only memories where the ethics seemed appropriate and the choices seemed to be the most suitable and comfortable at that moment. Doing that can make for a nice story, perhaps a saving story. I am challenged to push past smoothing stories and to return to the stories that are

not as smooth, the stories that cause tensions for me as they push against the tenuous ethical barometer that lives within me.

These challenges take me to a different narrative inquiry, one that is a resonating ripple of the U of A arts club. I often refer to Lugones' (1987) theoretical idea of "world-traveling"; yet this concept challenges me in the living when it is more difficult to "world-travel" and, at other times, seemingly impossible, times when I turn away from relationships.

I keep a note from a young person that I came to know through a research project. It is on a tattered wrinkled yellow sticky. The note simply reads "Macy Soccer Girl Was Here" with a happy face winking emoji neatly drawn in the right hand corner. This little yellow sticky was placed on my office computer after the youth from the research project had toured the university. The group stopped by my office as part of the tour. I found the yellow note days later. I have held it closely since finding it. It matters to me. I include the note as one of the slides at the beginning of invited speeches as I share stories of aboriginal youth and education. I know that somehow the note reminds me of how important, yet difficult, it is to maintain and hold spaces open for relationships. Now, as I turn to think about the challenges of engaging in the relational ethics of world-traveling and of opening spaces to allow youth to "world-travel" to my worlds, I think again of that tattered yellow note and what it signifies. I am wakeful to the challenges as well as the regrets when worlds and the possibilities of world-traveling seem to close off, when youth move on in different ways, sometimes out of anger, hurt, or other reasons.

I do not need the actual note to remind me of "Macy Girl" and my regrets about our time together. I wonder if I could have some way shifted how the story was lived out, how the relationship moved forward. I have spent time wondering what I could do to repair the relationship Macy and I have as I so want to continue to work alongside me in the research we still are composing. I can imagine the moment she left the gymnasium when she learned I was not there. She was angry as she moved between homes and she was lashing out as she asked where I was, why I was not in the gymnasium that day. Her anger at not finding me in the gymnasium was creating a difficult situation for my colleagues and the youth within the program.

I pause my writing and wonder if there was another way forward. What stopped the possibility in the relationship that we had been developing. What had happened that turned the optimistic emoji on the yellow sticky into something different. Many times she asked me to go for lunch and each time I really wanted to, as we would have been able to talk for hours or kick the soccer ball around like she, and I, so wanted. Somehow something stopped me from traveling to her world in this way at this time. Ethically I felt I had to stop I was no longer able to reach her parents or caregivers to gain their consent for me to engage in conversations with Macy. There were many legal entanglements that made seeing her difficult. Could I have picked her up from the club, picked her up from school, taken her to lunch or to play soccer on the school play ground? Somehow, without informed consent, that seemed wrong to me. Or was it more than not having informed consent? Who was I in her life, and who was she in mine. And mostly how would I be storied within social and institutional narratives. I stopped myself, as I wondered what others might see if they saw me, an older native man with a young aboriginal girl. I wondered about those larger social and cultural narratives within which lives

> are composed. I wondered how they shaped me, shaped her. The space closed for me and, as the possibilities closed for me, the space closed for us. All I have left is a yellow sticky note and the memories of good experiences, hoping that she too has the good memories and not the anger of me not being present in the club.

Challenges embedded in moving slowly

Our thinking about relational ethics draws attention to the importance of coming alongside slowly with attention to the life making of participants and researchers. Coming alongside slowly calls us to listen not only to the stories being told but also to the stories not told, to listen to the stories being lived but also to the stories that create narrative contexts for our lives. As Vera thinks about her experiences as a narrative inquirer, she recalls her time on Pender Island.

> It's been more than a year since we gathered on Pender Island and I am sitting at the kitchen table in Jean's house again writing. The weather is beautiful, the flowers in full bloom, and the birds are singing – it's hard to stay focused at times. In reading Jean's words about coming to her place, I am reminded about our time together. I remember all of the preparations, the carefully composed invitation letters and the energy that was present. While I remember less of Jean's worries, I do remember our conversations about how we might bring people together in ways that create a sense of opening, a sense of not knowing, and a sense of curiosity.
>
> Yet, what has stayed with me from that day was not the worry, or the laughter, or the sense of curiosity that settled in. What stayed with me that day was the walk I took with Isabelle – leaning across the railing by the local coffee place overlooking the small bay on Pender Island. Earlier on the Saturday morning, Isabelle and I had talked and agreed that it would be lovely to see at least a small part of the Island. We had seen the advertisement for the local farmers market and were set to adventure out, despite the tight time frames we were working with. If I knew then how much Jean had worried, I wonder if I would have agreed to the plan Isabelle and I had made. Jerry decided to join us.
>
> After visiting the local farmers market, we decided to follow some of the windy roads, which brought us to one of the local coffee places. While Jerry settled in for some quiet time, on a bench close to the coffee place, Isabelle and I wandered off. As we stood side by side, looking across the water, I turned to Isabelle. For weeks now I had carried with me deep worries about one of my research participants. As I talked, I realised how much I had been impacted by my worries. I had grown close to my research participant. Isabelle listened carefully to me that day, as I contemplated my ability to continue to walk slowly, to listen carefully to difficult and hard-to-comprehend life experiences.

The conversation with Isabelle that afternoon opened up many questions and made visible some of the challenges we have experienced in moving slowly in ways that allow for listening and living. While moving in this way allows us to build close relationships, it also opens up the possibilities to hear hard and difficult stories that are challenging to live with. Chris and Vera had been in conversations for several months both within the arts club and also outside of it in community settings. Vera had met his mother, and she knew several of Chris' friends. Chris shared with her many of the worries he had about his mother, his deep sense of loss after his father's and cousin's death, and also his struggle to find his place in the world. Vera also knew how deeply Chris cared for his mother, and how much his mother cared for him.

One day Chris came to Vera to ask what the process was for him to move out and access funding through social services to support himself. When Chris asked her about this process, Vera struggled, as she felt a loyalty to both him and his mother and as she imagined how difficult it would be for Chris to live on his own. She wondered out loud alongside Chris: What will happen to your mom when you leave? Will you be any less worried? Would you be able to manage? What would be the repercussions to have social services involved? Vera wondered about the complexity of Chris's life at the same time. She felt implicated in whatever decision Chris would make. By moving alongside Chris and listening carefully, she could not turn away in these moments.

When Vera turned to Isabelle that Saturday morning, she wondered how to make sense of who she was alongside Chris. Who had she become in his life? How would she navigate to walk slowly alongside Chris, and also alongside Chris' mother? How could she listen and hear amidst the ethical distress?

Challenges embedded in staying wakeful

In our understanding of relational ethics we highlight the importance of attending temporally, not only to what is, but to the ongoingness of life making, to the temporality of experience with wakefulness to the ways that lives are shifted and shaped over time and place and multiple relationships. Coming alongside the youth in the arts club we knew the importance of staying wakeful, of recognizing that they were in the midst of composing their lives. As we met Lane, Donovan, Chris, Jason, and other youth, we knew they were in their early teens and we saw the complexity of their unfolding lives as they began to compose their lives within the stories of junior high school. As we came alongside them in the arts club, we slowly came to know their stories of their experiences in their homes, communities, social media and so on. We also knew they were composing their lives in the complexities of school landscapes with courses, grades, and friendships. In Chapter 11 we described the weeks in the arts club when the youth were engaged in a play in which they were making visible their complex lives in their homes and their communities. And yet the play was being lived out in the arts club room and the adjoining foods classroom. We were in the place of school. While we saw the youth making visible the complexities of their unfolding lives lived within larger social and institutional narratives of the single stories (Adichie, 2009) of indigenous peoples and within the complexities of lives in urban settings and reservation settings, we and the youth were sharply reminded of where we were and how we were storied in the school when the school administrator entered the room. As we noted in Chapter 11 the play ended abruptly as we were reminded of school rules and discipline. In the improvised play, Jean had been cast as the police with a badge and sunglasses. While she was given no action role in the improvised play, with youth taking on the roles of security staff and police in pursuit, everything changed with the arrival of the administrator. As the "shoplifted items" (objects from the cooking stations in the room) fell out of the youths' clothing, the sharp words of the administrator, "What's going on here?" ruptured the play. Caught in the midst, this was the moment when Jean, still with her props, realized that in the ongoing action she could assume "the adult in charge" role in the real life drama unfolding. With a greeting to the administrator, Jean said: "We're working on a play here and making a film. The youth are playing out a script. Everything is fine." After a pause and a long look at Jean and the youth, the administrator said: "Make sure you clean up and put everything back when you finish." With assurances from Jean that all would be as it was, he turned and left. Play interrupted, the moment of composing the play ended. The youth and Jean began to quickly clean up the foods room and the youth dispersed.

The challenges of staying wakeful to the complexities of the school landscape and the youths' live composing within it were brought into sharp relief. We did not return to the play the next week or in any subsequent weeks, although Sean's role as Chief is still remembered by some of the youth these many years later. We wondered why the youth did not return to the play the next week. But somehow, perhaps with the sharp reminder that they were still in the place of school and storied as difficult youth in the school, was enough to keep them from making visible some of the contradictions and complexities of who they were. We wondered what we could have done to keep the work of play making going. And yet, perhaps, it was too difficult for the youth to make their lives so visible to each other and to us while we stayed in the school. As narrative inquirers we continue to live this ethical challenge, to continue to remind ourselves of the importance of wakefulness to the complexities of life making over time and multiple places.

Challenges in living with uncertainty

Relational ethics calls us to recognize that we live in, and co-create with participants, spaces of uncertainty or liminality, that both defy simple answers to questions of living and simultaneously acknowledge not knowing as part of living ethically in which we, as researchers, take care to position ourselves in places of dis/ease. Living with uncertainty requires us to put ourselves forward, we become, and are, part of the uncertainty. This is, at times, an exhausting process that pulls us to imagine otherwise.

Perhaps this dimension of relational ethics is the most challenging in relation to the writing of final research texts, where it is most significant to hold open "the consciousness of possibility . . . images of what could be or might be in their classrooms, their schools, their communities, and in some cases society as a whole" (Greene, 1988, p. 2). As we have shown in the beginning of this book, it was difficult to resist the labeling of Aboriginal youth, as less than, as problematic, as vulnerable. These struggles remain, as we are asked to label our work, as we speak more publicly about their lives. After a presentation Jean gave, that included aspects of our study alongside the youth, she was asked: Do you always study vulnerable people? As Jean, Sean, and Vera talked about the question, we noticed our struggles – that the question did not feel right, that the assumptions embedded in the question challenged how we experienced and lived alongside the youth (Lessard, Caine, and Clandinin, in progress).

In thinking with our struggles, we recall Greene's (1995) encouragement to engage in what she called "utopian thinking: thinking that refutes mere compliance, that looks down roads not yet taken to the shapes of a more fulfilling social order, to more vibrant ways of being in the world" (p. 5). Greene's call allows us to see our struggle as one in which our work and research texts can be constrained by the social contexts in which we and the work we do is situated. She calls on our imagination, in doing so invites us to remain uncertain. In writing final research texts, care has to be taken so that we can imagine others, so that we can create new possibilities to act differently, perhaps in this way writing with a sense of uncertainty allows us to challenge who the youth and we are and are becoming.

Challenges related to embodiment

Ethical relations are always lived embodiments, that is, they are always composed within our bodies, carrying the knowledge shaped by experiences lived in multiple places, over time and relationships. The knowledge that is embodied in each of us is the knowledge composed intergenerationally, the knowledge of our mothers and grandmothers, of fathers and grandfathers, stretching back. The knowledge that is embodied in us is the knowledge of the cultural, social, familial, and institutional narratives that we have lived within. The knowledge that is embodied in us is the knowledge that is written on our skins in shades and tones of colors, in features and shapes. We embody the knowledge of where we have come from and how we live this knowledge as narrative inquirers requires the attentiveness to who we are and who we are becoming, requires us to be silent and to contemplate who we and others are in each moment. That silent attentiveness to our own embodied knowledge and to the embodied knowledge of others becomes visible in Chapter 13 as Elder Francis shows us as he comes alongside Lane and Donovan.

As narrative inquirers it is challenging to be wakeful, aware of the knowledge we embody. As we came to the arts club and struggled to shape a space that would invite the youth to join us, some of us faced over and over again how our embodied knowledge shaped by teaching and schools was expressed in how we lived in the arts club space. We self-faced again and again, sometimes by studying photographs of how we stood, positioned ourselves, and looked at youth, sometimes by attending to how we laid out unfinished projects, how much we embodied who we were as teachers in the room. Those of us who were not Aboriginal self-faced to see how what was written on our skins shaped who we were in the stories of the youth. Sometimes the youth helped us in our self-facing by asking for "you know, the one who is a nurse" or "you know, the pretty one" and reminded us that their stories of us were shaped by what was written on our skins.

And yet, it was important to continue these processes of coming to know what we embodied by times of silent walking, by contemplating how we were shifting who we were, shifting the stories we live by. As the youth are not fixed and frozen as this way or that way, we as narrative inquirers are always also in the making, on our way. Learning to attend to our embodied knowledge is part of relational ethics as Elder Isabelle taught us through silent walking and stillness and silence.

Continuing challenges in relational ethics

As we turned considerations of relational ethics over and over in the conversations, we turned often to considerations of making sure we spoke to the relational ethics between people in the research but also relational ethics in the larger social/political contexts. For now, we engage in one last conversation about the challenges in relational ethics that remain.

JEAN: One continuing challenge around relational ethics in narrative inquiry emerges around writing final research texts. We, in some ways, move out of the relational ethical space of co-composing field texts and interim research texts when we begin to write final research texts that will become public – participants are no longer physically alongside us. When we are no longer physically alongside participants, how do we continue to live relational ethics?

VERA: It is interesting to think about what this means in terms of final research texts. How do we carry the relationships forward and make them visible in the texts, but also as we continue to live out our study. We, too, need to think about this in relation to others who joined the study as researchers initially. How do we continue to be responsible to each other? Sean, maybe thinking with your experience alongside Lane would help. I know you often talked about him.

SEAN: I think about how I am always trying to hold open an ethical space in the final writing of research texts – that multiple people continue to live in the space in the moments of composing research texts. You are right Vera, Lane and I really lived different life trajectories. We were so close during much of the time of my doctoral work and then our paths changed – Lane left school in a much more final way, he joined the circus and moved between communities and he began to travel with the circus. I, too, moved away and there was a physical separation. But in all of this I never forgot about Lane, the experiences he shared, and the experiences we lived together. I hold open a space for him, I could always go home to see him again. I could see Lane anywhere and my sense is that we could pick up our conversation. I look forward to the time when I will see Lane again, when he or his friends call me up for pizza.

JEAN: When we write final research texts, when we look across the threads that run across the narrative accounts, we need to write them in ways that keep open an ethical space in the writing and in future living.

SEAN: Lane and Donovan know that I will tell a good story, a thoughtful story, that I will be respectful and that I will hold open a space because in some ways I have to go back home to them with the stories that are shared. Both Lane and Donovan know that I talk about us and about them. They know they are part of a larger study in which they help us understand the experiences of Aboriginal youth.

VERA: In so many ways I think we negotiate these elements continuously. As Jean asked the question, I wondered what stories the youth tell about us. What stories does Lane tell of you and your relationship with him, Sean? What stories do they tell of us? They have agency in the stories they have lived alongside us. The stories stay alive in this way and the stories ask us to be respectful.

SEAN: There is a commitment that is called forth when we hold open the ethical space.

JEAN: We have to think about what it means to go home again. I think about Crow and Weasel (Lopez, 1990) and how the stories travel and how we live on storied landscapes. We are wakeful that the stories we tell have ripples; Thomas King (2003) reminds us that the stories we tell are loose in the world.

VERA: I have also been thinking about another challenge. In thinking with King (2003), I also think about the larger social political context in which our work can be taken up. Just recently I went with Chris to an educational institution to register for upgrading classes. He asked me to come with him. As we stood at the front desk, I could see how eyes followed me. I remember saying to Chris, "I wonder who they think I am."

SEAN: I can see how this is an important wonder about relational ethics. Our behaviors change as we, both the youth and I, are constructed and it shapes the way we go forward. It is a challenge to relational ethics because it changes us . . . whether we go silent, leave, or otherwise, it has changed us and subsequent events, perhaps in minor ways and perhaps in more major ways. What do the youth have to lose if we don't challenge constructions?

VERA: What happens to Chris if I challenge them? What happens to me? Sometimes it is to Chris's advantage if I am constructed as social service or an authority figure because we get better service or he receives more potential for access. However, it also could mean that Chris then can be constructed as one more deficit Aboriginal youth.

SEAN: I think about Lugones' (1987) world-traveling here and how we act on competing stories that might look different for different people. How do we negotiate our different loyalties? When I think about the competing stories I live in situations. I think about meeting the kids at West Edmonton mall when the kids were supposed to be in school . . . and the self-facing I did as I came to understand that one of the stories I live by is that school is good, valuable, important. In that moment I came to understand that my stories competed with what the kids wanted.

VERA: I don't think that living out relational ethics asks us to give up our beliefs, to not live out our stories to live by. But living relational ethics asks us to do more in other ways, to open up possibilities in order to live alongside the kids.

JEAN: I wonder what part response groups play in helping us to live out relational ethics. How do response groups help us stay wakeful to who we are in our relational work? Your talk about self-facing made me think about the people who come alongside us.

VERA: Perhaps it is important to think about how different response groups can be. In my work with both of you, I feel that we have become a very close response group, where we can raise the challenges, and ask each other to self-face – in these moments the ethical work is central.

SEAN: Yeah, I think that is important, but we have to situate ourselves each time and continue to do this. It's important that response groups are not layered in judgment. Relational ethics is not about right or wrong, but call us to think with our experiences. We need to continuously think about how we are changed, what we have silenced, what relationships we have perhaps not engaged in. It is important to know that we are part of response groups that challenge us – we are not in some kind of "high five" club, praising each other.

JEAN: What is important about response groups and how they help us to live out relational ethics is that we can help each other slow down, to say more, to count on others to help us tell a story differently, perhaps to understand an experience with more loving perception. Sometimes our embodied knowledge just seems to say "This is all I could do" or "This is the only way I could act" or "There was nothing I could do." Response helps us slow down, to ask about what Maxine Greene called otherwise, to imagine other possibilities forward.

VERA: And it allows us to act differently. For me, the work we do would not be possible without a sense of community and commitment to each other, as much as we live this way with participants, we also need to live this way with each other.

JEAN: What I learn through living within this response group has helped me in the ways I think about how to live in relationally ethical ways in the next study and the next, the idea of reverberations forward into what we do next.

SEAN: Living without a response community and trying to live relational ethics in narrative inquiry is like being lost in the woods!

References

Adichie, C. (2009, July). *The danger of a single story* [video file]. Retrieved from http://www.ted.com/talks/chimamanda_adichie_the_danger_of_a_single_story.html

Bateson, M. C. (1994). *Peripheral visions: Learning along the way*. New York: HarperCollins.

Bergum, V. (1999). Ethics as question. In T. Kohn & R. Mckechnic (Eds.), *Extending the boundaries of care: Medical ethics and caring practices* (pp. 167–180). New York: Oxford University Press.

Caine, V., Estefan, A., & Clandinin, D. J. (2013). A return to methodological commitment: Reflections on narrative inquiry. *Scandinavian Journal of Educational Research, 57*(6), 574–586, doi:10.1080/00313831.2013.798833

Charon, R., & Montello, M. (Eds.). (2002). *Stories matter: The role of narrative in medical ethics*. New York: Routledge.

Clandinin, D. J. (1985). Personal practical knowledge: A study of teachers' classroom images. *Curriculum Inquiry, 15*(4), 361–385.

Clandinin, D. J. (Ed.). (2007). *Handbook of narrative inquiry: Mapping a methodology*. Thousand Oaks, CA: Sage Publications.

Clandinin, D. J., & Caine, V. (2013). Narrative inquiry. In A. A. Trainor & E. Grace (Eds.), *Reviewing qualitative research in the social sciences* (pp. 166–179). New York: Routledge.

Clandinin, D. J., Caine, V., & Huber, J. (2016). Ethical considerations entailed by a relational ontology in narrative inquiry. In I. Goodson, A. Antikainen, M. Andrews, & P. Sikes (Eds.), *The Routledge international handbook on narrative and life history*. New York: Routledge.

Clandinin, D. J., & Connelly, F. M. (2000). *Narrative inquiry: Experience and story in qualitative research*. San Francisco, CA: Jossey-Bass.

Clandinin, D. J., & Rosiek, J. (2007). Mapping a landscape of narrative inquiry: Borderland spaces and tensions. In D. J. Clandinin (Ed.), *Handbook of narrative inquiry: Mapping a methodology* (pp. 35–75). Thousand Oaks, CA: Sage.

Connelly, F. M., & Clandinin, D. J. (1988). Studying teachers' knowledge of classrooms: Collaborative research, ethics, and the negotiation of narrative. *Journal of Educational Thought, 22*(2A), 269–282.

Connelly, F. M., & Clandinin, D. J. (1990). Stories of experience and narrative inquiry. *Educational Researcher, 19*(5), 2–14.

Greene, M. (1988). *The dialectic of freedom*. New York: Teachers College Press.

Greene, M. (1995). *Releasing the imagination: Essays on education, the arts, and social change*. San Francisco, CA: Jossey-Bass Publishers.

Huber, M., Clandinin, D. J., & Huber, J. (2006). Relational responsibilities of narrative inquirers. *Curriculum and Teaching Dialogue, 8*(2), 209–223.

King, T. (2003). *The truth about stories: A native narrative*. Toronto: House of Anansi Press.

Lessard, S., Caine, V., & Clandinin, J. (accepted). Exploring neglected narratives: understanding vulnerability in narrative inquiry. *Irish Educational Journal*.

Lopez, B. (1990). *Crow and weasel*. New York: North Point Press.

Lugones, M. (1987). Playfulness, "world"-travelling, and loving perception. *Hypatia, 2*(2), 3–19. doi:10.1111/j.1527-2001.1987.tb01062.x

Maclntyre, A. C. (1981). *After virtue: A study in moral theory*. Notre Dame, IN: University of Notre Dame Press.

Noddings, N. (1984). *Caring: A feminine approach to ethics and moral education*. Berkeleey and Los Angeles, CA: University of California Press.

18

LINGERING DEPARTURES

Reverberations through, and in, narrative inquiry response communities

Vera Caine, Sean Lessard, and D. Jean Clandinin

Beginning in the midst

> *Sitting together at Jean's kitchen table we talk about the work in the junior high arts club – we laugh about some of our experiences and recount the ongoing stories of the youth we remain in touch with – some of them now have families of their own, others are enrolled in educational programs, still others are finding their ways into jobs. We wonder about their unfolding lives. We remind each other that it has been more than 3 years since we filed the final reports with the funding agency and shared our findings with the school board and community partners.*
>
> *This conversation, long after we formally completed the study, is more than a reminiscence, more than the kind of happy talk that often becomes a bit too rosy when people gather to talk of times past. Sitting together opens into another dialogue as we pose questions about what we know about the youth's lives, our lives, and what we continue to learn from the study. Our conversation this morning turns away from the stories of the youth as we shift to contemplate how we have stayed in touch with each other, how we have continued to learn from, and with, not only the youth but each other.*
>
> *What brought us to the kitchen table with each other are wonders about the relational ethics of narrative inquiry alongside the youth. How, we wondered, do our experiences with the youth shape our ongoing work? But now as we look back on this conversation about the research with the youth, new wonders emerge about who we are in relation with each other. While we intentionally get together to engage in inquiry and writing, we also name ourselves as a response community. As we think with who we are as a response community, and as we think of other response communities, we ask ourselves about the reverberations of these communities. What sustains them? How do they hold possibility for lingering departures?*

Shaping questions about response communities

This book, and our chapter in it, explores ways to bring together metaphor and narrative, to bring together the ways that metaphors shape our living and telling of

Reprinted with permission. Acknowledgement; Caine, V., Lessard, S., & Clandinin, D. J. (2018). Lingering departures: reverberations through, and in, narrative inquiry response communities. In M. Hanne & A. A. Kaal (Eds.), *Narrative and metaphor in education: Look both ways* (Chapter 20, pp. 278–290). Abingdon and New York, NY: Routledge.

stories of experiences. As we begin, we play with the etymology of metaphor, from the Latin metaphora, a word that carries within it a sense of a transfer from one world to another, something carried over. We pause as we think about the centrality of response communities that allow us, as narrative inquirers, to carry over from one world to another, from one research project to another, in ways that open up new puzzles, and also allow us to ponder who we are, and are becoming, within these response communities. We begin this chapter in the midst of being embedded in a response community and in the midst of wondering about the place of response communities in narrative inquiry. We ask ourselves: How do response communities form? How do they function? What purposes do they serve in furthering research studies? How do they help us gain new insights?

Initially when we first began to imagine response communities, we conceptualized them as places where researchers working in a project met to discuss, share, and receive response to narrative accounts and final research texts we were writing (Clandinin, Steeves, & Caine, 2013). We have engaged in many such response communities with graduate students, colleagues, Elders, and, at times, community partners. We have encouraged the formation of many response communities (Clandinin & Connelly, 2000). We have seen tensions, and challenges in response communities, as well as possibilities; they are always spaces of ongoing negotiations. Perhaps, they are "both a safe space of coming home and starting new journeys" (Kubota, Menon, Redlich-Amirav, & Saleh, 2015, p. 161). However, we wondered about whether framing response communities in terms of safe spaces for homecomings, for returning and leaving again, was a robust enough way to think about the purposes response communities fulfilled for us and could serve for others.

As we considered the reverberations of our research programs where one study opens into another study (Clandinin, Lessard, & Caine, 2013), where ideas and insights continue past the end of one project and stretch into another, we began to explore the parts response communities play in furthering our, and others', always unfolding research programs. We began to explore how response communities keep us at further relationships, create possibilities to return to field texts, open further questions about participants' and our lives, and how they generate insights beyond those possible within defined research projects.

We turn again to our conversation at the kitchen table with which we open this paper and are reminded that as we engage in this ongoing research community, over time and place, we are reluctant to leave such a space that fosters such lively curiosity and dialogue. Embedded in this curiosity and dialogue is a sense of coming to know something different and coming to know something for the first time; it opens up possibilities. We turn again to considerations of the ways that response communities function in our research, both during a study, and in the spaces between studies where nascent puzzles begin to shape into new research studies, where the pursuit of ideas is critical.

As we think about the importance of slowing down, as one study leads into another, we see how these spaces, which are not determined by project timelines, allow us to return, to revisit, and to discuss again. Within these spaces we engage in re-search, searching again but searching with others. These response communities are formed and sustained intentionally; they are formed through ongoing negotiations of processes, of places, and of people coming together. As we consider ways of entering into, and opening up, the possibilities of response communities that stretch over time, we draw on two interwoven metaphors: a metaphor drawing on the ideas of response and responsibility, and a metaphor drawing on the ideas of lingering, of slowing down to stay longer than intended.

We remind ourselves that response is the root word of responsibility. The word response comes from the Latin *responsum* with its sense of 'something offered in return'. And while responsibility turns our attention to moral duties and obligations to satisfactorily perform or complete a task, response helps us see that responsibility also calls for something in return, something given in return for something offered. A metaphor of lingering draws our attention to the importance of something lasting over time, of being sustained over time, with a sense of reluctance to leave. These interwoven metaphors help us understand the purposes of response communities as places and people with whom we linger and with and to whom we owe response, a giving back of what we have been given but reshaped with new possibilities.

Jean, Sean, and Vera have been in conversation now for several years. Sean became connected during his graduate studies for a Masters Degree in Education. At that time we were just beginning to engage in a narrative inquiry into the experiences of youth who left school early (Clandinin, Steeves et al., 2013). The study had many research team members and participants from diverse settings were invited to participate through ongoing conversations stretched over months. We often think about this study; it was a starting place of a response community between Jean, Sean, and Vera. In reflecting on some of our early beginnings, we see what made this work for us. In part we worked counter to the often common university notion of around owning ideas, the idea of owning ideas and writing as individuals, as intellectual property. We did not live this sense of ownership of ideas, rather we started from a relational standpoint that made central the relationships we had with participants and with each other.

The early research that brought us together was a comprehensive inquiry into the experiences of Alberta youth who left school prior to graduation. The inquiry, undertaken in 2008–2010, involved both an extensive literature review and an empirical inquiry into the experiences of 19 youth who left school early. A strong relational stance was evident in how we worked with participants during our fieldwork, and became visible as we took turns around authorship of publications or presentations. What was particularly remarkable during the early years, and continuing into the future is the emphasis on curiosity and inquiry. What mattered most was that we figured things out together. Each coming together was marked by a sense of inquiry.

After our study alongside youth who left school early, we engaged in many conversations that led us to contemplate what sustains youth in school. Over time our interests became more focused and we became particularly interested in how indigenous youth and their families experienced education, both in and out of schools, and schooling (Clandinin, Caine, Lessard, & Huber, 2016, forthcoming). From 2010 to 2014, with the support of Social Sciences and Humanities Research Council of Canada (SSHRCC) and Alberta Centre for Children, Family and Community Research (ACCFCR) funding, we worked with indigenous youth in an afterschool club in a Canadian junior high school. New graduate students, scholars, and community agencies joined our team. Sean became a doctoral student whose work was embedded in this study. For two years we sustained the weekly after school club – it was a place filled with wonder and possibility. Outside of the club, Sean, Jean, and Vera engaged in many conversations – conversations that made visible their struggles with all aspects of experiences they encountered in the research, but their conversations became more than that. Over time, their ongoing conversations and commitment to each other and the research allowed them to come together as a response community. It was a slow process and one that called on their commitments to each other, as well as a commitment to who they are and are becoming.

As Sean, Jean, and Vera moved into new academic landscapes, they continued to write and inquire together. Their writings were fuelled by a desire to linger in past studies, to take 'one more look', to raise yet one more wonder. There were moments when they talked about new wonders, where they tried to make sense of the world around them. As they worked together, their conversations were also shaped by world events that marked recent migration patterns, that raised questions about the social inclusion of refugee populations, and that foreshadowed questions of their personal responsibilities in creating places that were marked by social inclusion. These conversations led us to propose a new SSHRC-funded study through which we could inquire into the experiences of refugee families with preschool children.

What makes a response community a response community?

As we engaged in a kind of autobiographical narrative inquiry (Clandinin, 2013) as we began to compose this chapter, we told stories of our experiences, one story calling forth another story, with a 'remember when?' or 'do you remember?' kind of sense to our stories. As we told, and then retold, stories of our experiences with an intention to understand more about the places, purposes, and intentions of response communities, we identified at least seven interwoven features of response communities that allow us to linger and to give response. Each feature needs to be present for a response community to be a space that sustains, that invites possibilities.

Feature 1: playfulness

> *We're gathered at the Centre table and we're talking about finding participants for the study with the youth who left school early. Without being able to somehow access participants through institutions like hospitals, schools or community agencies, we are stretching as we try to imagine ways to connect with potential participants. Sean volunteers that he could contact youth through facebook; Jean wonders about putting up posters at local grocery stores; Vera wonders about going through community centers that sponsor art displays. More ideas are tossed out: we laugh at what our suggestions tell us about our lives, laugh at our inability to get outside the boxes created by our skills at working with institutions to locate participants.*

The playfulness in this moment is remarkable and we see it as a key feature in our response community. While we could, at first glance, understand playfulness as humorous, our understandings of playfulness have been shaped by Lugones (1987) who wrote of playfulness in 'world'-travel. In her writing she pointed out that Gadamer's (1960) concept of play was an agonistic sense of play; she writes:

> an agonistic sense of play is one in which competence is supreme. [. . .] In agonistic play there is risk, there is uncertainty, but the uncertainty is about who is going to win and who is going to lose. There are rules that inspire hostility. The attitude of playfulness is conceived as secondary to or derivative from play. Since play is agon, then the only conceivable playful attitude is an agonistic one.
>
> *(Lugones, 1987, p. 15)*

This is not the idea of playfulness that Lugones sees as central to world traveling nor is it the one that we see as a key feature in response communities. We draw on Lugones' (1987) ideas of playfulness, where

> The playfulness that gives meaning to our activity includes uncertainty, but in this case the uncertainty is the openness to surprise. [. . .] We are not self-important, we are not fixed in particular constructions of ourselves, which is part of saying we are open to self-construction. We may not have rules, and when we do have rules, there are no rules that are to us sacred. We are not worried about competence [. . .] playfulness is, in part, an openness to being a fool, which is a combination of not worrying about competence, not being self-important, not taking norms as sacred and finding ambiguity and double edges a source of wisdom and delight.
>
> *(pp. 16–17)*

As we sat at the table, we were aware that we were struggling to get outside of our usual ways of easily finding participants: and, as we playfully engaged with each other, we were open to sharing who we were as visible in the ideas we held. This playfulness, this openness to playing the fool, that is, to not worrying about competence, self-importance or being seen as scholarly does not easily fit the dominant stories of engaging in research. And yet without this playful attitude the conversation would have been less productive, less filled with surprise at what we actually could come up with, and it would have been less sustaining. Abandoning the particular constructions of ourselves as researchers allowed us to see new possibilities. This playfulness is not marked by winning, or losing, or a sense of competition, rather it creates a sense of community where we become increasingly attentive to what we do not know, where we can gain a sense of "wisdom and delight" (Lugones, 1987, p. 17).

Feature 2: mutual responsibilities

The space that holds the possibility of playfulness is also marked by a sense of mutual responsibilities with research participants, as well as with each other. Mutual responsibilities open up spaces in relationships that are not always recognizable or clearly defined, they require wakefulness. The reshaping of relationships through mutuality suggests a back and forth commitment through our actions and attention to unfolding relationships. Sean recounts:

> *I think about an invitation from participants involved in the Early School Leavers study. Participants asked us (Sean, Jean, and Vera) to return to their junior high school with them, a school they had attended many years prior. I was a graduate student at this time, a beginning researcher who knew many students who had left school before graduation. My early experiences as a youth worker connected me to many youth, some of whom eventually became study participants. I was a connector in this study, somewhere between my relationships with the youth begun years earlier and in my relationships with the other researchers. My responsibilities rested within both places. The day we visited the junior high school, I recall walking slowly in the halls and listening to the youth tell many stories of school. They shared their experiences of classes and teachers, noting photographs and school sport banners displayed in the gymnasium, all memory markers*

of pride. Being alongside them that day in the school was a return to my own memories, as I recalled my time with the youth in the weekly after school program within this very school. I learned much from them and their families as we proudly called our after school group 'Mustang Pride'. Our group, named after the school team name, meant much more than that to us. Our school, a school where we first came to know each other, was in an urban setting, within the 'inner city'. It is was here youth taught me the importance of relationships and the importance of looking after one another. I look back and think about how relationships continue to shift and open up spaces to learn from one another.

Within this space of coming to know, and living alongside, participants, it is clear that we lived, and continue to live, the notion of mutual responsibilities, not only with participants, but also with each other. The youth participants took us to a place where their experiences were filled with good memories of school. Each of the participants had moved on to high school, but, over time, had left high school prior to graduation. Within the narrative inquiry they had the opportunity to return to memories and to teach us about what life looked like for them within this place and what they saw as important. For them, it was important to show us their junior high school. The mutual responsibilities in this relationship are defined by the willingness to travel to unexpected places, to open up memories and experiences. The mutual responsibilities between participants and between our relationships as researchers, opens up a space that is filled with uncertainty and not knowing, where participants lead the way and where knowledge shared is transactional and beyond what we had initially imagined. Mutual responsibilities live within the trusting processes of following, listening, and learning from participants, as well as from our experiences that push our understandings of each other.

Feature 3: understanding multiplicity of tensions

After spending several hours at Jean's kitchen table, it was time to take a walk to the local coffee shop. It was a welcome 20 minute walk down and back up a hill. Our side by side walking was accompanied by reflections and we had come to appreciate the rhythms that it called forth. Sean spoke of a young woman, a participant in another project with other youth. He spoke of the challenges of working across gender stereotypes. His struggles of working with the young girl led to a break in his relationship with the participant. Sean expressed sadness, as he wondered how Marie was doing. Walking slowly beside Sean, Vera turned towards him and asked, "Did you really not contact her again?" The tone in Vera's voice made Sean stop. He had been struggling with who he was in the stories others would potentially tell of him in relation with Marie. He was upset with Vera when she opened up that story, asking a question about what was a hard story for Sean to live and tell. A story perhaps best left alone with the hope that it would resolve itself, become easier to live within. Yet, silence as a response to this story was not a way to live our mutual responsibilities – tensions were present and the question Vera raised made these more visible. Our conversations continued, at first about Marie, and then about other things, but still centred around how we each are socially constructed. Weeks later Sean told Vera and Jean that he had written a letter to Marie.

Being part of a response community is sustaining and the mutual responsibilities are lived in ways that honor who participants are and who we each are and are becoming. Yet, over time, we also experience, and will continue to experience, not only tensions called forth within our relationships but tensions as we bump against institutional stories of efficiency, as we are called to claim ownership of ideas and as we are asked to pursue programs of research that place us individually at the centre of our work. The tensions have a living edge in that they help us stay awake to our lives and to the lives of participants. These tensions call us to wakefulness, not to resolution of tensions, but to trusting our responsibilities within response communities, to seeing the beauty and possibility in staying with inquiry edges.

These calls to wakefulness are sometimes challenges to who we are and are becoming, challenges to our stories to live by (Connelly and Clandinin, 1999). These challenges are based on knowing that we are always in the making, that we need to stay attentive to who we are becoming and wakeful to the stories that continue to, as Basso (1996) writes, work on us. These challenges often awaken us to previously smoothed over edges, creating places where we have learned to live with at least some ease. As we respond to each other, we are called to become vulnerable in ways that allow us to inquire further, to engage with ideas. At other times, response communities call us to explain why we behave in the world in certain ways.

In Sean's telling, and in Vera's response, we see how response opens up the story for further inquiry. In her response, Vera calls Sean to wakefulness about how he had become at ease in a socially constructed narrative in which he could not be otherwise with the young girl. The encounter is not a comfortable one for it opens up an inquiry edge that had been smoothed over, albeit in ways that Sean felt were not comfortable. Had he felt at ease with the story he would not have told it to Vera. The readiness to acknowledge tensions and to even, with care for the stories that we each live and tell, create tensions through our responses is part of what keeps us at response communities, keeps us at inquiry edges.

Feature 4: relational ethics: ethics of friendship

In the opening storied fragment of the paper we told of one of our kitchen table talks, of sharing what had happened in our lives since our last meeting. Each time we come together we spend some time in conversation about our lives, sharing stories of our recent travels, of encounters with people we know, of events with our children and families, of our health concerns, of our recent achievements, disappointments, and struggles. This takes some time, time that is not usually allotted on the agendas of research meetings. And yet we know that this attention to each other, this creation of, and lingering in, the relational spaces of who we are and who we are becoming is key to response communities.

The spaces of response communities do not have their first focus on outcomes, although much is accomplished, rather they focus first on who we are in relation to each other and to the research we are doing. It is a reminder that we need to focus on the ethics of everyday life, to see who we are, and are becoming, without layers of judgement, about not seeing within a binary of right or wrong but a seeing from within an other's worlds. This telling and retelling of our lives each time we come together is, in part, created by working within a relational ethics. These times spent living with each other within a space marked by relational ethics helps us to think about how we are changing, what we are silencing, what we are privileging.

These times remind us of the differences in our lives – in knowing that people's lives have different rhythms, are shaped by different concerns, are shaped by larger narratives. We are not all the same and yet, in our way of attending to ourselves and to each other within a relational ethics, we stay open to the possibilities and gifts we each bring. As experiences are shared, we each feel the energy and safety of knowing the embrace of the response community. For us, response communities are also influenced by our understanding of friendship as a marker of a good life. It is important that this sense of friendship implies that we are honest with each other, that we challenge what we have come to know and the ways in which we live our lives. We do not expect vacuous praise, a kind of general praise without substance.

The lingering time created by a relational ethics allows us to slow down, to say more, to count on each other to help us tell our stories differently, perhaps to understand an experience with more loving perception (Lugones, 1987). We then come to understandings that make visible complexities and layers previously unseen. We have certainty that we will always walk away as friends, with more wide awakeness about who we are in relation to each other, to ourselves, to participants, and to the research in which we are engaged.

Feature 5: imagination

In the story of Vera's questioning response to Sean's story, we saw the possibility of questioning who we are, and are becoming, within our response community. Within these questions about who we are, and in responses to think otherwise, we open questions around 'How do we live our social responsibilities to each other, to participants, and to the larger communities?' These larger questions within which smaller, more project-specific questions are nested, are not ones we stay away from in our response community.

These questions call us to imagine otherwise; taking up these questions requires that we think of "[i]magination [as] the capacity to think of things as if they could be otherwise" (Greene, 1988, p. 1). In times marked by uncertainty, increasing inequities, and a sense of global unrest, a sense of imagination is critical in our work and vitally important in our response community. Where else are we called to imagine otherwise as we face these necessarily troubling questions? According to Greene (1995), "[s]ocial imagination is the capacity to invent visions of what should be and what might be in our deficit society, in the streets where we live and our schools. Social imagination not only suggests but also requires that one take action to repair or renew" (p. 5). In this way imagination both lives within, and is brought to life in, response communities. We see this as Vera questions Sean and Sean begins to imagine a new story of being in relation with Marie, in spite of the larger social narrative that would place him in a single story in relation with a youth who is a girl. In Vera's questioning response to Sean's told story, she did not tell him what to do but drew him to his imagination, drew him to the larger narratives in which the single story of him and the youth were embedded. In Sean's response lived the possibility of otherwise, a way forward that allowed him to imagine ways to take action, to change how he and Marie might live the deficit story created by the social narrative.

For us, imagination is connected to playfulness and to world travelling in response communities. Playfulness and world travelling allow us to become vulnerable, to realize the sense of the other over time, in diverse places, and social contexts. This realization is also reflected when Arendt (1994) writes of the ways that imagination helps each of us make sense of the larger contexts and audiences with whom we want to share our research.

> Imagination alone enables us to see thing in their proper perspective, to be strong enough to put that which is too close at a certain distance so that we

> can see and understand it without bias and prejudice, to be generous enough to bridge abysses of remoteness until we can see and understand everything that is too far away from us as though it was our own affair.
>
> (*p. 323*)

We see Arendt's understandings of imagination as entwined with relational ethics. Her idea that it is imagination that allows researchers "to be generous enough to bridge abysses of remoteness" and to understand "as though it was our own affair" calls us to be attentive to the life in front of us, as well as to the social contexts in which experiences are shaped. Response communities hold the possibilities to raise questions, to imagine possibilities, and re-tell and re-live our experiences. Imagination is central to the joy we experience in being part of response communities.

Feature 6: safety

> *In the midst of the narrative inquiry alongside youth who left school early, Jean struggled with understanding the experiences of one particular youth, Andrew. Andrew, a star basketball player on an elite high school team, puzzled Jean and she knew she had not yet been able to come alongside Andrew, to understand why he had not remained in school even after he was removed from the team. "Sean", Jean asked, "could you please read this and help me understand Andrew". Sean, who worked in a high school and knew something of Andrew's life, read the account and together he and Jean talked. "In order to understand Andrew you need to understand the institutional narrative, you need to understand what it is like to be a star basketball player in a big high school, someone who has his locker with the team lockers, who wears a special school jacket, who is among the highest status youth in the school. Imagine what it is to lose that status and still have to go to school each day, without the jacket, the prestige, to still have to go to your locker where other team members have their lockers". As Sean talked, Jean was able to come alongside Andrew, to walk metaphorically with him into the school after he had been taken off the school team.*

Jean's action of turning to Sean to help her understand her experiences alongside Andrew gives a sense of the safety within the response community. Drawing attention to safe spaces in research has a bit of a clichéd sense as many researchers talk of the importance of trust and relationship in safe spaces as necessary preconditions for gathering interview or other qualitative research data. Just what this entails is not always clear as safety sounds like a stable condition where someone is safe from harm, danger or risk. In a response community, along with the other key features of playfulness and imagination, safety is connected to the experience of being accepted for who one is. While Jean felt safe in turning to Sean, knowing that he would come alongside her to help her figure out what she was missing, she also knew that her request would be met by Sean's sense of mutual responsibility. Here layers of institutional hierarchies and expertise, become less central and, while we are wakeful that they exist, we are intentional in dismantling them.

In acknowledging the importance of safety in a response community, we are not suggesting that there is protection from danger or risk. Rather we are suggesting that there is safety because we know that there will be response, that we will be met with playfulness, the openness to being otherwise that comes from imagination, and the surety of response situated in mutual responsibility. While we could focus on competence and the importance of being knowledgeable, in a response community we have learned that safety comes with understanding the nature of response communities that ask us to take risks, to imagine otherwise, and to share vulnerabilities. Safety within our response community creates a kind of dwelling place for each of us, a safety that the community will continue to respond in ways that ask us to consider otherwise, to consider what might be, that asks us to risk and to enter worlds (Lugones, 1987) where we feel dis/ease, not comfort. Safety comes with being asked to feel dis/ease – knowing that response communities will give back with possibilities.

Feature 7: staying with ideas

Memories of '*Mustang Pride*' come to mind as we sit as a response community at the Centre for Research for Teacher Education and Development on an unseasonably warm winter day in Alberta. We have sat at this table many times as colleagues and friends. Today we are writing and preparing for a future research study and upcoming presentation. We are discussing concepts woven throughout different research studies. Sean speaks:

> *I think about the ideas that have stayed with me and the experiences that are shaping influences in my life. I am thinking about my time as a youth worker and the 'Mustang Pride' moments and how they have shaped my teaching. Really, in many ways, they have shaped my life. These early experiences never quite left me and have guided me and sustained me in ways that I could not have imagined.*

Jean, Vera, and Sean look at each other, knowing that memories are being called forth, much in the same way thoughts turn to experience and to the sharing of stories that stay with us. The beginning points of learning about research, methodology, and design are important for all of us. However, what stands out is how we are rooted and committed to the relational ontology of narrative inquiry over time; we know this commitment is shared and shapes how we think about lives and what matters. We recall moments of past research studies, like the Early School Leavers study. And we look back now and see how it continues to shape future studies, like the study alongside urban aboriginal youth, the studies that are part of Growing Young Movers, and now a beginning study with Syrian Refugee families. While thinking about our research studies we acknowledge the theoretical connections to Dewey (1934) and how other scholars have also shaped narrative inquiry. The dialogue is rich, always going back to, and turning concepts over and over, in relationship and dialogue. The dialogue pushes in new directions and toward new possibilities over time. Sean slowly speaks again:

> *The importance of 'conversational spaces' in school resonates with me in particular. Vera makes me think about times when 'there are no conversational spaces'. These are important concepts and ideas that reverberate through, and trigger, discussions that both shape us and sustain us in our thinking. It is through the intentionality of design and actions within the field, we live a commitment to further understand experience.*

We move backwards to pull forward other concepts such as 'coming alongside' participants in the research and 'relational ethics' and 'world-travelling' as Lugones (1987) might say – these are concepts that shape, and are shaped, by our ideas. Okri (1997), King (2003), Anzaldúa (1990), Arendt (1958, 1994), Addams (1902), Baylor (1994) and other names are brought forth in the dialogue. We realize that while we have formed a close and lasting response community, we, too, are part of other response communities that have formed over time. These include the weekly research issues table (Clandinin et al., 2015) and a newly formed narrative inquiry reading group using video links where we engage with the ideas of pragmatists. It is our commitment to ideas and to each other that bind us.

Lingering in our response community

> *We're beginning a new project, one that takes us back to the stories of experience that first brought us together. We want to linger more, spend more time trying to understand what it means to compose a live in a place where you are not quite sure that you belong, not sure that you ever can belong. It takes us back to those who leave school early, to the importance of finding and creating conversational spaces. A returning to the idea of conversational spaces, an idea that comes back to mind as we consider our new puzzles alongside Syrian refugee families. Here we want to think with those coming to a new country, those who are leaving their homes because staying is not possible. We linger again with old ideas, ideas that see lives as always in the making. Seeing that we want to understand more, more about what seems foreign to us, but also more about our responsibilities. Always still wondering about what our responses can be.*

As we compose this chapter, we are beginning to draw together researchers who will work on a new project, a project which helps us puzzle through the experiences of young children and their families who are arriving from war-torn Syria. Our puzzle is around their experiences of coming to belong in a new country, a country very different from the one they are fleeing. And we puzzle around the ways their stories to live by will be reshaped, as their lives bump against the ways the larger social, cultural, institutional, familial, and linguistic narratives structure the local Canadian places into which they will move. We wonder about stories of families and family stories, about stories which welcome them, and stories which other them. And in the midst, we count on our response community to help us stay wakeful to who we are, to what we are learning about ourselves and others, about our responsibilities to them and to each other, about imagination, about playfulness, about tensions, about relational ethics and about staying with ideas. We each bring our unique stories to live by to these new research puzzles, stories shaped by difference, by moving from one place to another, stories shaped by belonging and not belonging. What we know is that we can count on a response community, one that may include new people, to allow us to engage in the ways we are now imagining.

References

Addams, J. (1902). *Democracy and social ethics*. New York. Macmillan Co.

Anzaldúa, G. (Ed.). (1990). *Making face, making soul/Haciendo caras: Creative and critical perspectives by feminists of color*. San Francisco, CA: Aunt Lute Books.

Arendt, H. (1958). *The human condition*. Chicago, IL: The University of Chicago Press.

Arendt, H. (1994). *Understanding and politics (the difficulties of understanding)*. In J. Kohn (Ed.), *Essays in understanding 1930–1954* (pp. 307–327). New York: Harcourt Brace & Company.

Basso, K. (1996) *Wisdom sits in places. Landscape and language among the Western Apache*. Albuquerque, NM: University of New Mexico Press.

Baylor, B. (1994). *The table where rich people sit.* New York: Aladdin Paperbacks.

Clandinin, D. J. (2013). *Engaging in narrative inquiry.* London: Routledge.

Clandinin, D. J., Caine, V., Estefan, A., Huber, J., Murphy, S., & Steeves, P. (2015). Places of practice: Learning to think narratively. *Narrative Works, 5*(1).

Clandinin, D. J., Caine, V., & Lessard, S. (forthcoming). *Relational ethics in narrative inquiry.* London: Routledge.

Clandinin, D. J., Caine, V., Lessard, S., & Huber, J. (2016). *Engaging in narrative inquiry with children and youth.* London: Routledge.

Clandinin, D. J., & Connelly, F. M. (2000). *Narrative inquiry: Experience and story in qualitative research.* San Francisco, CA: Jossey-Bass.

Clandinin, D. J., Lessard, S., & Caine, V. (2013). Reverberations of narrative inquiry: How resonant echoes of an inquiry with early school leavers shaped further inquiries. *Educação, Sociedade e Culturas, 36*, 7–24.

Clandinin, D. J., Steeves, P., & Caine, V. (Eds.). (2013). *Composing lives in transition: A narrative inquiry into the lives of early school leavers.* London: Emerald.

Connelly, F. M., & Clandinin, D. J. (1999). *Shaping a professional identity: Stories of educational practice.* New York: Teachers College Press.

Dewey, J. (1934). *Art as experience.* New York: Capricorn Books.

Gadamer, H. (1960). *Truth and method.* London: Continuum International Publishing Group.

Greene, M. (1988). *The dialectic of freedom.* New York: Teachers College Press.

Greene, M. (1995). *Releasing the imagination: Essays on education, the arts, and social change.* San Francisco, CA: Jossey-Bass Publishers.

King, T. (2003). *The truth about stories.* Toronto: Anansi Press.

Kubota, H., Menon, J., Redlich-Amirav, D., & Saleh, M. (2015). A narrative conception of professional development as a nested community. *Learning Landscapes, 9*(1).

Lugones, M. (1987). Playfulness, "world"-travelling, and loving perception. *Hypatia, 2*(2), 3–19. doi:10.1111/j.1527-2001.1987.tb01062.x

Okri, B. (1997). *A way of being free.* London: Phoenix House

19

EXPLORING NEGLECTED NARRATIVES

Understanding vulnerability in narrative inquiry

Sean Lessard, Vera Caine and D. Jean Clandinin

Beginning with a question

'Do you always work with vulnerable people?' is a question asked of Jean at the Contemporary Ethnographies Across the Disciplines conference in Cape Town, South Africa, in November 2016. In a plenary session, Jean had spoken of our narrative inquiry with the youth and families of Aboriginal heritage. She had not characterized the youth and their families as vulnerable so when the question was posed in a small group conversation after the keynote address, she was initially puzzled. Several weeks later, we – Jean, Sean, and Vera – sit together at Vera's kitchen table as Jean shares the question and her uncertainty about the question. The original question to Jean and her puzzlement call us to think again about our understandings of vulnerability, particularly in narrative inquiry. In thinking with this question, we call forth memories of earlier work, as well as new wonders, including Who gets to name vulnerability? What is vulnerability? How do we understand vulnerability in narrative inquiry? In thinking with the question asked of Jean at the conference, we return again to our study alongside indigenous youth and their families (Lessard, Caine, and Clandinin 2015; Clandinin et al. 2016).

Our thinking takes us back to the early days of the inquiry when we were writing proposals to obtain funding for this study. While we seldom make visible the work entailed in writing proposals for funding agencies, it was in writing the proposal that we began to think carefully with, and about, notions of vulnerability and to struggle with how to write about experiences of indigenous youth. As researchers, educators, and consultants for schools, we were aware of the challenges of sustaining indigenous students in schools: many indigenous students leave school prior to their high school graduation; and for many others, the transition between junior high school and high school marks their exit from the formal school system. We were aware of other evidence that appeared to forefront the

Reprinted with permission. Acknowledgement; Lessard, S., Caine, V., & Clandinin, D. J. (2018). Exploring neglected narratives: Understanding vulnerability in narrative inquiry. *Irish Educational Studies*, *37*(2), 191–204.

vulnerability of indigenous students. We made our struggle around constructing the youth as vulnerable visible stating:

> We will not repeat empirical data that portrays the experiences and achievements and, more often, the lack of achievement or deficit of Aboriginal youth in Canadian schools. Instead we focus on ways to make spaces for Aboriginal youth and families' experiences and to engage in telling more complex stories to ensure the voices of Aboriginal youth and their families have a place within Canadian education, beyond pictures in books, and school policies that far too often reflect a colonial curriculum.
>
> *(Battiste and Henderson 2000; Canadian Council on Learning 2007)*

At a later point in the proposal, we quoted LaFromboise, Trimble, and Mohatt (1990) who noted that Aboriginal youth 'live in a complex world of multiple loyalties – a world that challenges, sustains, and sometime destroys them but seldom removes their Indianness' (637). While we made our awareness of the complexities visible within the proposal, we struggled with positioning indigenous youth in particular ways, imposing categories and labels on them, or positioning our work as fixing them through interventions, or solving what was described as a problem of lower high school graduation rates for indigenous students in comparison to non-indigenous students.

Wonders about vulnerability

Returning to our proposal opens up questions of how we, as narrative inquirers, engage with indigenous youth, a population that is often considered inherently vulnerable because of their ethnicity and age. Many of the youth live, and have lived, complex lives in diverse geographical places. In Sean, Jean, and Vera's conversations over time, we wondered what happens when we reduce the complexities of their lives to a certainty that they are vulnerable, that is we label them as vulnerable and do not move beyond the naming of them as vulnerable to ask of, or about, their experiences. This also raised questions about how we ourselves, as researchers and people, are positioned in relation to, and with, vulnerability. Vera looked out the window as we sat at the kitchen table, and recalled for Sean and Jean:

> When we were writing the final report for the project, I returned to the proposal to see how the work we imagined many years prior had unfolded. I wondered if I would have seen Chris, Donovan, or Lane differently had I not struggled with the categories of school dropout, Indigenous, or male youth? Would it have been possible to disrupt these imaginings? Or to see who I could have become in relation to them?

Sometimes the concern about vulnerability becomes visible when researchers believe that someone else needs to speak for youth, that is, that youth themselves cannot be seen as research participants who are able to tell of, and inquire into, their experiences, or make decisions about the ways they are involved. Sometimes, implicitly or explicitly, researchers address the dangers that arise because of their belief in the youth's perceived vulnerability by not allowing them to speak, by co-opting their stories of experience, by writing over their stories, or by unintentionally minimizing the complexity of their experiences. In this paper, we take up the concerns around vulnerability to show how, as narrative inquirers, we are searching to find ways to think with vulnerability and with what others have called neglected narratives (Neglected Narratives Conference, 2015). We show how we come alongside youth in order to make their lives visible in the research and, consequently, to make their stories matter. We do this through maintaining a relational ethical stance (Clandinin et al. 2016; Clandinin, Caine, and Lessard 2018) throughout all aspects of each inquiry. In this way, we understand lives as always in the making, and, in that making, as holding the possibility to shift.

In the process of thinking with vulnerability, we cannot ignore who 'we' are. We see the intricate link, the entanglements of vulnerability, voice, and responsibility as we attend to who we are in relationships with participants. After three years of working alongside youth in the study, Sean wrote:

> I was trying to be much more attentive to who I was in relation to research participants I worked alongside (Clandinin and Connelly 2000). I was trying to slow down and think alongside – no diagnosis, no rush to conclusions. I was a work-in-progress. I was troubled as I thought about being a former youth worker, a teacher with the Aboriginal portfolio, a community worker, and a hopeful academic. These 'roles' pulled me towards 'knowing' what I thought might work with youth (Lugones 1987). I reminded myself that when I thought I had an answer or solution to the complexities in a life, there was a moment where I needed to spend time in deeper thought and consideration. It was as if I absorbed this approach through the lens of an interventionist or someone who tries to fix pieces of a life that are perhaps not mine to fix.
>
> *(Lessard 2013, 162)*

He considered:

> The relationships with Lane and Donovan [two participants in the study] took me back to days long ago when I used to spend most of my evenings working within the community. The titles and job descriptions were varied; some called me a youth worker, justice worker, mentor, or coach. In the moments of little formal education these are the jobs that I was drawn to. I was moved by the desire to lift a spirit even if sometimes selfishly the spirit was my own.
>
> *(214)*

As Sean reminded us of these considerations, we were drawn back again to attend to the multiplicity of who we are in each relationship, over time, and in multiple places. Who we are, and are becoming, is an ongoing challenge to how we are positioned in each narrative inquiry. And this careful attentiveness to who we are in relation shapes the ways we understand vulnerability in narrative inquiry.

What do we mean by narrative inquiry?

We work with a particular understanding of narrative inquiry, developed over many years, that draws on various theoretical resources such as Dewey's (1938) concept of experience, a concept that draws us toward a relational ontology. We use the following definition most often.

> People shape their daily lives by stories of who they and others are and as they interpret their past in terms of these stories. Story, in the current idiom, is a

> portal through which a person enters the world and by which their experience of the world is interpreted and made personally meaningful. Narrative inquiry, the study of experience as story, then, is first and foremost a way of thinking about experience. Narrative inquiry as a methodology entails a view of the phenomenon. To use narrative inquiry methodology is to adopt a particular view of experience as phenomenon under study.
>
> *(Connelly and Clandinin 2006, 375)*

Simply put, narrative inquiry is the study of experience understood narratively. Working with a narrative conception of experience, Clandinin and Rosiek (2007) pointed out that

> Framed within this view of experience, the focus of narrative inquiry is not only on individuals' experience but also on the social, cultural, and institutional narratives within which individuals' experiences are constituted, shaped, expressed, and enacted. Narrative inquirers study the individual's experience in the world, an experience that is storied both in the living and telling and that can be studied by listening, observing, living alongside one another and writing and interpreting texts.
>
> *(42–43)*

While understanding experience as a narrative phenomenon, inquiry is also an essential part of narrative inquiry. While both holding a particular narrative view of experience and attending to experience through the living and telling of stories are important, it is essential that we inquire into experiences, into the living and telling of stories, and into stories as lived and told. Narrative inquiry, the study of experience understood narratively, means much more than telling stories, much more than living stories.

It is Dewey's work that inspires the ways we bring experience alive in our narrative conception of experience. Dewey's theory of experience (1938), often cited as the philosophical underpinning of narrative inquiry (Clandinin and Connelly 2000), is central to our understandings of narrative inquiry. We see, for example, Deweyan foundations in the metaphorical three-dimensional narrative inquiry space with its dimensions of temporality, place, and sociality. Dewey's two criteria of experience – interaction and continuity enacted in situations – ground a narrative conception of experience. Clandinin and Connelly linked Dewey's criterion of interaction, that is, that a person is always in interaction with his/her world, to the dimension of sociality. The dimension of sociality asks that we attend to personal conditions and, simultaneously, to social conditions. By personal conditions, 'we mean the feelings, hopes, desires, aesthetic reactions and moral dispositions' (Connelly and Clandinin 2006, 480) of the inquirer and participants. Social conditions refer outward, to the milieu, the conditions within which people's experiences and events are unfolding. Clandinin and Connelly linked Dewey's second criterion of experience, continuity, to how a person's experience both takes up and moves from past experiences to present and future experiences with the dimension of temporality. The dimension of temporality draws attention to ways in which the past, present, and future of people, places, things, and events are interrelated, that is always in temporal transition, always on the way, in the making.

Clandinin and Connelly also drew attention to a third dimension, place (Basso 1996; Marmon Silko 1996), and linked it to Dewey's concept of situation. Within the three-dimensional narrative inquiry space, place is 'the specific concrete, physical, and topological boundaries of place or sequences of places where the inquiry and events take place' (Connelly and Clandinin 2006, 481). Working with Dewey's notion of situation allowed us to attend to the place or places where events occur.

Narrative inquiry with indigenous youth: contexts from which fragments are taken

In 2010 we, along with others, designed a narrative inquiry to inquire into the schooling and educational experiences of 12- to 15-year-old Aboriginal youth and their families. Aboriginal peoples are indigenous populations and, in Canada, are referred to by their legal status such as First Nations, Métis, or Inuit as constitutionally defined. In planning the narrative inquiry, we asked community members to help us frame a research puzzle that would allow us to hear multiple stories of the experiences of urban Aboriginal youth and their families outside of school. It was critically important to think with others within various communities in order to help us shape and reshape the research puzzle. These intentional processes of asking members of diverse communities acknowledged the larger personal and social contexts within the particular narrative inquiry and also kept us wakeful to the ways people's experiences are nested within larger social, institutional, linguistic, familial, and cultural narratives (Clandinin and Connelly 2000). Through these conversations during our design and proposal writing times, we built relationships and developed research partners, with Elders and Traditional Knowledge Keepers who guided the study, and shaped how we began to locate participants. We were attentive to how these opening considerations shaped, and shifted, the study and shaped how we found participants, and how we slowly came to realize, they found us (Clandinin et al. 2016).

As we engaged with communities about the research, we were mindful that we needed to satisfy the requirements of the university ethics board, which had particular ways of understanding vulnerabilities. The Canadian Tri-Council Research Ethics Policy focuses on respect for human dignity with special ethical obligations toward persons – or groups whose situation, diminished competence, and/or decision-making capacity make them vulnerable in the context of the research, and therefore unable to give full, free, and voluntary informed consent. The focus was on diminished competence and/or decision-making capacity and the need for special protections for people or groups who are vulnerable to abuse, exploitation, or discrimination. Within the Tri-Council guidelines, indigenous youth and their families are defined as vulnerable. We also sought approval through a local school district with its definition of vulnerabilities, which focuses on children and youth who, because of their age, a disability, or other circumstances, whether temporary or permanent, are in a position of dependence on others or are otherwise at a greater risk that the general population of being harmed by persons in a position of authority or trust relative to them. All children and youth are considered vulnerable because of their age and their relations with people in positions of trust and authority.

We eventually gained ethical approval from the university and institutional approval to work in a school. We began to establish what became known as the art club at a junior high school and began to invite students who were interested to join us in the club as the opening phase of coming alongside participants. We met each Wednesday afternoon after school, in the time allotted for school clubs, for approximately 90 minutes over a two-year period of time. We were very consistent in our participation in the art club. On any given Wednesday afternoon, at least two researchers were present. As we came to know youth in the art club, we gradually invited them, and people within their families, to participate in more intensive research conversations with us. It was as we began to work with the youth in the club that we again were called to consider vulnerability, particularly around the issue of naming the club and who the participants were who came to the club.

Names matter: considerations of vulnerability

Working within an afterschool place made us aware of working within a school with its overall rules and protocols but without attention to the requirements of the mandated curriculum. We asked for a place that was part of the school, a classroom, as it made participation more readily accessible to students after school hours. When youth, who we met in school hallways, or the front office, or the parking lot asked us where we were meeting, we often replied by saying, *the classroom at the end of the hall or the room the art teacher used last year.* Initially, the researchers named the club 'The U of A arts club'. Naming it came with challenges.

As we revisited field texts from the early beginnings of 'the U of A arts club', we were reminded of the importance of names, particularly in relation to vulnerability. What we mean by attending to the importance of names is the importance of attending to the names we carry with us, as well as the names we come to know each other by, and through, at various temporal points of the research. Attending closely to the names we each carry matters as we consider labelling and vulnerability. In our reflective turn, we noted that we designed a research study alongside members of diverse communities, paying careful attention to the definitions and categorizations that seemed to be present when engaging alongside Aboriginal youth and their families. Just what names and terms were used mattered as they evoked certain images and shaped dialogue that could minimize and categorize the lives of youth, their families, and their communities. Names mattered long before we started formal research conversations; names mattered when we first imagined a research study alongside Aboriginal youth, their families, and communities; names mattered when we began to live alongside the youth and their families.

Our research plan involved a specific geographic location within an urban setting, within a community, within a school district, and within a school that carried stories of all these places. We heard places labelled as West side or North side, as inner city, urban, and as reserve. While these are geographical markers, they are often misplaced and misguided when they are used in their categorical and systemic sorting functions. These names mattered because they called us to resist the singularity and simplicity of what these place name markers evoked.

As we began to work with the youth and their families, we were careful, mindful, and respectful that we were entering into the midst of relationships with intentions about what is possible and forward looking, and with intentions to not be defined by dominant scripts that shaped the experiences of researchers and participants in narrative inquiry. Drawing on our field notes, we wrote:

> Possible names for the after school 'club time' began to circulate as we first met youth within the school. While the time and place – an unused classroom – were set, the name of the club was open. The most simple of exercises, that is, naming the club, became complicated and nuanced. We, alongside some of the youth who began to attend the club from the first days, planned to develop a poster to let students know where we met and that, over time, we had a space

that could be recognized as a school club. We wondered, what could we possibly call this besides an 'art club', which had been our researcher name for the club? Surely we must be able to figure out a name alongside youth. As we talked in the club with the youth and with each other, names were presented: some with laughter; others with a more serious tone. Some names emerged as a possibility, with one standing out: 'The Neechie Club'. Neechie was presented by a student with a strong voice and presence. We did our best to seek consensus among the youth for a name, as they considered this classroom in this afterschool time period as their connecting space in the school. Neechie is a strong name, a name that simply means friend in Cree, a language that has strong indigenous roots in this part of western Canada. The name offered the opportunity to express an openness for friendship. Yet, the name met resistance and the immediate resistant reaction to this proposed name stayed with us as researchers. Attending carefully we learned that even the simple activity of choosing a name could signal inclusion, exclusion, vulnerability, strength, belonging or complex interweaving of all of the meanings. Names mattered, not just to the youth or to us, but also to their families.

Contemplating vulnerability as an ethical matter

We were wakeful that resistance to a name, which signalled for us friendship, signalled to some youth exclusion and called forth ethical considerations. Often when we think of ethical considerations in narrative inquiries with children and youth, we are reminded that vulnerability is a fluid concept, one that can be understood in multiple ways and one that is significant to all aspects of narrative inquiry. When the concept of vulnerability emerges in discussions around narrative inquiries with children and youth, we need to ask: What are children and/or youth vulnerable to? (Tronto 2014) Do these vulnerabilities lead us to consider different obligations and responsibilities and, if so, what are these obligations and responsibilities? When obligations and responsibilities call forth elements of care, there is a danger of pathogenic vulnerability, a vulnerability that arises from oppression or injustice, from a place of not respecting the choices of children and youth (Mackenzie, Rogers, and Dodds 2013). In these moments, we need to pause to carefully consider the connections between power and research (in the research processes, between participants and researchers, and also between participants). In the pause, what Arendt (1958) might call a stop and think, we also question: Who is responsible for dealing with vulnerabilities in children and youth's lives? Inherent vulnerability, a vulnerability intrinsic to the human condition, can neither be equated with a situational or contextual vulnerability nor be seen as a reason to call forth a sense of oppression or further victimization.

In the midst of considering these ethical matters, we return to contemplate the question with which we started this paper; *Do you always work with vulnerable people?* Again we wonder about possible understandings of vulnerability in this question. Is vulnerability part of the multiple contexts in which lives are embedded? Does vulnerability reside in the categories imposed on other people's lives? Does vulnerability stem from seeing a life from particular vantage points? How do we recognize and work with vulnerabilities that come to be because of the interactions between people?

These questions stayed with us as we began to work alongside the youth in the art club. We were mindful of the importance of working against a sense of oppression. Working against oppression was only possible with patience and perseverance, attending closely and carefully to the openings and spaces of possibility created through the art making with the youth, the meals and snacks shared together, and the gathering with friends in multiple places. We knew how easy it would be to be caught into oppression and victimization.

Revisiting naming as an ethical consideration interwoven with vulnerability

The naming of the arts club called forth community narratives composed around vulnerability and also resistance to these community narratives. These community narratives shaped stories, lived and told in the school, school district, and in the communities where the youth and families lived. They were, perhaps, created unintentionally, yet remained deeply problematic. Sean notes:

> One parent in particular balked strongly at the idea of naming the art club 'The Neechie Club', in some ways admonishing us for considering this name for the club. She reminded us that names carry with them different meanings in different places. Although the term Neechie could be considered a positive name in her Saulteaux community, in the same geographical region it also carried with it a connotation of slang and negativity, the exact opposite of possibility. Even when we turned back to youth and community members along the way, we began to further understand the complexity within names and the struggles within defined processes and categorizations that we can easily slip into with our actions and with a simple welcoming poster potentially gone wrong. The path forward took us back to the youth participants and with some kind of tacit and barely visible consensus they settled on a name similar to the one that the researchers had originally used, 'The U of A arts club'. We wondered about how the lack of acknowledging our research focus was on Aboriginal youth and families in the club name made it possible for some youth to attend, youth who might have been discouraged from attending if the club name had been otherwise. We wondered if naming the club the University of Alberta (U of A) art club made it possible for some youth to attend and to see themselves as studying with professors at the U of A. This wonder plays out in the more recent present when youth from the research study stay connected with us, ask us to help with resumes and reference letters, and in what is often noted in playful notations on their social media profiles indicating the youth have studied at the U of A.

The invitation to involve the youth in naming the club could easily have been a quick exercise with selections offered and a vote to select the most preferred name. However, as we awakened to the tensions around vulnerability and to the ethical considerations that became visible as we worked within the tensions, we learned from youth, families, Knowledge Keepers, and Elders that names do matter. Titles and categorizations are powerful influences both inside and outside of school as we resist colonial and systemic structures that shape youth, families, and communities in ways that limit possibilities for forward looking stories, ways that constrain what is possible in educative spaces. Attending to these experiences allowed us to attend to both actual and perceived vulnerabilities.

Living alongside: what becomes visible can create vulnerability

While being part of the arts club every week for two years, we learned of multiple ways in which youths' lives were shaped. During these years, we, as a research team, engaged in numerous conversations about the absence of some youth from school. When we designed the study and negotiated entry into the school, we agreed with the proviso that only students who were in attendance at the school could attend the club. At the time, we did not anticipate that many students would move to other schools during the temporal duration of the club but still want to attend the art club, that is, they were no longer registered at the school but wanted to still participate in the art club. This created a tension for us: we wanted to continue alongside youth who had moved to other schools, but we were not able to welcome them into the club because they no longer were registered students in the school. We had agreed to follow the school rules about which youth could be in the place.

Attendance at the school also emerged in other ways as we worked with the youth. While attendance seemed a straightforward constraint at the outset, we continually worked to create relationally ethical ways to honour both the youth who wanted to participate in the research with us and the school requirements. At times, this meant that we engaged with youth outside of the school during school hours. Sean (Lessard 2013) recalled one of those times when he met Donovan and Lane outside of school during school hours:

> While I had wondered why the boys decided to miss school on this day, I decided it was not going to be my starting point for a conversation. The shared companionship between the boys was evident. The sense of adventure, of ducking out on the formal structures, of taking a break from where they were supposed to be, was most definitely in the air. I imagined that the freedom of going on some rides and having a soda were all valid reasons in their minds. I did not ask.
>
> We found a seat in the food court and I ordered a juice for each of the boys. We talked as a group, deciding together that it probably was not the greatest idea to be cutting out on classes and having research conversations. We talked about the research project and how I wanted to discuss some parts of school and life more in depth with Lane. The boys all agreed, but with that they also said they wanted to share their stories. They talked mostly of being friends and that they felt comfortable sharing some parts of their stories together. It became apparent to me, in that moment, that the boys had so much to share and that they wanted a space to tell their stories. They shared fragments with me, bits and pieces, over the course of a couple hours, in-between sips of their drinks and the laughter that often entered the conversation. They shared stories of their families, places travelled, friendships, memories, and the beautiful things that come when thinking of places that they had been in their lives. Seldom did the talk of school, specific classes, or grades in our conversational space occur. Our time spent together focused on what they imagined for their lives in the future. On that day in the food court I visited with a future police officer, an actor, and a train engineer as they shared their stories, letting me into their worlds, glimpsing snapshots of what might be.
>
> *(168–169)*

As becomes evident in Sean's field notes, he, Lane, and Donovan discussed the importance of being in school during school hours rather than being engaged in research conversations outside of school during school hours. Both Sean and the youth were vulnerable during the conversation: Sean because he knew the youth were absent from school without excuse and the youth because they were absent from school. Rather than refuse to talk with them or to admonish them to return to school, Sean created a space that allowed them to engage in the research with an understanding that they would not engage in the research at this time on future occasions.

There were other moments created by the rules around school attendance that created other vulnerabilities interwoven with ethical matters. We also learned the importance of improvising ways forward in relationally ethical ways when youth, who had been absent from school for the day, wanted to come to the after-school art club. On one occasion, one youth, Craig, came to the art club through the back door of the school. The vice principal arrived in the arts club room looking for Craig. Craig was, in that moment, hiding in the room. Had the vice principal found him, he would have demanded he leave the school property because he had been absent from school for the day. Drawing on her field notes, Vera recalls:

> The footsteps of the vice principal were audible down the long corridor that led to the arts club. I do not recall hearing footsteps often, and was immediately wakeful that the steps came with a purpose and intent. Standing in the doorway, the vice principal called out: Has anyone seen Craig? There was silence in the room and I recall that everyone in the room looked at me. While Craig was in the room, carefully hunched underneath a desk, my answer to the vice principal was 'No we have not seen him today. Is there anything you would like us to tell him'? The vice principal made it clear that Craig had not been in school that day and that he was in trouble for being absent without an excuse. The vice principal left, his footsteps disappearing in the same way they had come. The art club was quiet – everyone knew I had lied to the vice principal. There was a palpable silence that was filled with worry. What if the vice principal came back? What if anyone found out one of us had lied? What would happen if Craig was discovered? What if Craig wanted to come to the arts club, but not to school? Slowly the chatter returned and, in the midst of the chatter, we knew we all needed to compose a forward looking story – one that acknowledged the school rules and one that also attended to the life of the youth.

Sean, Vera, and Jean recall these experiences of imagined vulnerabilities, where we, or others, imagined what might happen. We saw the layers of vulnerability for Craig, the other youth, for our selves, and for our research presence in the school and school district. In these moments, we risked calling forth a protectionist attitude, one in which we imagined possible things that could happen, triggering surveillance and/or care based on perceived needs or obligations to adhere to rules, rather than the experiences of participants, that is, experiences grounded in the midst of their lives. It is important to differentiate this kind of care from what we do as narrative inquirers, as traditional notions of care are different from the relational ethics of care we enact as narrative inquirers (Clandinin, Caine, and Lessard 2018). Vera thought often about the footsteps that brought the vice principal into the classroom that day. His footsteps shaped how we could live alongside the youth in the space, not just on the days when he entered the room 'at the end of the hall'. The footsteps were a reminder of imposed expectations – perhaps not unreasonable ones, but certainly ones that felt imposed.

Being wakeful to how our relationships with youth were shaped, we were attentive to the ways daily protocols of respect and mutuality shaped the ways vulnerability was understood as fluid and evolving. We lived these daily protocols of respect and mutuality as we attended to the food we provided, in both quantity and quality; as we created art-making activities that grew from the youth's interests; as we engaged in improvisatory ways in the art making when invited to do so. Living alongside the youth in the art club called us to continue to question the relational ethics around issues of vulnerability in the living.

Reverberations of vulnerability in moving from interim to final research texts

The ways in which Clandinin et al. (2010) portrayed tensions are resonant for us as we moved from co-composing field texts to representing our work in research texts. This view of tensions allows us to 'understand tensions in a more relational way, that is, tensions that live between people, events, or things, and are a way of creating a between space, a space which can exist in educative ways' (82). These are the spaces that are opened in the living alongside research participants. As we move into considerations of vulnerability in composing final research texts, we continue to wonder about the ways in which final research texts might hold open the possibilities of continuing to live alongside that exist in the actual living.

Moving from interim to final research texts is not a linear task. There is a back and forth movement that involves both extensive writing and also a return to the field and to co-composing more field texts in order to be able to write interim and final research texts attentive to participants' and our experiences. It is in these movements back and forth from field to field texts to interim and final research texts that tensions become visible and tangible. It is, as we struggle alongside participants with what to include in final research texts that we face questions once again of what, and how, we show to larger public audiences and how understandings of naming and vulnerability are always present, always in need of further wonders.

Questions of audience are with us throughout an inquiry but it seems they become more pressing as we consider writing research texts. While we, at times, may have a sense of who audiences are because of the journals, publishers, conferences, and/or funding agencies, we know the importance of staying wakeful to the uncertainties that exist around who audiences are for our work and how our research texts will be situated, particularly as we stay attentive to vulnerability. We wonder, for example, will those unfamiliar and distant from our work be able to travel the world in the ways Lugones (1987) suggests, so that their reading comes with loving perceptions? Calling on Frye (1983), Lugones explains, 'the loving eye is "the eye of one who knows that to know the seen, one must consult something other than one's own will and interests and fears and imagination"' (85). We must stay wakeful to the multiplicity of ways that our research texts can be read and positioned. It is at these points that response communities can be helpful as readers within those groups can provide insights that come embedded within loving perception, as well as within arrogant perception. Travelling to the youth's worlds with loving perception is important as vulnerability, by its etymological roots, is connected to a sense of woundedness.

It is only afterwards that we can see more clearly how we can rethink silences and see how silences are created and shaped by the labels, the single stories, the ways that people's stories create them as vulnerable people within particular contexts. This rethinking of silences stretches far beyond our research relationships and carries into who we are as people, as parents, as grandparents. We wonder about the places where silences can be broken, where the unsaid might be said.

Significance of narrative inquiries: the so what of vulnerability

As we consider the significance of narrative inquiries, the question of 'so what?' that always lives within our studies, becomes more overt again. When we return to the question of 'So what?' as we begin to compose research texts, this question sharpens our focus on what is important, what we may want to share with diverse audiences, and the ways in which we can do this. Most often we think of our narrative inquiries as holding personal, practical, and social significance. In many ways, what we offer as final research texts are meant to disrupt common understandings, perceptions, and practices. It is these disruptions that are intentionally part of the research texts we write. As we engage in considerations of how we understand, work with and against, understandings of vulnerability in narrative inquiry, these considerations necessarily become important considerations in the justifications of narrative inquiry. As we move from living alongside participants in the field and co-composing field texts, the issues around vulnerability appear again in representing narrative inquiries in research texts.

Issues of representation shaped by the design and living out of narrative inquiries

While it would be easy to separate issues of representation from the ongoing living out of a narrative inquiry, we need to be mindful of the ways we attend to participants, both as we invite them to live alongside and as we write their, and our, stories into research texts. Places, times, and relationships carry knowledge about participants' and our lives, and our vulnerabilities.

As we made visible at the outset, we see how important considerations of framing of participants was in proposal writing and in negotiating entry with the school and school district. These early framings, that is whether we saw the youth and their families as vulnerable as the media and policy documents too often did, would have shaped how we approached the youth and their families and how they understood our intentions. Attentive to the importance of obtaining funding, we highlighted our inquiry focus on attending to youth and families who fit within the broad category of Aboriginal youth and families. Even as we worked with labels of First Nations, Métis, and Inuit, we knew that such categories carried the possibility of having study participants being read as vulnerable, as marginal, as neglected. As we wrote against, and resisted the labels that we ourselves invoked, we argued for the importance of attending to the particular lives of youth and families as lived within, and shaped by, the larger cultural, social, institutional, and familial narratives. Resistance to seeing the experiences of the youth and their families from within a single story of vulnerability marked our work as narrative inquirers and was made visible by our final representations in research texts as we focused on the wholeness of each life in the making amidst the larger cultural, social, institutional, and familial narratives.

In writing research texts, we also needed to work against simplistic readings of youths' experiences as we considered how to first introduce participants. We resisted requests to write a brief précis or summary of each participant as a way to introduce participants. We saw the importance of resisting these requests for we realized that how we shape a summary introduction provides a kind of frame that sets readers up to focus on what we initially highlighted in the introduction. We saw how easily introductions too often created for readers a way to cast participants within labels, within single stories, and, in so doing, to see them as vulnerable. The importance of resisting the labels that lead to seeing participants as vulnerable is an ongoing issue throughout the inquiry from design to representation.

This concern about how we introduce participants is closely connected to the importance of disrupting and working against ways of telling that fix participants in particular ways or in chronological events. As writers, we need to 'remember that readers may freeze the narrative with the result that the restorying life quality intended by the writer may become fixed as a print portrait by the reader' (Connelly and Clandinin 1990, 9). We need to find ways to show that lives are always unfolding, are always in the midst, and that the tellings we create are 'for now' tellings. We see the possibilities of leaving openings in research texts that invite readers into our relationships with participants. We do this in order to create openings where readers can imagine future possibilities of lives unfolding and becoming, rather than holding on to a fixed story. We also draw the reader in so that their own lives may be shaped by what they come to know about the participants and themselves. This becomes particularly important in our representations of narrative inquiries with children and youth where, too often, readers want to be able to predict what will happen if programmes or interventions are provided. As our formal research was coming to a close alongside the youth, Sean (Lessard 2013) recalls:

> I think of Donovan in the present, as now I understand him differently. How, after the 2 years of research conversations I recognize more clearly who he was in that space and in the space between us. The gentle drumming is what I am reminded of when thinking of Donovan, and how the way he moved and interacted was with quiet presence, a gentle rhythm or beat that would guide . . . like that drum call Elder Isabelle Kootenay speaks of. It is a spirit or a way of living that is gentle and that is difficult to recognize if I am not listening carefully. Now, as I turn and gaze backward to my notes and memories, I see it differently. Donovan's quiet leadership, leading in a gentle way, is how he moves in relation. In those early moments in the club space, I didn't really recognize who was leading whom. I now see that the stories that I first told were not the stories I came to know when I began to hear, for the first time, Donovan playing that drum ever so softly.
>
> *(110–111)*

As we composed final research texts, we struggled as participants' and our silences, our abbreviated talks, and some experiences are difficult to represent in words. They, and we, struggle with notions of vulnerability that are placed on them, by labels and single stories. These assigned vulnerabilities lead to potential misinterpretations and fears that interpretations made with arrogant perceptions could create experiences of judgement. As we worked with the youth to create interim research texts that both disrupt what is known and yet create what might be acceptable as a research text, we returned again to the importance of making experiences visible, to shift understandings of who Aboriginal youth are and are becoming in a complex world that will not write over or 'erase their Indianness' nor their or our vulnerabilities. And we return again to the question we began with 'Do you always work with vulnerable people?' While we expect that the asker of the question expected a yes or no answer, we tried to show in this paper that questions of vulnerability are inextricably interwoven into narrative inquiry.

Acknowledgement

This work was supported by the Social Science and Humanities Research Council (SSHRC) [Grant no. 856–2009–0039] and Alberta Centre for Child, Family, and Community Research (ACCFCR) [Grant no. 091015TOP].

References

Arendt, H. 1958. *The Human Condition*. Chicago, IL: University of Chicago Press.

Basso, K. H. 1996. *Wisdom Sits in Places: Landscape and Language Among the Western Apache*. Albuquerque, NM: University of New Mexico Press.

Battiste, M. A., and J. Y. Henderson. 2000. *Protecting Indigenous Knowledge and Heritage: A Global Challenge*. Saskatoon: Purich

Canadian Council on Learning. 2007. *Redefining How Success Is Measured in First Nations, Inuit and Métis Learning*. Ottawa: Canadian Council on Learning. www.afn.ca/uploads/files/education/5._2007_redefining_how_success_is_measured_en.pdf.

Clandinin, D. J., V. Caine, and S. Lessard. 2018. *The Relational Ethics of Narrative Inquiry*. London: Routledge.

Clandinin, D. J., V. Caine, S. Lessard, and J. Huber. 2016. *Engaging in Narrative Inquiry with Children and Youth*. Walnut Creek, CA: Left Coast Press.

Clandinin, D. J., and F. M. Connelly. 2000. *Narrative Inquiry: Experience and Story in Qualitative Research*. San Francisco, CA: Jossey-Bass.

Clandinin, D. J., M. S. Murphy, J. Huber, and A. M. Orr. 2010. "Negotiating Narrative Inquiries: Living in a Tension-Filled Midst." *The Journal of Educational Research* 103 (2): 81–90. doi:10.1080/00220670903323404.

Clandinin, D. J., and J. Rosiek. 2007. "Mapping a Landscape of Narrative Inquiry: Borderland Spaces and Tensions." In *Handbook of Narrative Inquiry: Mapping a Methodology*, edited by D. J. Clandinin, 35–75. Thousand Oaks, CA: Sage.

Connelly, F. M., and D. J. Clandinin. 1990. "Stories of Experience and Narrative Inquiry." *Educational Researcher* 19: 2–14.

Connelly, F. M., and D. J. Clandinin. 2006. "Narrative Inquiry." In *Handbook of Complementary Methods in Education Research*, 3rd ed., edited by J. L. Green, G. Camilli, and P. B. Elmore, 477–487. Mahwah, NJ: Lawrence Erlbaum.

Dewey, J. 1938. *Experience and Education*. New York: Collier.

Frye, M. 1983. *The Politics of Reality: Essays in Feminist Theory*. Trumansburg, NY: Crossing Press.

LaFromboise, T. D., J. E. Trimble, and G. V. Mohatt. 1990. "Counseling Intervention and American Indian Tradition: An Integrative Approach." *The Counseling Psychologist* 18: 628–654.

Lessard, S. 2013. "Red Worn Runners: A Narrative Inquiry Into the Experiences of Aboriginal Youth and Families in Urban Settings." Unpublished doctoral diss., University of Alberta, Edmonton, Alberta, Canada.

Lessard, S., V. Caine, and D. J. Clandinin. 2015. "A Narrative Inquiry Into Familial and School Curriculum Making: Attending to Multiple Worlds of Aboriginal Youth and Families." *Journal of Youth Studies* 18 (2): 197–214. doi:10.1080/13676261.2014.944121.

Lugones, M. 1987. "Playfulness, 'World'-Travelling, and Loving Perception." *Hypatia* 2 (2): 3–19. www.jstor.org/stable/3810013.

Mackenzie, C., W. Rogers, and S. Dodds. 2013. *Vulnerability: New Essays in Ethics and Feminist Philosophy*. New York: Oxford University Press.

Marmon Silko, L. 1996. *Yellow Woman a Beauty of the Spirit: Essays on Native American Life Today*. New York: Simon and Schuster.

Negotiating Neglected Narratives. 2015. A Conference held at the University College of Bergen, Bergen, Norway, October 7, 2015.

Tronto, J. C. 2014. "Book Review of *Vulnerability: New Essays in Ethics and Feminist Philosophy*, edited by C. Mackenzie, W. Rogers, and S. Dodds." *Notre Dame Philosophical Reviews*. November 17, 2014. http://ndpr.nd.edu/news/53816-vulnerability-new-essays-in-ethics-and-feminist-philosophy/.